D1639721

KT-162-478
WITHDRAWN

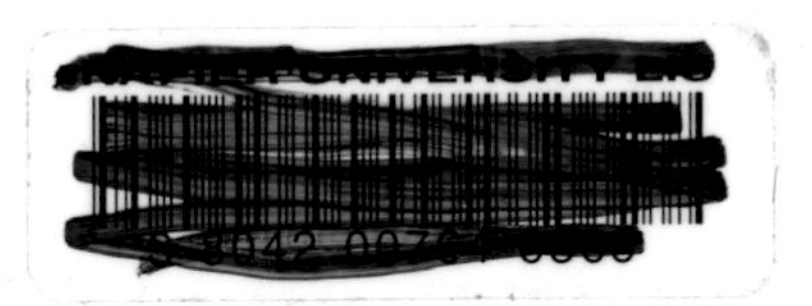

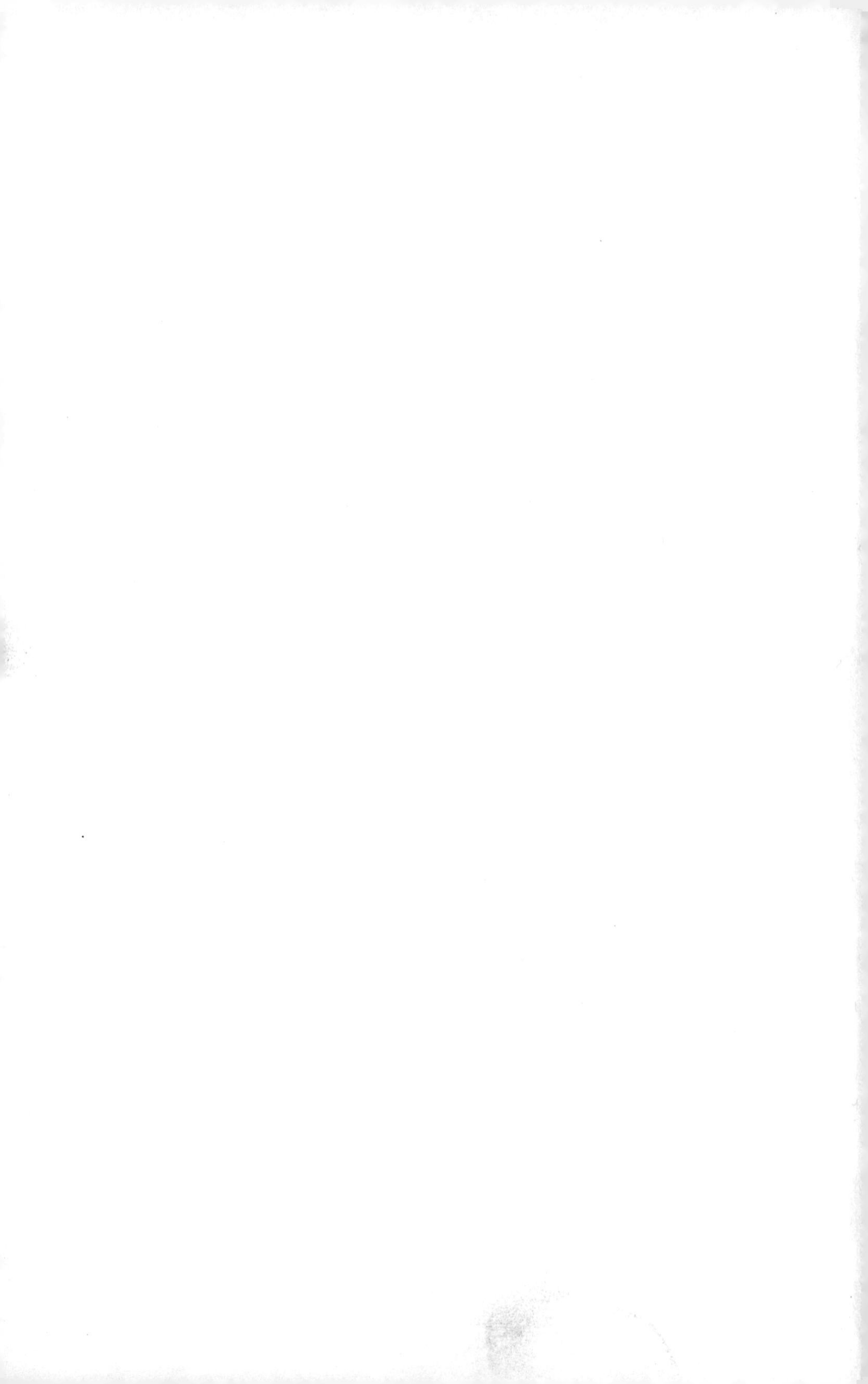

Neuroprotection in the Newborn

Guest Editors

ALAN R. SPITZER, MD
ROBERT D. WHITE, MD

CLINICS IN PERINATOLOGY

www.perinatology.theclinics.com

December 2008 • Volume 35 • Number 4

SAUNDERS an imprint of ELSEVIER, Inc.

W.B. SAUNDERS COMPANY
A Division of Elsevier Inc.

Elsevier, Inc. • 1600 John F. Kennedy Blvd. • Suite 1800 • Philadelphia, PA 19103-2899

http://www.theclinics.com

CLINICS IN PERINATOLOGY Volume 35, Number 4
December 2008 ISSN 0095-5108, ISBN-10: 1-4160-5801-X, ISBN-13: 978-1-4160-5801-4

Editor: Carla Holloway
Developmental Editor: Theresa Collier

Clinics in Perinatology (ISSN 0095-5108) is published in quarterly by Elsevier Inc., 360 Park Avenue South, New York, NY 10010-1710. Months of issue are March, June, September, and December. Business and Editorial offices: 1600 John F. Kennedy Blvd., Suite 1800, Philadelphia, PA 19103-2899. Customer Service Office: 6277 Sea Harbor Drive, Orlando, FL 32887-4800. Periodicals postage paid at New York, NY and additional mailing offices. Subscription prices are $217.00 per year (US individuals), $321.00 per year (US institutions), $255.00 per year (Canadian individuals), $408.00 per year (Canadian institutions), $314.00 per year (foreign individuals), $408.00 per year (foreign institutions) $105.00 per year (US students), and $153.00 per year (Canadian and foreign students). Foreign air speed delivery is included in all Clinics subscription prices. All prices are subject to change without notice. **POSTMASTER:** Send address changes to *Clinics in Perinatology*; Elsevier Periodicals Customer Service, 11830 Westline Industrial Drive, St. Louis, MO 63146. Customer Service (orders, claims, online, change of address): Elsevier Periodicals Customer Service, 11830 Westline Industrial Drive, St. Louis, MO 63146. Tel: 1-800-654-2452 (U.S. and Canada); 314-453-7041 (outside U.S. and Canada). Fax: 314-453-5170. E-mail: journalscustomerservice-usa@elsevier.com (for print support); journalsonlinesupport-usa@elsevier.com (for online support).

Reprints. For copies of 100 or more, of articles in this publication, please contact the Commercial Reprints Department, Elsevier Inc., 360 Park Avenue South, New York, NY 10010-1710. Tel. (212) 633-3812; Fax: (212) 482-1935; email: reprints@elsevier.com.

Clinics in Perinatology is also pubilshed in Spanish by McGraw-Hill Interamericana Editores S.A., P.O. Box 5-237, 06500 Mexico D.F., Mexico.

Clinics in Perinatology is covered in *MEDLINE/PubMed (Index Medicus) Current Contents, Excepta Medica, BIOSIS and ISI/BIOMED.*

Printed in the United States of America.

Contributors

GUEST EDITORS

ALAN R. SPITZER, MD
Senior Vice President and Director, The Center for Research and Education, Pediatrix Medical Group; Pediatrix Analytical Laboratory, Sunrise, Florida

ROBERT D. WHITE, MD
Director, Regional Newborn Program, Memorial Hospital, South Bend; Clinical Assistant Professor of Pediatrics, Indiana University School of Medicine, Indianapolis; Adjunct Professor of Psychology, University of Notre Dame, Notre Dame, Indiana

AUTHORS

JOHN D.E. BARKS, MD
Associate Professor of Pediatrics and Communicable Diseases, Neonatal-Perinatal Medicine, C.S. Mott Children's Hospital, University of Michigan Health System, Ann Arbor, Michigan

LAURA BENNET, PhD
Associate Professor, Department of Physiology, Faculty of Medical and Health Sciences, University of Auckland, Auckland, New Zealand

DONALD CHACE, PhD, MSFS
The Center for Research and Education, Pediatrix Medical Group; Director, Pediatrix Analytical Laboratory, Sunrise, Florida

ROBERT RYAN CLANCY, MD
Professor, Department of Neurology; Professor, Department of Pediatrics, The University of Pennsylvania School of Medicine; Director, Pediatric Regional Epilepsy Program, Division of Neurology, The Children's Hospital of Philadelphia, Philadelphia, Pennsylvania

OLAF DAMMANN, MD, SM
Research Professor of Pediatrics, Tufts University School of Medicine; Director of Clinical Research, Division of Newborn Medicine, Floating Hospital for Children at Tufts Medical Center, Boston, Massachusetts

LINDA S. DE VRIES, MD, PhD
Department of Neonatology, University Medical Center, Wilhelmina Children's Hospital, Utrecht, The Netherlands

ADRÉ J. DU PLESSIS, MBChB, MPH
Associate Professor in Neurology, Harvard Medical School; Director, Fetal-Neonatal Neurology, Department of Neurology, Children's Hospital Boston, Boston, Massachusetts

ALISTAIR JAN GUNN, MB, ChB, PhD
Professor, Department of Physiology, Faculty of Medical and Health Sciences; Professor, Department of Paediatrics, University of Auckland; Starship Children's Hospital, Auckland, New Zealand

TERRIE E. INDER, MD
Departments of Pediatrics, Neurology and Radiology, St. Louis Children's Hospital, Washington University, St. Louis, Missouri

RUSSELL K. LAWRENCE, MD
Department of Pediatrics, St. Louis Children's Hospital, Washington University, St. Louis, Missouri

JEREMY D. MARKS, PhD, MD
Associate Professor, Department of Pediatrics, Neurology, and The College Committees on Cell Physiology and Molecular Medicine, University of Chicago, Chicago, Illinois

HEATHER J. McCREA, PhD
MD Student, Yale University School of Medicine; Department of Cell Biology, Yale University, New Haven, Connecticut

LAURA R. MENT, MD
Professor and Associate Dean for Admissions, Department of Pediatrics; Department of Neurology, Yale University School of Medicine, New Haven, Connecticut

T. MICHAEL O'SHEA, MD, MPH
Professor of Pediatrics, Wake Forest University School of Medicine, Winston-Salem, North Carolina

RAKESH SAHNI, MD
Associate Professor of Clinical Pediatrics, Department of Pediatrics, College of Physicians and Surgeons, Columbia University, New York, New York

ULANA M. SANOCKA, MD
Associate Clinical Professor of Pediatrics, Department of Pediatrics, College of Physicians and Surgeons, Columbia University, New York, New York

MICHAEL D. SCHREIBER, MD
Professor, Department of Pediatrics and The College Committees on Cell Physiology and Molecular Medicine, University of Chicago, Chicago, Illinois

ALAN R. SPITZER, MD
Senior Vice President and Director, The Center for Research and Education, Pediatrix Medical Group; Pediatrix Analytical Laboratory, Sunrise, Florida

MARIANNE THORESEN, MD, PhD
Professor of Neonatal Neuroscience, Child Health, St. Michael's Hospital, University of Bristol, Bristol, United Kingdom

MONA C. TOET, MD, PhD
Department of Neonatology, University Medical Center, Wilhelmina Children's Hospital, Utrecht, The Netherlands

LINDA G.M. VAN ROOIJ, MD
Department of Neonatology, University Medical Center, Wilhelmina Children's Hospital, Utrecht, The Netherlands

Contents

Although inhaled nitric oxide–mediated decreases in chronic lung disease and severe intraventricular hemorrhage/periventricular leukomalacia undoubtedly contribute to improved neurodevelopmental outcomes, inhaled nitric oxide has an independent neuroprotective effect. Although these data are encouraging, additional studies are required before recommending the routine use of inhaled nitric oxide for neuroprotection in preterm infants.

Neonatal hypoxic-ischemic encephalopathy, prematurity, sepsis-meningitis, and serious forms of complex congenital heart disease requiring infant heart surgery are just a few examples of disorders that share high mortality and morbidity rates. Newborn heart surgery represents a period of planned and deliberate ischemia-reperfusion injury, which is obliged to occur to cure or palliate complex forms of congenital heart disease. Advances in cardiothoracic surgical and anesthetic techniques, including cardiopulmonary bypass and deep hypothermic circulatory arrest, have substantially decreased mortality, expanding the horizon to address functional neurologic and cardiac outcomes in long-term survivors. Interest in the functional status of survivors now stretches beyond the newborn period to childhood, adolescence, and adulthood.

GOAL STATEMENT

The goal of *Clinics in Perinatology* is to keep practicing neonatologists and maternal-fetal medicine specialists up to date with current clinical practice in perinatology by providing timely articles reviewing the state of the art in patient care.

ACCREDITATION

The *Clinics in Perinatology* is planned and implemented in accordance with the Essential Areas and Policies of the Accreditation Council for Continuing Medical Education (ACCME) through the joint sponsorship of the University of Virginia School of Medicine and Elsevier. The University of Virginia School of Medicine is accredited by the ACCME to provide continuing medical education for physicians.

The University of Virginia School of Medicine designates this educational activity for a maximum of 60 *AMA PRA Category 1 Credits*™. Physicians should only claim credit commensurate with the extent of their participation in the activity.

The American Medical Association has determined that physicians not licensed in the US who participate in this CME activity are eligible for *AMA PRA Category 1 Credits*™.

Credit can be earned by reading the text material, taking the CME examination online at http://www.theclinics.com/home/cme, and completing the evaluation. After taking the test, you will be required to review any and all incorrect answers. Following completion of the test and evaluation, your credit will be awarded and you may print your certificate.

FACULTY DISCLOSURE/CONFLICT OF INTEREST

The University of Virginia School of Medicine, as an ACCME accredited provider, endorses and strives to comply with the Accreditation Council for Continuing Medical Education (ACCME) Standards of Commercial Support, Commonwealth of Virginia statutes, University of Virginia policies and procedures, and associated federal and private regulations and guidelines on the need for disclosure and monitoring of proprietary and financial interests that may affect the scientific integrity and balance of content delivered in continuing medical education activities under our auspices.

The University of Virginia School of Medicine requires that all CME activities accredited through this institution be developed independently and be scientifically rigorous, balanced and objective in the presentation/discussion of its content, theories and practices.

All authors/editors participating in an accredited CME activity are expected to disclose to the readers relevant financial relationships with commercial entities occurring within the past 12 months (such as grants or research support, employee, consultant, stock holder, member of speakers bureau, etc.). The University of Virginia School of Medicine will employ appropriate mechanisms to resolve potential conflicts of interest to maintain the standards of fair and balanced education to the reader. Questions about specific strategies can be directed to the Office of Continuing Medical Education, University of Virginia School of Medicine, Charlottesville, Virginia.

The authors/editors listed below have identified no professional or financial affiliations for themselves or their spouse/partner:
Laura Bennet, PhD; Robert Boyle, MD (Test Author); Robert Ryan Clancy, MD; Olaf Dammann, MD, SM; Linda S. de Vries, MD, PhD; André J. du Plessis, MBChB, MPH; Alistair Jan Gunn, MB, ChB, PhD; Carla Holloway (Acquisitions Editor); Terrie E. Inder, MD; Russell K. Lawrence, MD; Heather J. McCrea, PhD; Laura R. Ment, MD; T. Michael O'Shea, MD, MPH; Rakesh Sahni, MD; Ulana M. Sanocka, MD; Marianne Thoresen, MD, PhD; Mona C. Toet, MD, PhD; and Linda G.M. van Rooij, MD.

The authors/editors listed below identified the following professional or financial affiliations for themselves or their spouse/partner:
John D.E. Barks, MD is a consultant for Brain Instruments.
Donald Chace, PhD, MSFS is employed by and owns stock in Pediatrix Medical Group.
Jeremy D. Marks, PhD, MD is a consultant for Ikaria.
Michael D. Schreiber, MD is an industry funded research/investigator and serves on the Speakers Bureau for Ikaria.
Alan R. Spitzer, MD (Guest Editor) owns stock in Pediatrix Medical Group.
Robert D. White, MD (Guest Editor) is employed and owns stock in Pediatrix Medical Group, owns stock and is a patent holder for White Briar Corp, and serves on the Speaker's bureau for GE Medical.

Disclosure of Discussion of Non-FDA Approved Uses for Pharmaceutical Products and/or Medical Devices.
The University of Virginia School of Medicine, as an ACCME provider, requires that all faculty presenters identify and disclose any off-label uses for pharmaceutical and medical device products. The University of Virginia School of Medicine recommends that each physician fully review all the available data on new products or procedures prior to clinical use.

TO ENROLL

To enroll in the Clinics in Perinatology Continuing Medical Education program, call customer service at 1-800-654-2452 or visit us online at www.theclinics.com/home/cme. The CME program is available to subscribers for an additional fee of $195.00

FORTHCOMING ISSUES

March 2009

Current Controversies in Perinatology

Michael R. Uhing, MD, Robert M. Kliegman, MD, *Guest Editors*

June 2009

Fetal Surgery

Hanmin Lee, MD, *Guest Editor*

September 2009

Fetal and Neonatal Neurology

Adré du Plessis, MD, *Guest Editor*

RECENT ISSUES

September 2008

Cesarean Delivery: Its Impact on the Mother and Newborn—Part II

Lucky Jain, MD, MBA, Ronald Wapner, MD, *Guest Editors*

June 2008

Cesarean Delivery: Its impact on the Mother and Newborn—Part I

Lucky Jain, MD, MBA, Ronald Wapner, MD, *Guest Editors*

March 2008

Iatrogenic Disease

Marcus C. Hermansen, MD, *Guest Editor*

RELATED INTEREST

Clinics in Perinatology, September 2006 (Vol. 33, Issue 3)
Brain Monitoring in the Neonate
Alan R. Spitzer, MD, and Robert D. White, MD, *Guest Editors*
www.perinatology.theclinics.com

Preface

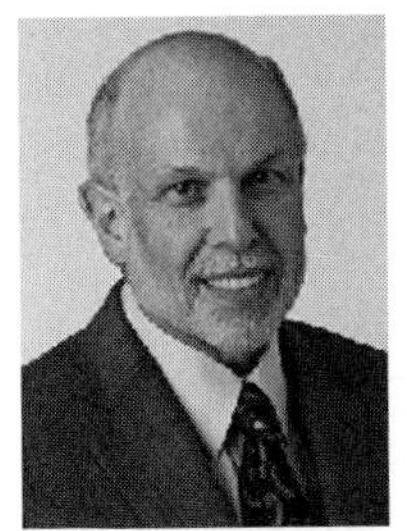
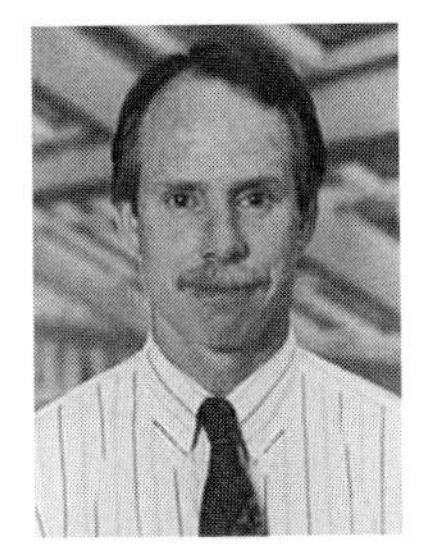

Alan R. Spitzer, MD Robert D. White, MD
Guest Editors

The current era in medicine represents an unusually exciting time for many reasons, an observation that is especially true in the area of neonatal brain injury. Without question, one of the most devastating problems in the neonatal period has traditionally been the newborn infant with brain injury: either the term baby born following a difficult delivery, or the premature infant with chronic hypoxia and ischemia. Until recently, the causes for these problems were not well understood, the sources of injury were difficult to diagnose, and the outcomes were refractory to treatment, resulting in a most depressing situation. Now, however, the prognosis is becoming increasingly brighter. Improvements in obstetrical monitoring and management have reduced the incidence and severity of perinatal hypoxemia, and fetal assessment and intervention are becoming more feasible each day. The rapidly emerging world of genomics, proteomics, and metabolomics indicates that we will soon have new diagnostic tests for a variety of disorders that often result in neurological injury in the fetus and newborn infant. Most importantly, trials of physiological approaches, such as brain and body cooling and new pharmacological therapies, have begun to suggest that brain injury as a clinical situation may, at last, be amenable to treatment and not an irrevocable circumstance.

This issue of *Clinics in Perinatology* is a follow-up to our issue published in September 2006 on brain monitoring in the neonate. We are again fortunate to have many of the world's leading experts in neonatal brain injury lend their knowledge and experience to create a state-of-the-art issue on the diagnosis of brain injury and the neuroprotective strategies that are currently available. We are most grateful to them for their

Clin Perinatol 35 (2008) xi–xii
doi:10.1016/j.clp.2008.09.001

thoughtful and thought-provoking contributions, and we hope that this issue is someday viewed as a summation of the story of how neonatal–perinatal medicine first began to eradicate neonatal brain injury as a NICU outcome.

Alan R. Spitzer, MD
Pediatrix Medical Group
1301 Concord Terrace
Sunrise, FL 33323, USA

Robert D. White, MD
Regional Newborn Program
Memorial Hospital
615 North Michigan Street
South Bend, IN 46601, USA

E-mail addresses:
alan_spitzer@pediatrix.com (A.R. Spitzer)
robert_white@pediatrix.com (R.D. White)

Cerebrovascular Injury in Premature Infants: Current Understanding and Challenges for Future Prevention

André J. du Plessis, MBChB, MPH

KEYWORDS

- Prematurity • Cerebral pressure autoregulation
- Carbon dioxide vasoreactivity • Oxygen vasoreactivity
- Brain injury

Cerebrovascular insults are a leading cause of brain injury in premature infants and contribute heavily to the high prevalence of motor, cognitive, and behavioral deficits in survivors.[1,2] The incidence and severity of ischemic and hemorrhagic lesions increase with decreasing gestational age, suggesting a fundamental role for circulatory immaturity in prematurity-related brain injury. Despite the enormous impact of cerebrovascular injury in the growing population of prematurity survivors, understanding of the complex pathways linking circulatory immaturity to brain injury in premature infants remains incomplete. These mechanisms, however, are significantly different from those causing injury in the mature brain, and management guidelines for sick premature infants cannot reliably be based on data derived from older subjects. If effective neuroprotection against cerebrovascular injury, in particular its prevention, is to become a clinical reality for premature infants, the enormous gaps in knowledge of normal and disturbed cerebral vasoregulation need to be addressed. The principal aims of this article are to review current understanding of cerebral perfusion and its control in general and in the sick premature infant in particular, to highlight the current deficiencies in understanding, and to discuss challenges that lie ahead.

Effective hemodynamic regulation is critical to satisfy the brain's dependence on a consistent and responsive supply of oxygen and glucose. Normally, the cardiorespiratory system provides the cerebral vasculature with a platform of oxygen-substrate support on which complex systems of intrinsic autoregulation act to preserve the structural and functional integrity of brain cells. The cerebrovascular autoregulatory systems serve in a compensatory capacity to maintain oxygen-substrate delivery

Department of Neurology, Children's Hospital Boston, 300 Longwood Avenue, Boston, MA 02115, USA
E-mail address: adre.duplessis@tch.harvard.edu

Clin Perinatol 35 (2008) 609–641
doi:10.1016/j.clp.2008.07.010
perinatology.theclinics.com

during fluctuations in systemic supply and to distribute blood flow according to regional demands within the brain. Without adequate cardiovascular support (eg, perfusion pressure and oxygenation), these intrinsic cerebral compensatory systems eventually fail and lead to brain injury.

Cerebral vascular responsiveness to a variety of stimuli begins to develop in the fetus during the latter half of gestation. Emergence of this intrinsic cerebral vasoreactivity coincides with the third-trimester acceleration in energy demand of the developing brain.[3–8] In infants born prematurely, this cerebrovascular responsiveness may be underdeveloped, leaving them poorly equipped to deal with the instability of the immature cardiopulmonary systems. The confluence of this systemic and cerebral immaturity peaks during the transition from fetal to extrauterine life when striking changes occur in circulating oxygen, in cerebral metabolic demand, and in the extrauterine cardiorespiratory system.[9] It is not surprising, therefore, that this period of circulatory transition is one of particularly high risk for prematurity-related brain injury.

Neonatal critical care has advanced dramatically in its ability to support the cardiorespiratory and other systems of the sick premature infant. Effective brain-oriented critical care in this population, however, remains impeded by two major obstacles: poor understanding of normal hemodynamics and the lack of clinically relevant bedside monitoring of cerebral function and blood flow. Given these limitations, this article does not prescribe guidelines for managing cerebral blood flow and hemodynamics but rather highlights the substantial gaps in current knowledge and the challenges waiting to be addressed before rational and informed brain-oriented care of the sick newborn becomes feasible.

THE SYSTEMIC CARDIOVASCULAR SYSTEM IN PREMATURE INFANTS

The cardiovascular system is responsible for providing the cerebral vasculature with an adequate cerebral perfusion pressure gradient between systemic blood pressure and central venous pressure. Given the immaturity of the cardiac and respiratory systems in sick premature infants, situations of decreased arterial blood pressure or increased central venous pressure are not uncommon and may lead to inadequate cerebral perfusion pressure. Recent reports have emphasized the inadequacies of current normal blood pressure criteria for preventing brain injury in premature infants,[10–13] although continuous cerebral venous pressure measurement is not readily accessible.

Normal control of cardiac output is dependent on heart rate and myocardial contractility and is maintained through opposing tonic and reflex input from the sympathetic and parasympathetic nervous systems. Control of peripheral vascular resistance, which is critical for maintaining blood pressure, is mediated through the sympathetic system. Development of the autonomic nervous system is asynchronous, with the sympathetic system developing earlier during gestation followed by parasympathetic maturation toward term.[14] In addition, the immature myocardium functions close to its maximum contractility in premature infants and has limited ability to increase its stroke volume. Consequently, during periods of low cardiac output, premature infants are particularly dependent on heart rate. Given the baseline sympathetic nervous system dominance, however, the ability to increase cardiac output by accelerating the heart rate is limited. With the sympathetic nervous system and the myocardium operating close to capacity, premature infants are poorly equipped to deal with the sudden transition from the low-resistance placental bed to the significantly higher extrauterine peripheral vascular resistance. Baroreflex and chemoreflex circuits are important for the normal regulation of oxygenated systemic and cerebral perfusion but are underdeveloped in premature infants who have decreased sensitivity and increased impulse-response time.[15,16] Finally, anatomic transition from the fetal to normal postnatal circulation is more prolonged in premature infants, with increased prevalence of persistent ductal patency.[17] For all these reasons, it is not surprising that a significant proportion of premature infants experience low cardiac output during the early postnatal hours.[12,18–21]

THE CEREBROVASCULAR ANATOMY IN PREMATURE INFANTS

Anatomic development of the cerebral vasculature is not complete in premature infants. Arterial ingrowth from the pial surface into the developing brain parenchyma occurs through long penetrating arteries destined for the deep periventricular white matter and short penetrators into the more superficial white matter.[22] Initially these vessels are sparse and poorly connected, leaving end zones vulnerable to decreases in perfusion.[22–26] Ongoing vascular proliferation reduces the vulnerability to hypoxic-ischemic injury in these areas with advancing gestation.[22,24,27,28]

In the mature brain, baseline blood flow exceeds the threshold for ischemic injury by fivefold.[29] In the premature brain, global[30–38] and regional cerebral blood flow are significantly lower,[39] especially in the white matter,[39,40] reflecting the underdeveloped vascular ingrowth into these regions. The markedly decreased white matter blood flow in these premature infants suggests a limited margin of safety for cerebral perfusion[41] and highlights the critical importance of a responsive cerebral vasoregulatory system. Recent studies suggest that premature infants are at significant risk for low systemic and cerebral blood flow during the first 12 to 24 hours of life.[18–21] The nadir and duration of this decreased cerebral blood flow are associated with acute brain injury germinal matrix–intraventricular hemorrhage (GM-IVH) and later neurodevelopmental disability.[18,19]

The ability of the cerebral vasculature to react to physiologic stimuli is dependent on a responsive smooth muscle cell (muscularis) layer in the cerebral resistance vessels. During brain maturation, the muscularis layer develops first around the surface pial vessels, then in the superficial penetrating arteries, and eventually in the precapillary resistance arterioles. Therefore, in premature infants, vasoregulation tends to occur mostly in the peripheral parenchyma, the deeper vessels being relatively passive.[42,43] During the early fetal period, the cerebral ventricular system is surrounded by a germinal neuroepithelium, the source of future neuronal and glial cells. The intense cellular proliferation in these regions is supported by a profuse but transient and fragile vascular system.[44–50] As neuroglial cells migrate out of the germinal matrix layer, it undergoes progressive involution which is largely complete by the late third trimester.[51] In premature infants, however, residual germinal matrix is present in the caudothalamic groove adjacent to the lateral ventricles. This fragile vasculature lies within an arterial end zone, exposing it to ischemic insults during periods of hypoperfusion and to rupture during fluctuations in perfusion pressure.[44–46,52–54]

INTRINSIC CEREBROVASCULAR AUTOREGULATION IN THE MATURE AND PREMATURE BRAIN

The concept of cerebral vasoreactivity to physiologic stimuli originated with Roy and Sherrington, in 1890,[55] who proposed a coupling between neuronal activity and cerebral blood flow. Subsequent studies demonstrated cerebral vasoreactivity to a variety of other stimuli, including changes in circulating blood gases[56] and blood pressure.[57] Over time, the term, *cerebral autoregulation*, has become largely synonymous with cerebral pressure-flow autoregulation. In this article, the term, *cerebral autoregulation*, is used to include, more broadly, the reactivity of the cerebral resistance vessels to a variety of physiologic stimuli. A distinguishing feature of all cerebral autoregulatory systems is that the sensor, transducer, and effector components of their response are intrinsic to the brain. Therefore, although activation of the baroreflex may have an impact on cerebral perfusion through pathways in the brainstem, because the sensors and effector mechanisms are outside the brain, this neural circulatory reflex is not considered part of the cerebral autoregulatory system.

BASIC CELLULAR MECHANISMS OF CEREBRAL AUTOREGULATION

Cerebral autoregulation normally is mediated by a complex integrated system of myogenic, neurogenic, and metabolic mechanisms. The final common pathway for all forms of cerebral vasoreactivity, however, is a change in smooth muscle tone and caliber of the cerebral resistance vessels. Basal tone in the resistance vessel muscularis is maintained by a tonic rate of membrane depolarization-repolarization, primarily through changes in ionic (mainly potassium) channel conductance. These potassium channels are pivotal components of pathways mediated by vasoactive substances, because modulating their conductance allows regulation of calcium influx through voltage-sensitive channels.[58–60] In the cerebral circulation, different paracrine signals to the smooth muscle cells of the resistance vessels originate from one or more points within the neurovascular unit (ie, neurons, astrocytes, pericytes, and endothelium), whereas autocrine signals may be triggered within the smooth muscle cells themselves.[61,62] Myogenic (pressure-active) reactivity is mediated directly at the smooth muscle cell, independent of endothelial or neural input in response to a intravascular pressure change.[63] Understanding of the precise mechanisms underlying the myogenic response remains unclear,[64–66] in particular its sensor-transduction mechanism.[67–70] Vasoactive paracrine substances include the vasodilators, nitric oxide (NO), prostanoids, adenosine, and carbon monoxide (CO), and the vasoconstrictors, endothelin, thromboxane, and others. The vasodilators are produced and released in response to stimuli, such as hypotension, hypoxemia, and hypercarbia, and share a complex and often permissive relationship.[71–75] The paracrine substances stimulate formation of cyclic nucleotides, such as cGMP (by NO and CO) and cAMP (by prostacyclin), within the smooth muscle cells,[76,77] which in turn influence calcium channel conductivity.

NO is generated by constitutive NO synthase (NOS) in the endothelium (eNOS) and neurons (nNOS). NO generated by eNOS plays an important role in resting cerebral vascular tone and autoregulation at rest[78–82] and the vasoreactivity triggered by flow-shear mechanisms. nNOS is the major source of NO during hypotension and hypoxemia (ie, stimuli that cause tissue hypoxia).[83–85] The vasodilator prostanoids (eg, prostacyclin), are generated by the cyclooxygenase pathways[86,87] and activate adenylate cyclase to increase cAMP in the smooth muscle cells; this in turn opens potassium channels, leading to hyperpolarization and vasorelaxation.[76,77] In a newborn, prostanoids are the principal endothelial vasodilators.[88–90] With maturation, however, NO becomes increasingly important and is the dominant endothelial vasodilator in the adult brain.[91,92] Adenosine is a vasodilator and breakdown product of high-energy phosphates,[93] allowing it to increase perfusion in regions of increased ATP use, as during neuronal activity and anaerobic metabolism. CO is a rapidly acting gasotransmitter produced by the constitutive enzyme, heme oxygenase-2, which is activated by, among other stimuli, increased extracellular glutamate and seizures.[94,95]

Endothelin is a potent endothelium-derived vasoconstrictor of large and small cerebral arteries[96,97] that does not contribute to basal cerebral vasoregulation but is activated during pathologic states, such as hypoxia-ischemia[98,99] and hyperoxia.[100]

SPECIFIC CEREBRAL AUTOREGULATORY SYSTEMS

Although a variety of physiologic and pathologic stimuli are capable of eliciting a cerebral vascular response, this discussion is confined to autoregulatory responses to five specific stimuli (ie, changes in cerebral perfusion pressure, changes in circulating oxygen, carbon dioxide [CO_2] and glucose, and neuronal activation). Regardless of the stimulus, the efficacy of these pathways is influenced by the resting tone and diameter of the cerebral arteries at the onset of the stimulus,[101,102] such that vessels previously dilated by baseline hypotension, hypercarbia, or hypoxia have a limited vasodilatory response to an acute hypotensive episode, for example.[103,104]

CEREBRAL BLOOD PRESSURE-FLOW AUTOREGULATION

The notion of myogenic vascular reactivity to changing perfusion pressure emerged more than a century ago,[105–108] followed 50 years later by Lassen's[57] seminal description of the cerebral pressure-flow autoregulatory plateau. This plateau refers to a range of cerebral perfusion pressures (the gradient between mean arterial pressure and cerebral venous pressure) over which cerebral blood flow is normally maintained relatively constant by intrinsic cerebrovascular mechanisms. At perfusion pressures outside the limits of the autoregulatory plateau, cerebral blood flow tracks perfusion pressure and the cerebral circulation becomes pressure passive. The limits of the autoregulatory plateau are not fixed and may be shifted by any stimulus that changes the caliber of the resistance vessels.[109]

Characteristics of Cerebral Pressure-Flow Autoregulation

The features of pressure-flow autoregulation are influenced by multiple factors, including maturation, nature of the pressure change, coexisting systemic and cerebral factors, and the ambient cerebral physiology. Understanding of pressure-flow autoregulation has evolved with the development of new techniques for estimating cerebral perfusion. Earlier studies applied the Fick principle to isolated cerebral blood flow measurements (eg, with inert tracers such as xenon),[110–112] which provided so-called static cerebral autoregulatory measurements. Although these static measurements yielded valuable insights into cerebral pressure-flow autoregulation, they could not adequately capture its dynamic and evolving nature. More recently, techniques, such as Doppler flow velocity and near-infrared spectroscopy (NIRS), have been used to study cerebral pressure-flow autoregulation.[113–122] Although these approaches allow longer continuous and repeated estimations, the results of these studies have been less than consistent.

In adults, the autoregulatory plateau ranges between 50 and 150 mm Hg and becomes narrower and lower with decreasing age. Although controversy persists, the lower limit of the autoregulatory plateau in stable preterm infants has been estimated at approximately 25 to 30 mm Hg.[38,123] The temporal features of cerebral pressure-flow autoregulation depend on the nature of the pressure stimulus, the brain maturation state, and the species studied.[124–134] Doppler studies have described a biphasic dynamic pressure-flow response in the brain to a step change in blood pressure,[113] with a brief initial passive phase, followed by a slower, longer, active vascular response. The efficacy of pressure autoregulation is measured by the transition from passive to active phase, the latency between these phases being the impulse-response time. Although there is significant variation between studies in animals,[133,135] healthy adult humans,[114] and premature infants[115] the impulse-response time has ranged from 3 to 15 seconds.[114,135] In the frequency domain, pressure autoregulation behaves like a high-pass filter with a threshold above 0.07 Hz.[136]

Studies in animal models have provided valuable insights into the role of maturation in cerebrovascular regulation.[7,137–151] With decreasing gestational age, the blood pressure range of the autoregulatory plateau is narrower and lower.[152,153] In addition, with decreasing gestational age, the normal resting blood pressures approach the lower threshold of autoregulation,[7,138,145] rendering the immature brain critically dependent on a consistent perfusion pressure and vulnerable to injury during even minor pressure decreases.

Cerebral pressure-flow autoregulation is well characterized in children and adults[57,65,154,155] but not in human newborns,[156] least of all in sick premature infants.[38,120,121,157–161] In early studies,[156] cerebral pressure autoregulation was more effective in term than in preterm infants, although pressure passivity was less likely in clinically stable[157,162–164] than in sick, ventilated premature infants.[30,31,118,156,164–167]

Using continuous cerebral NIRS and blood pressure measurements over more prolonged periods, the author's research group have been able to focus on the prevalence of cerebral pressure passivity over time.[120,121,168] In these studies[120,121] the group used frequency-based coherence and transfer function analyses to identify periods of cerebral pressure passivity. Tsuji and colleagues[120] demonstrated that a pressure-passive cerebral circulation could be identified by NIRS in more than half of mechanically ventilated premature infants and that these infants were at high risk of brain injury detected by cranial ultrasound (US). A subsequent larger study[121] with longer recording periods found that cerebral pressure passivity was almost uniformly present in sick premature infants at different times, most prevalent among the most premature infants. Furthermore, cerebral pressure passivity was not an all-or-none phenomenon but fluctuated over time, with infants spending an average of 20% of the recording period in this state.[121] More recent studies have focused on the magnitude of pressure passivity, as measured by the transfer gain between blood pressure and cerebral perfusion, and have shown that the magnitude of pressure passivity is associated with GM-IVH (H. O'Leary, BSc, personal communication, 2008).

Mechanisms of Normal Cerebral Pressure-Flow Autoregulation

Pressure-flow autoregulation likely is mediated by several different mechanisms whose activation depends on the rate, duration, and nature of the stimulus.[136,169] The rapid response, which is initiated within seconds of a pressure change,[135] suggests that the initial mechanism is an intrinsic myogenic effect, with responses to more sustained stimuli being mediated by other mechanisms, including metabolic signals.[170,171] The role of endothelial-derived vasoactive substances in pressure autoregulation remains unresolved.[170,172–175] Prostacyclin contributes to vasodilation in severe hypotension.[175] In sustained hypotension, cerebral tissue oxygen delivery may become impaired and vasoactive products of anaerobic metabolism may become important contributors to cerebral vasodilation.[176–178] The vasodilator adenosine is known to increase rapidly with even modest decreases in blood pressure due to accelerated high-energy phosphate breakdown.[179] Neuronally derived NO[84] and CO seem to play an important role in hypotensive vasodilation.[180]

The role of blood flow in pressure autoregulation remains poorly understood.[181,182] Animal studies using isolated pial vessels[127] suggest that small resistance vessels respond to blood flow, independent of changes in transmural pressure. Specifically, at low pressures, the onset of flow is associated with vasodilation, with vessels returning to their preflow diameter when flow stops. Conversely, at high transmural pressure, the onset of flow triggers vasoconstriction, with dilation to the original diameter when flow stops. The role of blood flow in cerebral vasoreactivity is in need of further study.

Does "Abnormal" Blood Pressure Play a Role in Brain Injury in Premature Infants?

Hypotension is diagnosed in up to 20% to 45% of premature infants during the early newborn period,[183–185] and the high rate of pressor-inotrope use in some centers suggests that this diagnosis is entertained even more frequently. Conversely, sustained hypertension is far less common in premature infants.[185]

Systemic blood pressure changes have been implicated in hemorrhagic and hypoxic-ischemic prematurity-related brain injury.[186–189] GM-IVH has been a particular focus in these studies, perhaps because it is easily diagnosed acutely by bedside cranial US. Early animal studies focused on the beagle puppy because it has a germinal matrix similar to the human preterm infant.[144,190–198] These early studies described an association between hypertension and GM-IVH, especially after a period of hypotension. Gronlund and colleagues[189] described a significant association between hypertension during the first 24 hour of life and GM-IVH in premature humans. Overall, hypotension has been implicated more commonly in premature infants as an antecedent to GM-IVH.[187,188,199,200] Other investigators have found, however, no association between systemic hypotension[10,121,201] (as defined by different commonly used criteria)[10] or its duration and the development of GM-IVH. Fluctuations in blood pressure (and cerebral blood flow velocity) were associated with GM-IVH in an earlier study of ventilated premature infants.[202] In a more recent study, however, there was no relationship between frequency domain measures of blood pressure variability and GM-IVH.[121] A role for hypotension in the pathogenesis of periventricular leukomalacia, another major form of prematurity-related brain injury, has been proposed in immature animals and preterm infants.[187,188,201,203] Other studies were unable to confirm this relationship, however, in premature infants.[10,204–209]

In summary, the role of blood pressure, hypotension, and impaired cerebral pressure-flow autoregulation in prematurity-related brain injury is far from resolved. There are several possible reasons for the disparities between studies. First, the diagnosis of hypotension often is made based on intermittent blood pressure measurements and inconsistent definitions. Given that cerebral blood flow measurement is difficult in sick premature infants, indirect inferences often are made about the integrity of cerebral pressure-flow autoregulation. In addition, recent studies suggest that during the early period after premature birth, blood pressure may be a poor indicator of cerebral blood flow and its pressure autoregulation.

Evans and colleagues[18–21,210] have used functional echocardiography to measure cardiac output and superior vena caval (SVC) flow as a surrogate for cerebral blood flow to show that during the first 12 hours of life a substantial minority of premature infants develop low-flow states in the systemic and cerebral circulations. These low-flow states are poorly associated with blood pressure[210] and are not improved by the use of pressor-inotropes.[21] These investigators suggest that cardiac output may be a more relevant measure for cerebral perfusion and oxygenation than blood pressure. Similar findings are described by Kusaka and colleagues[211] who report a significant positive relationship between cardiac output (but not blood pressure) and cerebral blood flow. Other studies have corroborated the poor relationship between cerebral perfusion and systemic blood pressure in the early premature period.[121,212] Using continuous cerebral NIRS and arterial blood pressure measurements, Soul and colleagues[121] showed an association between the prevalence of hypotension and cerebral pressure passivity in premature infants; however, the ability to predict cerebral pressure passivity from the blood pressure was poor.

Furthermore, low SVC flow, but not blood pressure, was associated with brain injury in premature infants.[18,19,213–215] The nadir and duration of this low-flow state during the first 24 hours was predictive of GM-IVH[213–215] and later adverse neurologic outcome.[18,19] Specifically, the recovery of SVC flow is associated with severe GM-IVH,[18–21,210] suggesting a hypoperfusion-reperfusion mechanism, as proposed in earlier animal studies of GM-IVH.[191–193] Meek and colleagues[216] found that low cerebral blood flow, but not hypotension, on the first day of life was associated with severe GM-IVH.

Advancing the understanding of these complex hemodynamics during the transitional period is of critical importance. First, widespread use of pressor-inotropes in premature infants persists, despite the lack of clear evidence that they significantly decrease brain injury.[13,185,217] Management of the low cardiac output state is complicated by the fact that pressor-inotropes may increase the peripheral vascular resistance, further challenging the immature myocardium and increasing left-to-right ductal shunting.[11,218]

CEREBRAL CARBON DIOXIDE VASOREACTIVITY

Characteristics of Cerebral Carbon Dioxide Vasoreactivity

Since the original description of cerebral vasoreactivity to changes in arterial CO_2 (CVR-CO_2) by Kety and Schmidt in 1948,[56] a complex relationship has emerged between changes in circulating CO_2 and cerebral hemodynamics.[219–223]

The response of the cerebral circulation to changes in circulating CO_2 can be categorized into early, delayed, and late phases. The initial response to a decreasing arterial CO_2 is vasoconstriction whereas increasing CO_2 causes vasodilation. The response is initiated within 0.5 to 2 minutes[102] and reaches a steady state after 5 to 10 minutes.[224] During the delayed phase, there is a gradual waning over 3 to 6 hours of the cerebrovascular response to a sustained CO_2 change.[222,223,225,226] During the late phase, a secondary hyperemia develops to persistent hypercapnea, which is slow in reversing after return to normocapnea.[222,223] For all these reasons, the cerebrovascular response to an acute change in CO_2 depends not only on the degree and direction of change but also on the pre-existing CO_2 conditions. An understanding of these evolving hemodynamic changes has become more important with the widespread use of permissive hypercapnea in premature infants.

Of clinical importance, the cerebral vessels are responsive to CO_2 changes within the range commonly encountered in sick premature infants. Vasoconstriction to hypocapnea is progressive until CO_2 reaches 20 mm Hg, below which no further vasoconstriction occurs.[102] The cerebral vasomotor effects of CO_2 occur at all levels from the resistance arterioles to the larger circle of Willis, pial, and parenchymal arteries.[102,227,228]

CVR-CO_2 has important maturational features. Although the cerebral vasculature responds in the same way to CO_2 in neonates and adults, the underlying mechanisms may differ.[229,230] Vasoreactivity to CO_2 has been demonstrated in immature animal models[231,232] and in human newborns, with a reduced response magnitude compared with the mature brain.[229,233,234] Stable preterm infants have an active CVR-CO_2[235] whereas in ventilated premature infants, CVR-CO_2 may be markedly reduced, particularly during the first 24 hours.[166] Such loss of CVR-CO_2 during the first 36 hours of life may be an important predictor of hypoxic-ischemic injury and poor neurodevelopmental outcome in very premature infants.[167]

Mechanisms of Normal Cerebral Carbon Dioxide Vasoreactivity

Although the subsequent pathways may differ,[236,237] acute and delayed responses to CO_2 seem to be pH dependent.[226,238,239] The initial vascular responses to changes in

CO_2 are initiated by changes in extracellular pH after CO_2 crosses the blood-brain barrier.[238–240] Similarly, the subsequent waning in vascular response to sustained CO_2 changes is associated with gradual restoration of extracellular,pH.[110,222] These pH-mediated changes in vascular tone result from direct hyperpolarization of smooth muscle cells, inhibition of voltage dependent Ca-channels,[238] and activation of secondary vasoactive substances.[102,241–243] During acute hypercapneic vasodilation, prostanoid[90,241] and NO levels are elevated[90,244] but wane during the delayed restoration of vascular caliber with sustained hypercapnea.[226] In the mature brain, NO[79,245–255] and prostanoids[252] play important roles in CVR-CO_2. In the immature animal and human brain, NO oxide plays a minimal role in CO_2 vasodilation.[249,256] Conversely, endothelium-derived prostaglandins seem to play an important role in CVR-CO_2 in the immature brain, although the inconsistent cerebrovascular response to different cyclooxygenase inhibitors[257,258] and human newborn[259–262] has been difficult to explain. The mechanisms for the late secondary hyperemia with sustained hypercapnea[226,263–265] remain poorly understood. The mechanism seems to be triggered early, however, through an acidosis-mediated release of endothelial prostanoids[226,266] which then trigger the delayed activation of endothelial NOS transcription.[226]

Do Circulating Carbon Dioxide Levels Play a Role in Prematurity-Related Brain Injury?

Both extremes of circulating CO_2 levels have been implicated in prematurity-related brain injury.[267] There are several potential mechanisms by which abnormal CO_2 levels might cause brain injury in premature infants. Hypercapneic hyperemia may trigger hemorrhagic lesions through vasodilation and engorgement of the microvasculature. Hypercapnea during the first 3 days of life increased the risk for severe GM-IVH.[268] In addition, hypercapnea may limit the normal response to stimuli, such as hypotension and hypoxemia, predisposing to hypoxic-ischemic insults. Doppler studies showed that permissive hypercapnea at relatively modest increases in CO_2, approximately 45 to 55 mm Hg, are associated with impaired pressure autoregulation.[269] Conversely, severe hypocapnea may cause sustained vasoconstriction and an increase in oxygen-hemoglobin affinity thereby limiting cerebral oxygen delivery.[270,271] Moderate hypocapnea decreases cerebral blood flow without affecting cerebral oxygen metabolism,[56,272,273] but more severe hypocapnea decreases cerebral oxygen metabolism,[274,275] whereas increasing cerebral glucose metabolism and cerebrospinal lactate levels,[276,277] together suggesting anaerobic metabolism. Severe hypocapnea has been associated with brain injury in premature infants, particularly in the immature white matter.[278–286] A recent large study of premature infants found a strong association between a high score on a cumulative index of hypocarbia over the first 7 days of life and the development of cystic periventricular leukomalacia on cranial US.[286]

CEREBRAL OXYGEN VASOREACTIVITY

Because a fundamental goal of the cerebral circulation and its regulatory systems is to maintain an appropriate oxygen supply responsive to cerebral demands, it is not surprising that hypoxemia is a particularly potent and robust vasodilatory stimulus.[287,288] Any form of reduced arterial oxygen content—a reduction in hemoglobin,[162,289] oxyhemoglobin affinity, or partial pressure of oxygen—increases cerebral blood flow. Cerebral vasoreactivity to hypoxemia during low oxygen inhalation was first described by Wolff and Lennox[290] and corroborated in many subsequent studies.[110,142,291,292] Conversely, hyperoxemia was shown to trigger vasoconstriction and a decrease in cerebral blood flow in an immature canine model[293] and may be most prominent in early postnatal life.

Characteristics of Cerebral Oxygen Vasoreactivity

In the mature brain the oxygen-hemoglobin dissociation curve maintains arterial oxygen content relatively constant until arterial oxygen pressure reaches 50 mm Hg, below which oxygen extraction increases. At this same threshold, cerebral vasodilation is triggered, usually within 30 to 60 seconds,[294–296] reaching steady state within 5 to 10 minutes.[57,102,297–299] Below this threshold the relationship between cerebral arterial oxygen content and cerebrovascular tone is almost linear.[130,287,297,300] Cerebral oxygen vasoreactivity differs in several ways from CO_2 vasoreactivity. First, unlike the response to CO_2, cerebral vasoreactivity to changes in arterial oxygenation occurs outside the physiologic range usually experienced by premature infants. Second, the vasodilation response to hypoxemia is more potent and overrides hypocapneic vasoconstriction. Finally, unlike hypercapnea, hypoxemic vasodilation persists during sustained hypoxemia,[301] and vasodilation to acute and chronic hypoxia is rapidly reversed with restoration of normoxia.

Cerebral oxygen vasoreactivity (CVR-O_2) is present in fetal, neonatal, and adult animals and humans[5,137,294,302–305] with a magnitude of vessel response that appears similar across maturation. Some studies suggest a faster rate and greater response magnitude in the more immature brain.[306,307]

Data are limited for hyperoxemic vasoconstriction and its mechanisms remain incompletely understood. Studies in an immature canine model suggest a decreasing sensitivity to hyperoxemia with increasing maturation.[293] Studies in premature infants show an increase in cerebral vascular resistance and decrease in cerebral blood volume and flow with hyperoxemia.[235,308–310] Cerebral vasoconstriction does not occur until high levels of arterial oxygenation are reached.[308] This vasoconstriction may be sustained for several hours, however, after relatively brief periods of hyperoxia at birth.[308]

Mechanisms of Cerebral Oxygen Vasoreactivity

The complex mechanisms underlying CVR-O_2, in particular hyperoxemic vasoconstriction, remain incompletely understood. Earlier studies in isolated cerebral arteries suggest that hypoxemia has a direct effect on vascular smooth muscle.[311–314] In vivo, hypoxia may release vasoactive tissue metabolites directly from the endothelium or muscularis layer[301]; the role of the endothelium in hypoxemic vasodilation remains controversial.[315,316] Finally, potent vasoactive substances may be released from the brain parenchymal cells during hypoxia,[317] with a decrease in extracellular pH and increase in potassium, adenosine, prostanoids, NO, and CO.[84,102,318–325] Endogenous opioids also may play a role in hypoxemic vasodilation.[318,319,326–328] In the mature brain,[83] NO generated by nNOS is important for hypoxemic vasodilation[329–331] but seems less important in premature infants.[256] It is likely that different stimuli are active during different phases of hypoxemic vasodilation. Significant changes in extracellular pH[332] and lactate[333] are more gradual, suggesting a more delayed role for extracellular acidosis during sustained hypoxemia.During early tissue hypoxia, however, extracellular potassium[102] and adenosine[323,334,335] accumulate rapidly, therefore likely playing an early role in hypoxemic vasodilation. Theophylline, a competitive inhibitor of adenosine, markedly attenuates the initial cerebral hypoxemic vasodilation.[336,337]

CEREBRAL GLUCOSE VASOREACTIVITY

Coupling between circulating glucose levels and cerebral blood flow, specifically hypoglycemia-triggered vasodilation, has been described in the mature and immature brain.[35,36,157,338,339] Unlike other vasoactive stimuli (eg, CO_2), the temporal evolution of cerebrovascular changes during sustained glucose deprivation is not well understood. In one study of healthy adults, hypoglycemic vasodilation was transient, starting to wane after 60 minutes of sustained glucose deprivation.[339]

As with other cerebral autoregulatory systems, there are important maturational differences in the cerebral vasodilation to glucose deprivation. Unlike hypotension and hypercarbia, however, the response to hypoglycemia is greater in immature than mature brains. In mature animals, hypoglycemic vasodilation seems to have a threshold effect[340] with an abrupt increase in cerebral blood flow at glucose levels associated with the onset of decreasing ATP.[341] Hypoglycemic cerebral vasodilation develops in the mature brain only after the electroencephalogram (EEG) becomes isoelectric[342–345] and consciousness is lost. In mature animals, moderate hypoglycemia increases blood flow in the cerebral cortex and thalamus, and only during severe hypoglycemia is a global increase in cerebral blood flow elicited.[346] Cerebral hemodynamic data from hypoglycemic human newborns are sparse. In premature infants, cerebral vasodilation develops at glucose levels below 30 mg/dL, before the EEG becomes significantly abnormal or major mental status changes develop.[36] This vasodilation is rapidly reversed by glucose administration.[35,36,157] Several reasons are proposed for these maturational differences in activation of hypoglycemic vasodilation. First, the blood-to-brain glucose gradient is significantly steeper in the immature brain as a result of the reduced glucose transporter proteins in the immature blood-brain barrier and neuroglial cell membranes.[347–349] In addition, there is a greater tendency toward anaerobic metabolism in the immature brain, which increases glucose demands. Together, these factors may increase the sensitivity of the immature brain's vasodilatory response to a fall in brain glucose delivery.

The mechanisms and mediators of hypoglycemic vasodilation remain poorly defined. Because glucose deprivation to the brain cells causes vasodilation in response to insulin-induced hypoglycemia and to 2-deoxyglucose administration, which increases circulating glucose levels, neither blood glucose nor insulin levels seem to play a direct role. Animal data do not suggest a significant role for changes in extracellular pH or potassium concentration in hypoglycemic vasodilation.[340,350] In piglets with hypoglycemia severe enough to cause an isoelectric EEG, NO seems to play little if any role in cerebral vasodilation.[351] Severe hypoglycemia disrupts pressure-flow autoregulation and increases systemic blood pressure; however, this mechanism does play a significant role in cerebral vasodilation.[350] Alternatively, adenosine may be an important mediator of hypoglycemic vasodilation, because blockade of adenosine receptors decreases and eventually blocks this response.[352]

NEURONAL ACTIVATION-FLOW AUTOREGULATION

Although neuronal activation-perfusion coupling first was proposed more than a century ago,[55] significant advances in understanding the nature of this response only became possible with the advent of techniques, such as PET and functional MRI, that allow measurement of regional cerebral perfusion changes.[65,66,353,354]

Characteristics of Neuronal Activation-Blood Flow Coupling

A tight temporal and spatial coupling exists between neuronal activation and blood flow in the normal mature brain.[143,176,355–357] The hyperemic response to neuronal activation is extremely fast and highly localized, occurring within 1 second and remaining confined to a 250 mm^2 area.[358] The hyperemic response may anticipate and exceed the initial metabolic demand, with a transient increase in oxyhemoglobin. Although the vast majority of data for neurovascular coupling originate from mature subjects, this phenomenon has been clearly described in young children and in healthy term, stable, and unstable preterm newborn infants.[359–367] Because the age of these infants does not permit predictable repetitive motor activity, NIRS measurements of cerebral oxyhemoglobin changes in response to several different modalities of sensory activation have been used to detect neurovascular coupling in the newborn. Types of stimuli have included visual,[361,362] auditory,[363,365] olfactory,[366] and painful.[364] Yamada and colleagues[360] described rapid neurovascular coupling with visual stimulation and detected by functional MRI in young infants, with an age-related difference in response. In premature infants, coupling has been described between the normal bursts in the discontinuous background EEG pattern and oxyhemoglobin changes by NIRS;[367] in these studies a brief decrease in cerebral oxyhemoglobin preceded the EEG burst, which was followed by an overshoot in oxyhemoglobin. The temporal response of these patterns was different between normal and neurologically stressed infants.[367] The cerebral hemodynamic responses to the abnormal neuronal activation of seizures are discussed later.

Mechanisms of Neuronal Activation-Blood Flow Coupling

Mechanisms proposed to underlie neurovascular coupling include neuronal electrochemical events, accumulation of metabolic products, or a local decrease in tissue oxygenation from increased use. It is generally believed that the endothelium plays little or no role in neurovascular coupling.[62] With neuronal activation, extracellular potassium accumulates and stimulates the Na/K-ATPase pump[356,368] which restores transmembrane ionic gradients, a process responsible for approximately 60% of cerebral oxygen use. The acute initiating stimulus for local vasodilation has been debated, with some suggesting an initial local accumulation of extracellular potassium hyperpolarizing the smooth muscle membrane.[369–376] Sufficient extracellular potassium takes approximately 5 to 10 seconds to accumulate, however, which is too slow to activate the acute phase hyperemic response.[377] The rate of accumulation and removal of adenosine, the product of high-energy phosphate breakdown,[378] also is too slow to reconcile with the rapidity of the initial neurovascular response.[93]

Although these and other metabolic paracrine substances (eg, NO and prostanoids)[379] seem unlikely to trigger the initial vasodilation, they may play an important role in supporting sustained neurovascular coupling during prolonged periods of activation.[380] More recently, the importance of perivascular astrocytes as mediators of this rapid neurovascular response has been highlighted.[381,382]

CEREBRAL AUTOREGULATION SYSTEMS MAY BE DISRUPTED BY BRAIN INSULTS

Cerebral autoregulation fails at the physiologic extremes and if persistent, impairment of cerebral hemodynamics may be sustained, extending the risk for brain injury. Insults, such as cerebral hypoxia-ischemia/reperfusion (HI/R), may cause direct injury not only to the cerebral parenchyma but also to systems that regulate cerebrovascular control.[142,383–388] The effects of HI/R insults on subsequent cerebral hemodynamics and autoregulatory function have been studied in many experimental models[307,385,389–393] and clinical studies in newborn infants.[394,395] With reperfusion after severe asphyxia, there is a delayed phase of vasodilation and hyperemia possibly related to the delayed activation of inducible NOS with sustained production of NO.[396] After global HI/R in newborn animals, there is a marked and selective loss of prostanoid-dependent vasodilation,[386,397] probably a result of depletion of membrane arachidonic acid pools required for generation of vasodilating prostanoids.[398,399] Prostanoid-independent responses,[392] however (eg, hypocapneic or hyperoxemic vasoconstriction),[308] are preserved, with potentially important repercussions for resuscitation after HI/R insults. A hierarchic vulnerability of cerebral vasoreactivity to HI/R insults has been described,[356,400] with pressure-flow autoregulation disrupted more readily than CVR-CO_2 and with CVR-O_2 being the most robust response.

Seizures are caused by repetitive uncontrolled neuronal discharges and commonly have systemic hemodynamic effects resulting from sympathetic activation with initial tachycardia and hypertension. Seizures also cause major increases in cerebral blood flow[401] and severe cerebrovascular dysfunction that persists for many hours into the postictal period;[150] during this time, reactivity to a variety of important vasodilators is impaired. In a small series of seizures in human newborns, seizures triggered an increase in cerebral blood flow velocity, even when acute blood pressure changes did not accompany the seizure.[402] In neonatal piglets, seizures increase cerebral blood flow by increasing local CO through activation of heme oxygenase;[403–405] others have shown that the prolonged hemodynamic dysfunction after seizures could be prevented by augmenting heme oxygenase activity.[404] Other experimental studies have shown NO of neuronal origin[406] and prostanoids[407] may be involved in seizure-related vasodilation.

SUMMARY

There has been significant progress in understanding normal and disrupted cerebral hemodynamic regulation. The vast majority of data have come, however, from experimental and clinical studies in mature subjects. The dominant form of brain injury responsible for the enormous burden of neurodevelopmental dysfunction in survivors of prematurity is mediated by cerebrovascular insults. If effective neuroprotection, in particular primary prevention, against these potentially devastating forms of prematurity-related brain injury is to become a reality, there are major challenges that need to be overcome. This review attempts to outline the progress to date to better understand these challenges for the future.

REFERENCES

1. Shalak L, Perlman JM. Hemorrhagic-ischemic cerebral injury in the preterm infant: current concepts. Clin Perinatol 2002;29(4):745–63.
2. Khwaja O, Volpe JJ. Pathogenesis of cerebral white matter injury of prematurity. Arch Dis Child Fetal Neonatal Ed 2008;93(2):F153–61.
3. Gleason CA, Hamm C, Jones MD Jr. Cerebral blood flow, oxygenation, and carbohydrate metabolism in immature fetal sheep in utero. Am J Physiol 1989;256 (6 Pt 2):R1264–8.
4. Jones MD Jr, Rosenberg AA, Simmons MA, et al. Oxygen delivery to the brain before and after birth. Science 1982;216(4543):324–5.
5. Jones MD Jr, Traystman RJ. Cerebral oxygenation of the fetus, newborn, and adult. Semin Perinatol 1984;8(3):205–16.
6. Ashwal S, Majcher JS, Longo LD. Patterns of fetal lamb regional cerebral blood flow during and after prolonged hypoxia: studies during the posthypoxic recovery period. Am J Obstet Gynecol 1981;139(4):365–72.
7. Papile LA, Rudolph AM, Heymann MA. Autoregulation of cerebral blood flow in the preterm fetal lamb. Pediatr Res 1985;19(2):159–61.
8. Rudolph AM. Distribution and regulation of blood flow in the fetal and neonatal lamb. Circ Res 1985;57(6):811–21.
9. Richardson BS, Carmichael L, Homan J, et al. Regional blood flow change in the lamb during the perinatal period. Am J Obstet Gynecol 1989;160(4):919–25.

10. Limperopoulos C, Bassan H, Kalish LA, et al. Current definitions of hypotension do not predict abnormal cranial ultrasound findings in preterm infants. Pediatrics 2007;120(5):966–77.
11. Seri I, Evans J. Controversies in the diagnosis and management of hypotension in the newborn infant. Curr Opin Pediatr 2001;13(2):116–23.
12. Evans N, Osborn D, Kluckow M. Preterm circulatory support is more complex than just blood pressure. Pediatrics 2005;115(4):1114–5 [author reply 5–6].
13. Dempsey EM, Barrington KJ. Treating hypotension in the preterm infant: when and with what: a critical and systematic review. J Perinatol 2007;27(8):469–78.
14. Chatow U, Davidson S, Reichman BL, et al. Development and maturation of the autonomic nervous system in premature and full-term infants using spectral analysis of heart rate fluctuations. Pediatr Res 1995;37(3):294–302.
15. Drouin E, Gournay V, Calamel J, et al. Assessment of spontaneous baroreflex sensitivity in neonates. Arch Dis Child Fetal Neonatal Ed 1997;76(2):F108–12.
16. Andriessen P, Koolen AMP, Berendsen RCM, et al. Cardiovascular fluctuations and transfer function analysis in stable preterm infants. Pediatr Res 2003;53(1):89–97.
17. Clyman RI. Mechanisms regulating the ductus arteriosus. Biol Neonate 2006;89(4):330–5.
18. Kluckow M, Evans N. Low superior vena cava flow and intraventricular haemorrhage in preterm infants. Arch Dis Child Fetal Neonatal Ed 2000;82(3):F188–94.
19. Hunt RW, Evans N, Rieger I, et al. Low superior vena cava flow and neurodevelopment at 3 years in very preterm infants. J Pediatr 2004;145(5):588–92.
20. Kluckow M, Evans N. Low systemic blood flow and hyperkalemia in preterm infants. J Pediatr 2001;139(2):227–32.
21. Osborn D, Evans N, Kluckow M. Randomized trial of dobutamine versus dopamine in preterm infants with low systemic blood flow. J Pediatr 2002;140(2):183–91.
22. Rorke LB. Anatomical features of the developing brain implicated in pathogenesis of hypoxic-ischemic injury. Brain Pathol 1992;2(3):211–21.
23. De Reuck JL. Cerebral angioarchitecture and perinatal brain lesions in premature and full-term infants. Acta Neurol Scand 1984;70(6):391–5.
24. Takashima S, Armstrong DL, Becker LE. Subcortical leukomalacia. Relationship to development of the cerebral sulcus and its vascular supply. Arch Neurol 1978;35(7):470–2.
25. De Reuck J. The human periventricular arterial blood supply and the anatomy of cerebral infarctions. Eur Neurol 1971;5(6):321–34.
26. De Reuck J. The cortico-subcortical arterial angio-architecture in the human brain. Acta Neurol Belg 1972;72(5):323–9.
27. Ballabh P, Braun A, Nedergaard M. Anatomic analysis of blood vessels in germinal matrix, cerebral cortex, and white matter in developing infants. Pediatr Res 2004;56(1):117–24.
28. Miyawaki T, Matsui K, Takashima S. Developmental characteristics of vessel density in the human fetal and infant brains. Early Hum Dev 1998;53(1):65–72.
29. Powers WJ, Grubb RL Jr, Darriet D, et al. Cerebral blood flow and cerebral metabolic rate of oxygen requirements for cerebral function and viability in humans. J Cereb Blood Flow Metab 1985;5(4):600–8.
30. Greisen G. Cerebral blood flow in preterm infants during the first week of life. Acta Paediatr Scand 1986;75(1):43–51.
31. Greisen G. Cerebral blood flow in mechanically ventilated, preterm neonates. Dan Med Bull 1990;37(2):124–31.

32. Greisen G. Thresholds for periventricular white matter vulnerability in hypoxia-ischemia. In: Lou H, Greisen G, Larsen J, editors. Brain lesions in the newborn. Copenhagen (Denmark): Munksgaard; 1994. p. 222–9.
33. Greisen G, Johansen K, Ellison PH, et al. Cerebral blood flow in the newborn infant: comparison of Doppler ultrasound and 133xenon clearance. J Pediatr 1984;104(3):411–8.
34. Greisen G, Pryds O. Low CBF, discontinuous EEG activity, and periventricular brain injury in ill, preterm neonates. Brain Dev 1989;11:164–8.
35. Pryds O, Christensen NJ, Friis HB. Increased cerebral blood flow and plasma epinephrine in hypoglycemic, preterm neonates. Pediatrics 1990;85(2):172–6.
36. Pryds O, Greisen G, Friis-Hansen B. Compensatory increase of CBF in preterm infants during hypoglycaemia. Acta Paediatr Scand 1988;77(5):632–7.
37. Pryds O, Greisen G, Johansen KH. Indomethacin and cerebral blood flow in premature infants treated for patent ductus arteriosus. Eur J Pediatr 1988;147(3): 315–6.
38. Pryds O, Andersen GE, Friis-Hansen B. Cerebral blood flow reactivity in spontaneously breathing, preterm infants shortly after birth. Acta Paediatr Scand 1990; 79(4):391–6.
39. Altman DI, Powers WJ, Perlman JM, et al. Cerebral blood flow requirement for brain viability in newborn infants is lower than in adults. Ann Neurol 1988;24: 218–26.
40. Borch K, Greisen G. Blood flow distribution in the normal human preterm brain. Pediatr Res 1998;43(1):28–33.
41. Volpe JJ. Hypoxic-ischemic encephalopathy: biochemical and physiological aspects. Neurology of the newborn. 5th edition. Philadelphia: Saunders Elsevier; 2008. p. 247–24.
42. Kuban KC, Gilles FH. Human telencephalic angiogenesis. Ann Neurol 1985; 17(6):539–48.
43. Nelson MD Jr, Gonzalez-Gomez I, Gilles FH. Dyke Award. The search for human telencephalic ventriculofugal arteries. AJNR Am J Neuroradiol 1991;12(2): 215–22.
44. Larroche JC. Intraventricular hemorrhage in the premature neonate. In: Korobkin R, Guilleminault C, editors, Advances in perinatal neurology, vol. 1. New York: S.P. Medical and Scientific Books; 1979. p. 115.
45. Hambleton G, Wigglesworth JS. Origin of intraventricular haemorrhage in the preterm infant. Arch Dis Child 1976;51(9):651–9.
46. Rorke LB. Pathology of perinatal brain injury. New York: Raven Press; 1982.
47. Nakamura Y, Okudera T, Fukuda S, et al. Germinal matrix hemorrhage of venous origin in preterm neonates. Hum Pathol 1990;21(10):1059–62.
48. Moody DM, Brown WR, Challa VR, et al. Alkaline phosphatase histochemical staining in the study of germinal matrix hemorrhage and brain vascular morphology in a very-low-birth-weight neonate. Pediatr Res 1994;35:424–30.
49. Ghazi-Birry HS, Brown WR, Moody DM, et al. Human germinal matrix: venous origin of hemorrhage and vascular characteristics. AJNR Am J Neuroradiol 1997;18(2):219–29.
50. Anstrom JA, Brown WR, Moody DM, et al. Subependymal veins in premature neonates: implications for hemorrhage. Pediatr Neurol 2004;30(1):46–53.
51. Szymonowicz W, Schafler K, Cussen LJ, et al. Ultrasound and necropsy study of periventricular haemorrhage in preterm infants. Arch Dis Child 1984;59:637–42.
52. Yakovlev PI, Rosales RK. Distribution of the terminal hemorrhages in the brain wall in stillborn premature and nonviable neonates. In: Angle CR,

Bering EA Jr, editors. Physical trauma as an etiologic agent in mental retardation. Washington, DC: U.S. Government Printing Office; 1970. p. 67.
53. Gruenwald P. Subependymal cerebral hemorrhage in premature infants, and its relation to various injurious influences at birth. Am J Obstet Gynecol 1951;61: 1285–92.
54. Leech RW, Kohnen P. Subependymal and intraventricular hemorrhages in the newborn. Am J Pathol 1974;77(3):465–75.
55. Roy C, Sherrington C. On the regulation of the blood supply of the brain. J Physiol 1890;11:85–108.
56. Kety SS, Schmidt CF. The effects of altered arterial tensions of carbon dioxide and oxygen on cerebral blood flow and cerebral oxygen consumption of normal young men. J Clin Invest 1948;27(4):484–92.
57. Lassen NA. Cerebral blood flow and oxygen consumption in man. Physiol Rev 1959;39(2):183–233.
58. Harder DR. A cellular mechanism for myogenic regulation of cat cerebral arteries. Ann Biomed Eng 1985;13(3–4):335–9.
59. Harder DR, Kauser K, Roman RJ, et al. Mechanisms of pressure-induced myogenic activation of cerebral and renal arteries: role of the endothelium. J Hypertens Suppl 1989;7(4):S11–5 [discussion S6].
60. Meininger GA, Zawieja DC, Falcone JC, et al. Calcium measurement in isolated arterioles during myogenic and agonist stimulation. Am J Physiol 1991;261 (3 Pt 2):H950–9.
61. Girouard H, Iadecola C. Neurovascular coupling in the normal brain and in hypertension, stroke, and Alzheimer disease. J Appl Physiol 2006;100(1):328–35.
62. Andresen J, Shafi NI, Bryan RM Jr. Endothelial influences on cerebrovascular tone. J Appl Physiol 2006;100(1):318–27.
63. Davis MJ, Hill MA. Signaling mechanisms underlying the vascular myogenic response. Physiol Rev 1999;79(2):387–423.
64. McCarron JG, Crichton CA, Langton PD, et al. Myogenic contraction by modulation of voltage-dependent calcium currents in isolated rat cerebral arteries. J Physiol 1997;498(Pt 2):371–9.
65. Heistad DD, Kontos HA. Cerebral circulation. In: Shepherd JT, Abboud FM, editors, Handbook of physiology, vol. 3. Bethesda (MD): American Physiological Society; 1983. p. 137–82.
66. Daffertshofer M, Hennerici M. Cerebrovascular regulation and vasoneuronal coupling. J Clin Ultrasound 1995;23(2):125–38.
67. Osol G, Laher I, Cipolla M. Protein kinase C modulates basal myogenic tone in resistance arteries from the cerebral circulation. Circ Res 1991;68(2):359–67.
68. Hill MA, Falcone JC, Meininger GA. Evidence for protein kinase C involvement in arteriolar myogenic reactivity. Am J Physiol 1990;259(5 Pt 2):H1586–94.
69. Henrion D, Laher I. Effects of staurosporine and calphostin C, two structurally unrelated inhibitors of protein kinase C, on vascular tone. Can J Physiol Pharmacol 1993;71(7):521–4.
70. Narayanan J, Imig M, Roman RJ, et al. Pressurization of isolated renal arteries increases inositol trisphosphate and diacylglycerol. Am J Physiol 1994;266 (5 Pt 2):H1840–5.
71. Ingi T, Cheng J, Ronnett GV. Carbon monoxide: an endogenous modulator of the nitric oxide-cyclic GMP signaling system. Neuron 1996;16(4):835–42.
72. Leffler CW, Balabanova L. Mechanism of permissive prostacyclin action in cerebrovascular smooth muscle. Prostaglandins Other Lipid Mediat 2001;66(3): 145–53.

73. Leffler CW, Nasjletti A, Johnson RA, et al. Contributions of prostacyclin and nitric oxide to carbon monoxide-induced cerebrovascular dilation in piglets. Am J Physiol Heart Circ Physiolsiol 2001;280(4):H1490–5.
74. Leffler CW, Balabanova L, Fedinec AL, et al. Nitric oxide increases carbon monoxide production by piglet cerebral microvessels. Am J Physiol Heart Circ Physiol 2005;289(4):H1442–7.
75. Leffler CW, Fedinec AL, Parfenova H, et al. Permissive contributions of NO and prostacyclin in CO-induced cerebrovascular dilation in piglets. Am J Physiol Heart Circ Physiol 2005;289(1):H432–8.
76. Faraci FM, Brian JE Jr. Nitric oxide and the cerebral circulation. Stroke 1994; 25(3):692–703.
77. Parfenova H, Shibata M, Zuckerman S, et al. CO2 and cerebral circulation in newborn pigs: cyclic nucleotides and prostanoids in vascular regulation. Am J Physiol 1994;266(4 Pt 2):H1494–501.
78. Atochin DN, Demchenko IT, Astern J, et al. Contributions of endothelial and neuronal nitric oxide synthases to cerebrovascular responses to hyperoxia. J Cereb Blood Flow Metab 2003;23(10):1219–26.
79. Wang Q, Pelligrino DA, Baughman VL, et al. The role of neuronal nitric oxide synthase in regulation of cerebral blood flow in normocapnia and hypercapnia in rats. J Cereb Blood Flow Metab 1995;15(5):774–8.
80. Jones SC, Radinsky CR, Furlan AJ, et al. Cortical NOS inhibition raises the lower limit of cerebral blood flow-arterial pressure autoregulation. Am J Physiol 1999; 276(4 Pt 2):H1253–62.
81. Kajita Y, Takayasu M, Dietrich HH, et al. Possible role of nitric oxide in autoregulatory response in rat intracerebral arterioles. Neurosurgery 1998;42(4):834–41 [discussion 41–2].
82. Kajita Y, Takayasu M, Suzuki Y, et al. Regional differences in cerebral vasomotor control by nitric oxide. Brain Res Bull 1995;38(4):365–9.
83. Hudetz AG, Shen H, Kampine JP. Nitric oxide from neuronal NOS plays critical role in cerebral capillary flow response to hypoxia. Am J Physiol 1998;274 (3 Pt 2):H982–9.
84. Bauser-Heaton HD, Bohlen HG. Cerebral microvascular dilation during hypotension and decreased oxygen tension: a role for nNOS. Am J Physiol Heart Circ Physiol 2007;293(4):H2193–201.
85. Domoki F, Perciaccante JV, Shimizu K, et al. N-methyl-D-aspartate-induced vasodilation is mediated by endothelium-independent nitric oxide release in piglets. Am J Physiol Heart Circ Physiol 2002;282(4):H1404–9.
86. Smith WL, Garavito RM, DeWitt DL. Prostaglandin endoperoxide H synthases (cyclooxygenases)-1 and -2. J Biol Chem 1996;271(52):33157–60.
87. Kis B, Snipes JA, Busija DW. Acetaminophen and the cyclooxygenase-3 puzzle: sorting out facts, fictions, and uncertainties. J Pharmacol Exp Ther 2005;315(1): 1–7.
88. Zuckerman SL, Armstead WM, Hsu P, et al. Age dependence of cerebrovascular response mechanisms in domestic pigs. Am J Physiol 1996;271(2 Pt 2): H535–40.
89. Armstead WM, Zuckerman SL, Shibata M, et al. Different pial arteriolar responses to acetylcholine in the newborn and juvenile pig. J Cereb Blood Flow Metab 1994;14(6):1088–95.
90. Willis AP, Leffler CW. NO and prostanoids: age dependence of hypercapnia and histamine-induced dilations of pig pial arterioles. Am J Physiol 1999;277(1 Pt 2): H299–307.

91. Bryan RM Jr, You J, Golding EM, et al. Endothelium-derived hyperpolarizing factor: a cousin to nitric oxide and prostacyclin. Anesthesiology 2005;102(6):1261–77.
92. You J, Golding EM, Bryan RM Jr. Arachidonic acid metabolites, hydrogen peroxide, and EDHF in cerebral arteries. Am J Physiol Heart Circ Physiol 2005;289(3): H1077–83.
93. Winn HR, Morii S, Berne RM. The role of adenosine in autoregulation of cerebral blood flow. Ann Biomed Eng 1985;13(3–4):321–8.
94. Parfenova H, Fedinec A, Leffler CW. Ionotropic glutamate receptors in cerebral microvascular endothelium are functionally linked to heme oxygenase. J Cereb Blood Flow Metab 2003;23(2):190–7.
95. Leffler CW, Parfenova H, Fedinec AL, et al. Contributions of astrocytes and CO to pial arteriolar dilation to glutamate in newborn pigs. Am J Physiol Heart Circ Physiol 2006;291(6):H2897–904.
96. Faraci FM. Effects of endothelin and vasopressin on cerebral blood vessels. Am J Physiol 1989;257(3 Pt 2):H799–803.
97. Sagher O, Jin Y, Thai QA, et al. Cerebral microvascular responses to endothelins: the role of ETA receptors. Brain Res 1994;658(1–2):179–84.
98. Matsuo Y, Mihara S, Ninomiya M, et al. Protective effect of endothelin type A receptor antagonist on brain edema and injury after transient middle cerebral artery occlusion in rats. Stroke 2001;32(9):2143–8.
99. Petrov T, Rafols JA. Acute alterations of endothelin-1 and iNOS expression and control of the brain microcirculation after head trauma. Neurol Res 2001;23(2–3): 139–43.
100. Armstead WM. Role of endothelin-1 in age-dependent cerebrovascular hypotensive responses after brain injury. Am J Physiol 1999;277(5 Pt 2):H1884–94.
101. Busija D. Sympathetic nerves reduce cerebral blood flow during hypoxia in awake rabbits. Am J Physiol 1984;247:H446–51.
102. Busija D, Heistad D. Factors involved in the physiological regulation of the cerebral circulation (Pt 1). Rev Physiol Biochem Pharmacol 1984;101:161–211.
103. Haggendal E, Johansson B. Effects of arterial carbon dioxide tension and oxygen saturation on cerebral blood flow autoregulation in dogs. Acta Physiol Scand Suppl 1965;258:27–53.
104. Nilsson B, Agardh C, Ingvar M, et al. Cerebrovascular response during and following severe insulin-induced hypoglycemia: CO2-sensitivity, autoregulation, and influence of prostaglandin synthesis inhibition. Acta Physiol Scand 1981; 111:455–63.
105. Bayliss W. On the local reactions of the arterial wall to changes of internal pressure. J Physiol (Lond) 1902;28:220–31.
106. Fog M. Cerebral circulation. The reaction of the pial arteries to a fall in blood pressure. Arch Neurol Psychiatry 1937;37:351–64.
107. Fog M. The relationship between the blood pressure and the tonic regulation of the pial arteries. J Neurol Psychiatry 1938;1:187–97.
108. Fog M. Cerebral circulation II. The reaction of the pial arteries to an increase in blood pressure. Arch Neurol Psychiatry 1939;41:260–8.
109. Edvinsson L, MacKenzie ET, McCulloch J. Autoregulation. In: Edvinsson L, MacKenzie ET, McCulloch J, editors. Cerebral blood flow and metabolism. New York: Raven Press; 1993. p. 553–80.
110. Lassen NA. Control of cerebral circulation in health and disease. Circ Res 1974; 34(6):749–60.

111. Younkin DP, Reivich M, Jaggi J, et al. Noninvasive method of estimating human newborn regional cerebral blood flow. J Cereb Blood Flow Metab 1982;2(4): 415–20.
112. Greisen G, Pryds O. Intravenous 133Xe clearance in preterm neonates with respiratory distress. Internal validation of CBF infinity as a measure of global cerebral blood flow. Scand J Clin Lab Invest 1988;48(7):673–8.
113. Anthony MY, Evans DH, Levene MI. Neonatal cerebral blood flow velocity responses to changes in posture. Arch Dis Child 1993;69(3 Spec No):304–8.
114. Aaslid R, Lindegaard KF, Sorteberg W, et al. Cerebral autoregulation dynamics in humans. Stroke 1989;20(1):45–52.
115. Panerai RB, Kelsall AW, Rennie JM, et al. Cerebral autoregulation dynamics in premature newborns. Stroke 1995;26(1):74–80.
116. Panerai RB, Kelsall AW, Rennie JM, et al. Analysis of cerebral blood flow autoregulation in neonates. IEEE Trans Biomed Eng 1996;43(8):779–88.
117. Panerai RB, Kelsall AW, Rennie JM, et al. Mechanism of cerebral autoregulation in neonates. Early Hum Dev 1997;47:206–7.
118. Boylan GB, Young K, Panerai RB, et al. Dynamic cerebral autoregulation in sick newborn infants. Pediatr Res 2000;48(1):12–7.
119. von Siebenthal K, Beran J, Wolf M, et al. Cyclical fluctuations in blood pressure, heart rate and cerebral blood volume in preterm infants. Brain Dev 1999;21(8): 529–34.
120. Tsuji M, Saul JP, du Plessis A, et al. Cerebral intravascular oxygenation correlates with mean arterial pressure in critically ill premature infants. Pediatrics 2000;106(4):625–32.
121. Soul JS, Hammer PE, Tsuji M, et al. Fluctuating pressure-passivity is common in the cerebral circulation of sick premature infants. Pediatr Res 2007;61(4): 467–73.
122. Lemmers PM, Toet M, van Schelven LJ, et al. Cerebral oxygenation and cerebral oxygen extraction in the preterm infant: the impact of respiratory distress syndrome. Exp Brain Res 2006;173(3):458–67.
123. van de Bor M, Walther FJ. Cerebral blood flow velocity regulation in preterm infants. Biol Neonate 1991;59(6):329–35.
124. Mueller SM, Heistad DD, Marcus ML. Total and regional cerebral blood flow during hypotension, hypertension, and hypocapnia. Effect of sympathetic denervation in dogs. Circ Res 1977;41(3):350–6.
125. Sadoshima S, Thames M, Heistad D. Cerebral blood flow during elevation of intracranial pressure: role of sympathetic nerves. Am J Physiol 1981;241(1): H78–84.
126. Baumbach G, Heistad D. Regional, segmental, and temporal heterogeneity of cerebral vascular autoregulation. Ann Biomed Eng 1985;13:303–13.
127. Garcia-Roldan JL, Bevan J. Flow-induced constriction and dilation of cerebral resistance vessels. Circulation Research 1990;66:1445–8.
128. Yoshida K, Meyer JS, Sakamoto K, et al. Autoregulation of cerebral blood flow. Electromagnetic flow measurements during acute hypertension in the monkey. Circ Res 1966;19(4):726–38.
129. Symon L, Crockard HA, Dorsch NW, et al. Local cerebral blood flow and vascular reactivity in a chronic stable stroke in baboons. Stroke 1975;6(5):482–92.
130. Kontos H, Wei E, Navari R, et al. Responses of cerebral arteries and arterioles to acute hypotension and hypertension. Am J Physiol 1978;3(4):H371–83.

131. Busija DW, Heistad DD, Marcus ML. Effects of sympathetic nerves on cerebral vessels during acute, moderate increases in arterial pressure in dogs and cats. Circ Res 1980;46(5):696–702.
132. Baumbach GL, Heistad DD. Effects of sympathetic stimulation and changes in arterial pressure on segmental resistance of cerebral vessels in rabbits and cats. Circ Res 1983;52(5):527–33.
133. Symon L, Held K, Dorsch NWC. A study of regional autoregulation in the cerebral circulation to increased perfusion pressure in normocapnea and hypercapnea. Stroke 1973;4(2):139–47.
134. Bell BA, Symon L, Branston NM. CBF and time thresholds for the formation of ischemic cerebral edema, and effect of reperfusion in baboons. J Neurosurg 1985;62(1):31–41.
135. Florence G, Seylaz J. Rapid autoregulation of cerebral blood flow: a laser-Doppler flowmetry study. J Cereb Blood Flow Metab 1992;12(4):674–80.
136. Zhang R, Zuckerman JH, Giller CA, et al. Transfer function analysis of dynamic cerebral autoregulation in humans. Am J Physiol 1998;274:H233–41.
137. Jones MD Jr, Sheldon RE, Peeters LL, et al. Regulation of cerebral blood flow in the ovine fetus. Am J Physiol 1978;235(2):H162–6.
138. Hernandez MJ, Brennan RW, Bowman GS. Autoregulation of cerebral blood flow in the newborn dog. Brain Res 1980;184(1):199–202.
139. Camp D, Kotagal UR, Kleinman LI. Preservation of cerebral autoregulation in the unanesthetized hypoxemic newborn dog. Brain Res 1982;241(2):207–13.
140. Tweed WA, Cote J, Wade JG, et al. Preservation of fetal brain blood flow relative to other organs during hypovolemic hypotension. Pediatr Res 1982;16(2):137–40.
141. Tweed WA, Cote J, Pash M, et al. Arterial oxygenation determines autoregulation of cerebral blood flow in the fetal lamb. Pediatr Res 1983;17(4):246–9.
142. Tweed A, Cote J, Lou H, et al. Impairment of cerebral blood flow autoregulation in the newborn lamb by hypoxia. Pediatr Res 1986;20:516–9.
143. Armstead WM, Leffler CW. Neurohumoral regulation of the cerebral circulation. Proc Soc Exp Biol Med 1992;199(2):149–57.
144. Pasternak JF, Groothuis DR. Autoregulation of cerebral blood flow in the newborn beagle puppy. Biol Neonate 1985;48(2):100–9.
145. Szymonowicz W, Walker AM, Yu VY, et al. Regional cerebral blood flow after hemorrhagic hypotension in the preterm, near-term, and newborn lamb. Pediatr Res 1990;28(4):361–6.
146. Hohimer AR, Bissonnette JM. Effects of cephalic hypotension, hypertension, and barbiturates on fetal cerebral flood flow and metabolism. Am J Obstet Gynecol 1989;161(5):1344–51.
147. Young RS, Hernandez MJ, Yagel SK. Selective reduction of blood flow to white matter during hypotension in newborn dogs: a possible mechanism of periventricular leukomalacia. Ann Neurol 1982;12(5):445–8.
148. Arnold BW, Martin CG, Alexander BJ, et al. Autoregulation of brain blood flow during hypotension and hypertension in infant lambs. Pediatr Res 1991;29:110–5.
149. Monin P, Stonestreet BS, Oh W. Hyperventilation restores autoregulation of cerebral blood flow in postictal piglets. Pediatr Res 1991;30(3):294–8.
150. Hascoet JM, Monin P, Vert P. Persistence of impaired autoregulation of cerebral blood flow in the postictal period in piglets. Epilepsia 1988;29(6):743–7.
151. Del Toro J, Louis PT, Goddard-Finegold J. Cerebrovascular regulation and neonatal brain injury. Pediatr Neurol 1991;7(1):3–12.

152. van Os S, Liem D, Hopman J, et al. Cerebral O2 supply thresholds for the preservation of electrocortical brain activity during hypotension in near-term-born lambs. Pediatr Res 2005;57(3):358–62.
153. Van Os S, Klaessens J, Hopman J, et al. Cerebral oxygen supply during hypotension in near-term lambs: a near-infrared spectroscopy study. Brain Dev 2006; 28(2):115–21.
154. Lassen N, Christensen M. Physiology of cerebral blood flow. Br J Anaesth 1976; 48:719–34.
155. Gebremedhin D, Lange AR, Lowry TF, et al. Production of 20-HETE and its role in autoregulation of cerebral blood flow [see comments]. Circ Res 2000;87(1):60–5.
156. Lou HC, Lassen NA, Friis-Hansen B. Impaired autoregulation of cerebral blood flow in the distressed newborn infant. J Pediatr 1979;94(1):118–21.
157. Pryds O. Control of cerebral circulation in the high-risk neonate. Ann Neurol 1991;30:321–9.
158. Milligan DW. Failure of autoregulation and intraventricular haemorrhage in preterm infants. Lancet 1980;1(8174):896–8.
159. Miall-Allen VM, de Vries LS, Dubowitz LM, et al. Blood pressure fluctuation and intraventricular hemorrhage in the preterm infant of less than 31 weeks' gestation. Pediatrics 1989;83(5):657–61.
160. Ramaekers VT, Casaer P, Daniels H, et al. Upper limits of brain blood flow autoregulation in stable infants of various conceptional age. Early Hum Dev 1990; 24(3):249–58.
161. Verma PK, Panerai RB, Rennie JM, et al. Grading of cerebral autoregulation in preterm and term neonates. Pediatr Neurol 2000;23(3):236–42.
162. Younkin DP, Reivich M, Jaggi JL, et al. The effect of hematocrit and systolic blood pressure on cerebral blood flow in newborn infants. J Cereb Blood Flow Metab 1987;7(3):295–9.
163. Tyszczuk L, Meek J, Elwell C, et al. Cerebral blood flow is independent of mean arterial blood pressure in preterm infants undergoing intensive care. Pediatrics 1998;102:337–41.
164. Pryds O, Edwards AD. Cerebral blood flow in the newborn infant. Arch Dis Child 1996;74:F63–9.
165. Greisen G, Trojaborg W. Cerebral blood flow, PaCO2 changes, and visual evoked potentials in mechanically ventilated, preterm infants. Acta Paediatr Scand 1987;76(3):394–400.
166. Pryds O, Greisen G, Lou H, et al. Heterogeneity of cerebral vasoreactivity in preterm infants supported by mechanical ventilation. J Pediatr 1989;115(4):638–45.
167. Muller AM, Morales C, Briner J, et al. Loss of CO2 reactivity of cerebral blood flow is associated with severe brain damage in mechanically ventilated very low birth weight infants. Eur J Paediatr Neurol 1997;1(5–6):157–63.
168. Bassan H, Gauvreau K, Newburger JW, et al. Identification of pressure passive cerebral perfusion and its mediators after infant cardiac surgery. Pediatr Res 2005;57:35–41.
169. Giller CA. The frequency-dependent behavior of cerebral autoregulation. Neurosurgery 1990;27(3):362–8.
170. Harder D. Pressure-induced myogenic activation of cat cerebral arteries is dependent on intact endothelium. Circ Res 1987;60:102–7.
171. Wahl M, Schilling L. Regulation of cerebral blood flow—a brief review. Acta Neurochir Suppl (Wien) 1993;59:3–10.
172. Eidson TH, Edrington JL, Albuquerque ML, et al. Light/dye microvascular injury eliminates pial arteriolar dilation in hypotensive piglets. Pediatr Res 1995;37(1):10–4.

173. Falcone JC, Davis MJ, Meininger GA. Endothelial independence of myogenic response in isolated skeletal muscle arterioles. Am J Physiol 1991;260(1 Pt 2): H130–5.
174. Rubanyi G. Endothelium-dependent pressure-induced contraction of isolated canine carotid arteries. Am J Physiol 1988;255:H783–8.
175. Leffler CW, Busija DW, Beasley DG, et al. Maintenance of cerebral circulation during hemorrhagic hypotension in newborn pigs: role of prostanoids. Circ Res 1986;59(5):562–7.
176. Raichle ME, Grubb RL Jr, Gado MH, et al. Correlation between regional cerebral blood flow and oxidative metabolism. In vivo studies in man. Arch Neurol 1976; 33(8):523–6.
177. Powers W. Hemodynamics and metabolism in ischemic cerebrovascular disease. Neurol Clin 1992;10(1):31–48.
178. Powers W. Cerebral hemodynamics in ischemic cerebrovascular disease. Ann Neurol 1991;29:231–40.
179. Winn HR, Welsh JE, Rubio R, et al. Brain adenosine production in rat during sustained alteration in systemic blood pressure. Am J Physiol 1980;239(5): H636–41.
180. Kanu A, Whitfield J, Leffler CW. Carbon monoxide contributes to hypotension-induced cerebrovascular vasodilation in piglets. Am J Physiol Heart Circ Physiol 2006;291(5):H2409–14.
181. Fujii K, Heistad DD, Faraci FM. Flow-mediated dilatation of the basilar artery in vivo. Circ Res 1991;69(3):697–705.
182. Koller A, Sun D, Kaley G. Role of shear stress and endothelial prostaglandins in flow-and viscosity-induced dilation of arterioles in vitro. Circ Res 1993;72(6): 1276–84.
183. Gill AB, Weindling AM. Randomised controlled trial of plasma protein fraction versus dopamine in hypotensive very low birthweight infants. Arch Dis Child 1993;69(3 Spec No):284–7.
184. Al-Aweel I, Pursley DM, Rubin LP, et al. Variations in prevalence of hypotension, hypertension, and vasopressor use in NICUs. J Perinatol 2001;21(5):272–8.
185. Fanaroff JM, Fanaroff AA. Blood pressure disorders in the neonate: hypotension and hypertension. Semin Fetal Neonatal Med 2006;11(3):174–81.
186. Ment LR, Duncan CC, Ehrenkranz RA, et al. Intraventricular hemorrhage in the preterm neonate: timing and cerebral blood flow changes. J Pediatr 1984; 104(3):419–25.
187. Miall-Allen VM, de Vries LS, Whitelaw AG. Mean arterial blood pressure and neonatal cerebral lesions. Arch Dis Child 1987;62(10):1068–9.
188. Watkins AM, West CR, Cooke RW. Blood pressure and cerebral haemorrhage and ischaemia in very low birthweight infants. Early Hum Dev 1989;19(2): 103–10.
189. Gronlund JU, Korvenranta H, Kero P, et al. Elevated arterial blood pressure is associated with peri-intraventricular haemorrhage. Eur J Pediatr 1994;153(11): 836–41.
190. Ment LR, Stewart WB, Duncan CC, et al. Beagle puppy model of intraventricular hemorrhage. J Neurosurg 1982;57(2):219–23.
191. Goddard-Finegold J, Michael LH. Cerebral blood flow and experimental intraventricular hemorrhage. Pediatr Res 1984;18(1):7–11.
192. Goddard J, Lewis RM, Alcala H, et al. Intraventricular hemorrhage—an animal model. Biol Neonate 1980;37(1):39–52.

193. Goddard-Finegold J, Armstrong D, Zeller RS. Intraventricular hemorrhage following volume expansion after hypovolemic hypotension in the newborn beagle. J Pediatr 1982;100(5):796–9.
194. Pasternak JF, Groothuis DR, Fischer JM, et al. Regional cerebral blood flow in the newborn beagle pup: the germinal matrix is a "low-flow" structure. Pediatr Res 1982;16(6):499–503.
195. Pasternak JF, Groothuis DR, Fischer JM, et al. Regional cerebral blood flow in the beagle puppy model of neonatal intraventricular hemorrhage: studies during systemic hypertension. Neurology 1983;33(5):559–66.
196. Pasternak JF, Groothuis DR. Regional variability of blood flow and glucose utilization within the subependymal germinal matrix. Brain Res 1984;299(2):281–8.
197. Ment LR, Stewart WB, Petroff OA, et al. Thromboxane synthesis inhibitor in a beagle pup model of perinatal asphyxia. Stroke 1989;20(6):809–14.
198. Goddard-Finegold J, Donley DK, Adham BI, et al. Phenobarbital and cerebral blood flow during hypertension in the newborn beagle. Pediatrics 1990;86(4):501–8.
199. Bada HS, Korones SB, Perry EH, et al. Frequent handling in the neonatal intensive care unit and intraventricular hemorrhage. J Pediatr 1990;117(1):126–31.
200. Bada HS, Korones SB, Perry EH, et al. Mean arterial blood pressure changes in premature infants and those at risk for intraventricular hemorrhage. J Pediatr 1990;117(4):607–14.
201. Weindling AM, Wilkinson AR, Cook J, et al. Perinatal events which precede periventricular haemorrhage and leukomalacia in the newborn. Br J Obstet Gynaecol 1985;92(12):1218–23.
202. Perlman JM, McMenamin JB, Volpe JJ. Fluctuating cerebral blood-flow velocity in respiratory-distress syndrome: relation to the development of intraventricular hemorrhage. N Engl J Med 1983;309:204–9.
203. Low JA, Froese AB, Galbraith RS, et al. The association between preterm newborn hypotension and hypoxemia and outcome during the first year. Acta Paediatr 1993;82(5):433–7.
204. Dammann O, Allred EN, Kuban KC, et al. Systemic hypotension and white-matter damage in preterm infants. Dev Med Child Neurol 2002;44(2):82–90.
205. Cunningham S, Symon AG, Elton RA, et al. Intra-arterial blood pressure reference ranges, death and morbidity in very low birthweight infants during the first seven days of life. Early Hum Dev 1999;56(2–3):151–65.
206. Perlman JM, Risser R, Broyles RS. Bilateral cystic periventricular leukomalacia in the premature infant: associated risk factors. Pediatrics 1996;97(6 Pt 1):822–7.
207. Baud O, d'Allest AM, Lacaze-Masmonteil T, et al. The early diagnosis of periventricular leukomalacia in premature infants with positive rolandic sharp waves on serial electroencephalography. J Pediatr 1998;132(5):813–7.
208. Trounce JQ, Shaw DE, Levene MI, et al. Clinical risk factors and periventricular leucomalacia. Arch Dis Child 1988;63(1):17–22.
209. Bejar RF, Vaucher YE, Benirschke K, et al. Postnatal white matter necrosis in preterm infants. J Perinatol 1992;12(1):3–8.
210. Kluckow M, Evans N. Relationship between blood pressure and cardiac output in preterm infants requiring mechanical ventilation. J Pediatr 1996;129(4):506–12.
211. Kusaka T, Okubo K, Nagano K, et al. Cerebral distribution of cardiac output in newborn infants. Arch Dis Child Fetal Neonatal Ed 2005;90(1):F77–8.

212. Weindling AM, Kissack CM. Blood pressure and tissue oxygenation in the newborn baby at risk of brain damage. Biol Neonate 2001;79(3–4):241–5.
213. Kissack CM, Garr R, Wardle SP, et al. Cerebral fractional oxygen extraction in very low birth weight infants is high when there is low left ventricular output and hypocarbia but is unaffected by hypotension. Pediatr Res 2004;55(3):400–5.
214. Evans N, Kluckow M, Simmons M, et al. Which to measure, systemic or organ blood flow? Middle cerebral artery and superior vena cava flow in very preterm infants. Arch Dis Child Fetal Neonatal Ed 2002;87(3):F181–4.
215. Osborn DA, Evans N, Kluckow M. Hemodynamic and antecedent risk factors of early and late periventricular/intraventricular hemorrhage in premature infants. Pediatrics 2003;112(1 Pt 1):33–9.
216. Meek JH, Tyszczuk L, Elwell CE, et al. Low cerebral blood flow is a risk factor for severe intraventricular haemorrhage. Arch Dis Child Fetal Neonatal Ed 1999;81(1):F15–8.
217. Barrington KJ, Dempsey EM. Cardiovascular support in the preterm: treatments in search of indications. J Pediatr 2006;148(3):289–91.
218. Seri I. Cardiovascular support in the preterm: treatments in search of indications. J Pediatr 2007;150(2):e31–3 [author reply e3].
219. Raichle M, Posner J, Plum F. Cerebral blood flow during and after hyperventilation. Arch Neurol 1970;23:394–403.
220. Dahlgren N, Ingvar M, Siesjo BK. Effect of propranolol on local cerebral blood flow under normocapnic and hypercapnic conditions. J Cereb Blood Flow Metab 1981;1(4):429–36.
221. Brian JE Jr. Carbon dioxide and the cerebral circulation. Anesthesiology 1998;88(5):1365–86.
222. Warner D, Turner D, Kassel N. Time-dependent effects of prolonged hypercapnea on cerebrovascular parameters: acid-base chemistry. Stroke 1987;18:142–9.
223. Yang SP, Krasney JA. Cerebral blood flow and metabolic responses to sustained hypercapnia in awake sheep. J Cereb Blood Flow Metab 1995;15(1):115–23.
224. Edvinsson L, MacKenzie ET, McCulloch J. Changes in arterial gas tensions. In: Edvinsson L, MacKenzie ET, McCulloch J, editors. Cerebral blood flow and metabolism. New York: Raven Press; 1993. p. 524–52.
225. Brubakk AM, Oh W, Stonestreet BS. Prolonged hypercarbia in the awake newborn piglet: effect on brain blood flow and cardiac output. Pediatr Res 1987;21(1):29–33.
226. Najarian T, Marrache AM, Dumont I, et al. Prolonged hypercapnia-evoked cerebral hyperemia via K(+) channel- and prostaglandin E(2)-dependent endothelial nitric oxide synthase induction [In Process Citation]. Circ Res 2000;87(12):1149–56.
227. Heistad DD, Marcus ML, Abboud FM. Role of large arteries in regulation of cerebral blood flow in dogs. J Clin Invest 1978;62(4):761–8.
228. Sadoshima S, Fujishima M, Tamaki K, et al. Response of cortical and pial arteries to changes of arterial CO2 tension in rats—a morphometric study. Brain Res 1980;189(1):115–20.
229. Wyatt JS, Edwards AD, Cope M, et al. Response of cerebral blood volume to changes in arterial carbon dioxide tension in preterm and term infants. Pediatr Res 1991;29:553–7.
230. Greenberg J, Alavi A, Reivich M, et al. Local cerebral blood volume response to carbon dioxide in man. Circ Res 1978;43(2):324–31.

231. Shapiro HM, Greenberg JH, Naughton KV, et al. Heterogeneity of local cerebral blood flow-PaCO2 sensitivity in neonatal dogs. J Appl Physiol 1980;49(1): 113–8.
232. Haaland K, Orderud W, Thoresen M. The piglet as a model for cerebral circulation: an angiographic study. Biol Neonate 1995;68:75–80.
233. Yamashita N, Kamiya K, Nagai H. CO2 reactivity and autoregulation in fetal brain. Childs Nerv Syst 1991;7:327–31.
234. Dietz V, Wolf M, Keel M, et al. CO2 reactivity of the cerebral hemoglobin concentration in healthy term newborns measured by near infrared spectrophotometry. Biol Neonate 1999;75(2):85–90.
235. Leahy FA, Cates D, MacCallum M, et al. Effect of CO2 and 100% O2 on cerebral blood flow in preterm infants. J Appl Physiol 1980;48(3):468–72.
236. Leffler CW, Mirro R, Shanklin DR, et al. Light/dye microvascular injury selectively eliminates hypercapnia-induced pial arteriolar dilation in newborn pigs. Am J Physiol 1994;266(2 Pt 2):H623–30.
237. Mirro R, Karanth S, Armstead WM, et al. Alterations in cerebrovascular reactivity after positive pressure ventilation. Pediatr Res 1992;32(1):114–7.
238. Aalkjaer C, Poston L. Effects of pH on vascular tension: which are the important mechanisms? J Vasc Res 1996;33(5):347–59.
239. Arvidsson S, Haggendal E, Winso I. Influence on cerebral blood flow of infusion of sodium bicarbonate during respiratory acidosis and alkalosis in the dog. Acta Anaesthesiol Scand 1981;25(2):146–52.
240. Lassen NA. Brain extracellular pH: the main factor controlling cerebral blood flow. Scand J Clin Lab Invest 1968;22(4):247–51.
241. Wagerle L, Mishra O. Mechanisms of CO2 response in cerebral arteries of the newborn pig: role of phospholipase, cyclooxygenase and lipoxygenase. Circ Res 1988;62:1019–26.
242. Hermansen MC, Kotagal UR, Kleinman LI. The effect of metabolic acidosis upon autoregulation of cerebral blood flow in newborn dogs. Brain Res 1984;324(1): 101–5.
243. Laptook AR. The effects of sodium bicarbonate on brain blood flow and O2 delivery during hypoxemia and acidemia in the piglet. Pediatr Res 1985;19(8): 815–9.
244. Harada M, Fuse A, Tanaka Y. Measurement of nitric oxide in the rat cerebral cortex during hypercapnoea. Neuroreport 1997;8(4):999–1002.
245. Hormann C, Schmidauer C, Haring H, et al. Hyperventilation reverses the nitrous oxide-induced increase in cerebral blood flow velocity in human volunteers. Br J Anaesth 1995;74:616–8.
246. Keyeux A, Ochrymowicz-Bemelmans D, Charlier A. Induced response to hypercapnia in the two-compartment total cerebral blood volume: influence on brain vascular reserve and flow efficiency. J Cereb Blood Flow Metab 1995;15: 1121–31.
247. McPherson RW, Kirsch JR, Ghaly RF, et al. Effect of nitric oxide synthase inhibition on the cerebral vascular response to hypercapnia in primates. Stroke 1995; 26:682–7.
248. Meng W, Tobin J, Busija D. Glutamate-induced cerebral vasodilation is mediated by nitric oxide through N-methyl-D-aspartate receptors. Stroke 1995;26: 857–63.
249. Takei Y, Edwards A, Lorek A, et al. Effects of N-w-Nitro-L-Arginine methyl ester on the cerebral circulation of newborn piglets quantified in vivo by near-infrared spectroscopy. Pediatr Res 1993;34(3):354–9.

250. Thompson B, Pluta R, Girton M, et al. Nitric oxide mediation of chemoregulation but not autoregulation of cerebral blood flow in primates. J Neurosurg 1996;84: 71–8.
251. Hindman B, Dexter F, Cutkomp J, et al. Hypothermic acid-base management does not affect cerebral metabolic rate for oxygen at 27°C. A study during cardiopulmonary bypass in rabbits. Anesthesiology 1993;79:580–7.
252. Apkon M, Boron W. Extracellular and intracellular alkalinization and the constriction of rat cerebral arterioles. J Physiol 1995;484:743–53.
253. Iadecola C, Pelligrino D, Moskowitz M, et al. Nitric oxide synthase inhibition and cerebrovascular regulation. J Cereb Blood Flow Metab 1994;14(2):175–92.
254. Iadecola C, Zhang F. Nitric oxide-dependent and -indepedent components of cerebrovasodilation elicited by hypercapnea. Am J Physiol 1994;266(2): R546–52.
255. Iadecola C, Zhang F. Permissive and obligatory roles of NO in cerebrovascular responses to hypercapnea and acetylcholine. Am J Physiol 1996;271(4): R990–1001.
256. Patel J, Pryds O, Roberts I, et al. Limited role for nitric oxide in mediating cerebrovascular control of newborn piglets. Arch Dis Child 1996;75(2):F82–6.
257. Leffler CW, Busija DW, Beasley DG, et al. Effects of indomethacin on cardiac output distribution in normal and asphyxiated piglets. Prostaglandins 1986; 31(2):183–90.
258. Mirro R, Leffler CW, Armstead W, et al. Indomethacin restricts cerebral blood flow during pressure ventilation of newborn pigs. Pediatr Res 1988;24(1):59–62.
259. Edwards AD, Wyatt JS, Richardson C, et al. Effects of indomethacin on cerebral haemodynamics in very preterm infants. Lancet 1990;335(8704):1491–5.
260. Patel J, Roberts I, Azzopardi D, et al. Randomized double-blind controlled trial comparing the effects of ibuprofen with indomethacin on cerebral hemodynamics in preterm infants with patent ductus arteriosus [see comments]. Pediatr Res 2000;47(1):36–42.
261. McCormick DC, Edwards AD, Brown GC, et al. Effect of indomethacin on cerebral oxidized cytochrome oxidase in preterm infants. Pediatr Res 1993;33(6): 603–8.
262. Pellicer A, Aparicio M, Cabanas F, et al. Effect of the cyclo-oxygenase blocker ibuprofen on cerebral blood volume and cerebral blood flow during normocarbia and hypercarbia in newborn piglets. Acta Paediatr 1999;88(1):82–8.
263. Dumont I, Hou X, Hardy P, et al. Developmental regulation of endothelial nitric oxide synthase in cerebral vessels of newborn pig by prostaglandin E(2). J Pharmacol Exp Ther 1999;291(2):627–33.
264. Dumont I, Hardy P, Peri KG, et al. Regulation of endothelial nitric oxide synthase by PGD(2) in the developing choroid. Am J Physiol Heart Circ Physiol 2000; 278(1):H60–6.
265. Leffler CW, Mirro R, Thompson C, et al. Activated oxygen species do not mediate hypercapnia-induced cerebral vasodilation in newborn pigs. Am J Physiol 1991;261(2 Pt 2):H335–42.
266. Hsu P, Shibata M, Leffler CW. Prostanoid synthesis in response to high CO2 in newborn pig brain microvascular endothelial cells. Am J Physiol 1993;264 (5 Pt 2):H1485–92.
267. Fabres J, Carlo WA, Phillips V, et al. Both extremes of arterial carbon dioxide pressure and the magnitude of fluctuations in arterial carbon dioxide pressure are associated with severe intraventricular hemorrhage in preterm infants. Pediatrics 2007;119(2):299–305.

268. Kaiser JR, Gauss CH, Pont MM, et al. Hypercapnia during the first 3 days of life is associated with severe intraventricular hemorrhage in very low birth weight infants. J Perinatol 2006;26(5):279–85.
269. Kaiser JR, Gauss CH, Williams DK. The effects of hypercapnia on cerebral autoregulation in ventilated very low birth weight infants. Pediatr Res 2005;58(5): 931–5.
270. Wilson DF, Pastuszko A, DiGiacomo JE, et al. Effect of hyperventilation on oxygenation of the brain cortex of newborn piglets. J Appl Physiol 1991;70(6):2691–6.
271. Kennealy JA, McLennan JE, Loudon RG, et al. Hyperventilation-induced cerebral hypoxia. Am Rev Respir Dis 1980;122(3):407–12.
272. Reivich M, Brann AW Jr, Shapiro H, et al. Reactivity of cerebral vessels to CO2 in the newborn rhesus monkey. Eur Neurol 1971;6(1):132–6.
273. Grubb RL Jr, Raichle ME, Eichling JO, et al. The effects of changes in PaCO2 on cerebral blood volume, blood flow, and vascular mean transit time. Stroke 1974; 5(5):630–9.
274. Reuter JH, Disney TA. Regional cerebral blood flow and cerebral metabolic rate of oxygen during hyperventilation in the newborn dog. Pediatr Res 1986;20(11): 1102–6.
275. Hansen NB, Nowicki PT, Miller RR, et al. Alterations in cerebral blood flow and oxygen consumption during prolonged hypocarbia. Pediatr Res 1986;20(2): 147–50.
276. Plum F, Posner JB. Blood and cerebrospinal fluid lactate during hyperventilation. Am J Physiol 1967;212(4):864–70.
277. Granholm L, Siesjo BK. The effects of hypercapnia and hypocapnia upon the cerebrospinal fluid lactate and pyruvate concentrations and upon the lactate, pyruvate, ATP, ADP, phosphocreatine and creatine concentrations of cat brain tissue. Acta Physiol Scand 1969;75(3):257–66.
278. Graziani LJ, Spitzer AR, Mitchell DG, et al. Mechanical ventilation in preterm infants: neurosonographic and developmental studies. Pediatrics 1992;90(4): 515–22.
279. Calvert SA, Hoskins EM, Fong KW, et al. Etiological factors associated with the development of periventricular leukomalacia. Acta Paediatr Scand 1987;76(2): 254–9.
280. Greisen G, Munck H, Lou H. May hypocarbia cause ischaemic brain damage in the preterm infant? Lancet 1986;2(8504):460.
281. Greisen G, Munck H, Lou H. Severe hypocarbia in preterm infants and neurodevelopmental deficit. Acta Paediatr Scand 1987;76(3):401–4.
282. Greisen G, Vannucci RC. Is periventricular leucomalacia a result of hypoxic-ischaemic injury? Hypocapnia and the preterm brain. Biol Neonate 2001;79(3–4): 194–200.
283. Fujimoto S, Togari H, Yamaguchi N, et al. Hypocarbia and cystic periventricular leukomalacia in premature infants. Arch Dis Child 1994;71(2):F107–10.
284. Wiswell T, Graziani L, Kornhauser M, et al. Effects of hypocarbia on the development of cystic periventricular leukomalacia in premature infants treated with high-frequency jet ventilation. Pediatrics 1996;98:918–24.
285. Okumura A, Hayakawa F, Kato T, et al. Hypocarbia in preterm infants with periventricular leukomalacia: the relation between hypocarbia and mechanical ventilation. Pediatrics 2001;107(3):469–75.
286. Shankaran S, Langer JC, Kazzi SN, et al. Cumulative index of exposure to hypocarbia and hyperoxia as risk factors for periventricular leukomalacia in low birth weight infants. Pediatrics 2006;118(4):1654–9.

287. Jones M, Traystman R, Simmons M, et al. Effects of changes in arterial O2 content on cerebral blood flow in the lamb. Am J Physiol 1981;240:H209–15.
288. Hudak ML, Koehler RC, Rosenberg AA, et al. Effect of hematocrit on cerebral blood flow. Am J Physiol 1986;251(1 Pt 2):H63–70.
289. Pryds O, Greisen G. Effect of $PaCO_2$ and haemoglobin concentration on day to day variation of CBF in preterm neonates. Acta Paediatr Scand Suppl 1989; 360(1S):33–6.
290. Wolff J, Lennox K. Cerebral circulation; effect on pial vessels of variations in oxygen and carbon dioxide content of blood. Arch Neurol Psychiatry 1930;23: 1097–120.
291. Kety SS, Hafkenschiel JH, Jeffers WA, et al. The blood flow, vascular resistance, and oxygen consumption of the brain in essential hypertension. J Clin Invest 1948;27(4):511–4.
292. Johannsson H, Siesjo BK. Cerebral blood flow and oxygen consumption in the rat in hypoxic hypoxia. Acta Physiol Scand 1975;93(2):269–76.
293. Kennedy C, Grave GD, Sokoloff L. Alterations of local cerebral blood flow due to exposure of newborn puppies to 80–90 per cent oxygen. Eur Neurol 1971;6(1): 137–40.
294. Busija DW, Heistad DD. Effects of cholinergic nerves on cerebral blood flow in cats. Circ Res 1981;48(1):62–9.
295. Craigen ML, Jennett S. Pial arterial response to systemic hypoxia in anaesthetised cats. J Cereb Blood Flow Metab 1981;1(3):285–96.
296. Nilsson B, Nordberg K, Nordstrom CH, et al. Influence of hypoxia and hypercapnia in rats. In: Harper M, Jennett B, Miller R, et al, editors. Blood flow and metabolism in brain. Edinburgh (United Kingdom): Churchill Livingstone; 1975. p. 9.19–9.23.
297. Borgstrom L, Johannsson H, Siesjo BK. The relationship between arterial po2 and cerebral blood flow in hypoxic hypoxia. Acta Physiol Scand 1975;93(3):423–32.
298. Shimojyo S, Scheinberg P, Kogure K, et al. The effects of graded hypoxia upon transient cerebral blood flow and oxygen consumption. Neurology 1968;18(2): 127–33.
299. Kogure K, Scheinberg P, Reinmuth O, et al. Mechanisms of cerebral vasodilation in hypoxia. J Appl Physiol 1970;29:223–9.
300. Kogure K, Scheinberg P, Fujishima M, et al. Effects of hypoxia on cerebral autoregulation. Am J Physiol 1970;219(5):1393–6.
301. Longo LD, Pearce WJ. Fetal and newborn cerebral vascular responses and adaptations to hypoxia. Semin Perinatol 1991;15(1):49–57.
302. Ashwal S, Dale PS, Longo LD. Regional cerebral blood flow: studies in the fetal lamb during hypoxia, hypercapnia, acidosis, and hypotension. Pediatr Res 1984;18(12):1309–16.
303. Szymonowicz W, Walker AM, Cussen L, et al. Developmental changes in regional cerebral blood flow in fetal and newborn lambs. Am J Physiol 1988; 254(1 Pt 2):H52–8.
304. Koehler RC, Traystman RJ, Jones MD. Regional blood flow and O2 transport during hypoxic and CO hypoxia in neonatal and adult sheep. Am J Physiol 1985;248(1 Pt 2):H118–24.
305. Cavazzuti M, Duffy T. Regulation of local cerebral blood flow in normal and hypoxic newborn dogs. Ann Neurol 1982;11:247–57.
306. Pearce WJ, Ashwal S. Developmental changes in thickness, contractility, and hypoxic sensitivity of newborn lamb cerebral arteries. Pediatr Res 1987;22(2): 192–6.

307. Gilbert R, Pearce W, Ashwal S, et al. Effects of hypoxia on contractility of isolated fetal lamb cerebral arteries. J Dev Physiol 1990;13:199–203.
308. Lundstrom K, Pryds O, Greisen G. Oxygen at birth and prolonged cerebral vasoconstriction in preterm infants. Arch Dis Child 1995;73:F81–6.
309. Niijima S, Shortland DB, Levene MI, et al. Transient hyperoxia and cerebral blood flow velocity in infants born prematurely and at full term. Arch Dis Child 1988;63(10 Spec No):1126–30.
310. Greisen G, Skov L. Changing inspired oxygen fraction may alter cerebral hemoglobin concentration as detected by near-infrared spectroscopy. In: Lafeber H, editor. Fetal and neonatal physiological measurements. Amsterdam: Elsevier Science Publishers; 1991. p. 83–6.
311. Detar R, Bohr DF. Oxygen and vascular smooth muscle contraction. Am J Physiol 1968;214(2):241–4.
312. Pittman RN, Duling BR. Oxygen sensitivity of vascular smooth muscle. I. In vitro studies. Microvasc Res 1973;6(2):202–11.
313. Chang AE, Detar R. Oxygen and vascular smooth muscle contraction revisited. Am J Physiol 1980;238(5):H716–28.
314. Simeone F, Vinall P, Pickard J. Response of extraparenchymal cerebral arteries to biochemical environment of cerebrospinal fluid. In: Wood J, editor, Neurobiology of cerebrospinal fluid, vol. 1. New York: Plenum; 1980. p. 303–11.
315. Coburn RF, Eppinger R, Scott DP. Oxygen-dependent tension in vascular smooth muscle. Does the endothelium play a role? Circ Res 1986;58(3):341–7.
316. Pearce WJ. Role of endothelial relaxing and contracting factors in rabbit cranial artery responses to hypoxia. Proc West Pharmacol Soc 1989;32:239–45.
317. Kontos HA, Wei EP, Ellis EF, et al. Prostaglandins in physiological and in certain pathological responses of the cerebral circulation. Fed Proc 1981;40(8): 2326–30.
318. Shankar V, Armstead WM. Opioids contribute to hypoxia-induced pial artery dilation through activation of ATP-sensitive K+ channels. Am J Physiol Heart Circ Physiol 1995;38:H997–1002.
319. Armstead WM. Opioids and nitric oxide contribute to hypoxia-induced pial arterial vasodilation in newborn pigs. Am J Physiol 1995;268(1 Pt 2):H226–32.
320. Coyle MG, Oh W, Stonestreet BS. Effects of indomethacin on brain blood flow and cerebral metabolism in hypoxic newborn piglets. Am J Physiol 1993; 264(1 Pt 2):H141–9.
321. Fredricks KT, Liu Y, Rusch NJ, et al. Role of endothelium and arterial K + channels in mediating hypoxic dilation of middle cerebral arteries. Am J Physiol 1994;267(2 Pt 2):H580–6.
322. Pelligrino DA, Wang Q, Koenig HM, et al. Role of nitric oxide, adenosine, N-methyl-D-aspartate receptors, and neuronal activation in hypoxia-induced pial arteriolar dilation in rats. Brain Res 1995;704(1):61–70.
323. Winn HR, Rubio R, Berne RM. Brain adenosine concentration during hypoxia in rats. Am J Physiol 1981;241(2):H235–42.
324. Berger C, von Kummer R. Does NO regulate the cerebral blood flow response in hypoxia? Acta Neurol Scand 1998;97(2):118–25.
325. Kanu A, Leffler CW. Carbon monoxide and Ca2+-activated K+ channels in cerebral arteriolar responses to glutamate and hypoxia in newborn pigs. Am J Physiol Heart Circ Physiol 2007;293(5):H3193–200.
326. Armstead WM. Role of activation of calcium-sensitive K+ channels in NO- and hypoxia-induced pial artery vasodilation. Am J Physiol 1997;272(4 Pt 2): H1785–90.

327. Armstead WM. The contribution of delta 1- and delta 2-opioid receptors to hypoxia-induced pial artery dilation in the newborn pig. J Cereb Blood Flow Metab 1995;15(3):539–46.
328. Armstead WM. Contribution of kca channel activation to hypoxic cerebrovasodilation does not involve NO. Brain Res 1998;799(1):44–8.
329. Dreier JP, Korner K, Gorner A, et al. Nitric oxide modulates the CBF response to increased extracellular potassium. J Cereb Blood Flow Metab 1995;15:914–9.
330. Wilderman MJ, Armstead WM. Relationship between nitric oxide and opioids in hypoxia-induced pial artery vasodilation. Am J Physiol 1996;270(3 Pt 2):H869–74.
331. Armstead WM. Role of ATP-sensitive K+ channels in cGMP-mediated pial artery vasodilation. Am J Physiol 1996;270(2 Pt 2):H423–6.
332. Astrup J, Heuser D, Lasser NA, et al. Evidence against H + and K + as the main factors in the regulation of cerebral blood flow during epileptic discharges, acute hypoxia, amphetamine intoxication, and hypoglycemia. A microelectrode study. In: Betz E, editor. Ionic actions on vascular smooth muscle. New York: Springer; 1976. p. 110–5.
333. Norberg K, Siesjo BK. Cerebral metabolism in hypoxic hypoxia. I. Pattern of activation of glycolysis: a re-evaluation. Brain Res 1975;86(1):31–44.
334. Wahl M, Kuschinsky W. The dilatatory action of adenosine on pial arteries of cats and its inhibition by theophylline. Pflugers Arch 1976;362(1):55–9.
335. Heistad DD, Marcus ML, Gourley JK, et al. Effect of adenosine and dipyridamole on cerebral blood flow. Am J Physiol 1981;240(5):H775–80.
336. Morii S, Ngai A, Ko K, et al. Role of adenosine in regulation of cerebral blood flow: effects of theophylline during normoxia and hypoxia. Am J Physiol 1987; 253:H165–75.
337. Emerson TE Jr, Raymond RM. Involvement of adenosine in cerebral hypoxic hyperemia in the dog. Am J Physiol 1981;241(2):H134–8.
338. Kennan RP, Takahashi K, Pan C, et al. Human cerebral blood flow and metabolism in acute insulin-induced hypoglycemia. J Cereb Blood Flow Metab 2005; 25(4):527–34.
339. Elman I, Sokoloff L, Adler CM, et al. The effects of pharmacological doses of 2-deoxyglucose on cerebral blood flow in healthy volunteers. Brain Res 1999; 815(2):243–9.
340. Horinaka N, Artz N, Jehle J, et al. Examination of potential mechanisms in the enhancement of cerebral blood flow by hypoglycemia and pharmacological doses of deoxyglucose. J Cereb Blood Flow Metab 1997;17(1):54–63.
341. Bryan RM Jr, Keefer KA, MacNeill C. Regional cerebral glucose utilization during insulin-induced hypoglycemia in unanesthetized rats. J Neurochem 1986;46(6): 1904–11.
342. Abdul-Rahman A, Agardh CD, Siesjo BK. Local cerebral blood flow in the rat during severe hypoglycemia, and in the recovery period following glucose injection. Acta Physiol Scand 1980;109(3):307–14.
343. Agardh CD, Kalimo H, Olsson Y, et al. Hypoglycemic brain injury: metabolic and structural findings in rat cerebellar cortex during profound insulin-induced hypoglycemia and in the recovery period following glucose administration. J Cereb Blood Flow Metab 1981;1(1):71–84.
344. Hernandez MJ, Vannucci RC, Salcedo A, et al. Cerebral blood flow and metabolism during hypoglycemia in newborn dogs. J Neurochem 1980;35(3):622–8.
345. Siesjo BK, Ingvar M, Pelligrino D. Regional differences in vascular autoregulation in the rat brain in severe insulin-induced hypoglycemia. J Cereb Blood Flow Metab 1983;3(4):478–85.

346. Bryan RM Jr, Hollinger BR, Keefer KA, et al. Regional cerebral and neural lobe blood flow during insulin-induced hypoglycemia in unanesthetized rats. J Cereb Blood Flow Metab 1987;7(1):96–102.
347. Vannucci RC, Nardis EE, Vannucci SJ, et al. Cerebral carbohydrate and energy metabolism during hypoglycemia in newborn dogs. Am J Physiol 1981;240(3): R192–9.
348. Vannucci R, Yager J, Vannucci S. Cerebral glucose and energy utilization during the evolution of hypoxic-ischemic brain damage in the immature rat. J Cereb Blood Flow Metab 1994;14:279–88.
349. Vannucci RC, Yager JY. Glucose, lactic acid, and perinatal hypoxic-ischemic brain damage. Pediatr Neurol 1992;8(1):3–12.
350. Breier A, Crane AM, Kennedy C, et al. The effects of pharmacologic doses of 2-deoxy-D-glucose on local cerebral blood flow in the awake, unrestrained rat. Brain Res 1993;618(2):277–82.
351. Ichord RN, Helfaer MA, Kirsch JR, et al. Nitric oxide synthase inhibition attenuates hypoglycemic cerebral hyperemia in piglets. Am J Physiol 1994; 266(3 Pt 2):H1062–8.
352. Horinaka N, Kuang TY, Pak H, et al. Blockade of cerebral blood flow response to insulin-induced hypoglycemia by caffeine and glibenclamide in conscious rats. J Cereb Blood Flow Metab 1997;17(12):1309–18.
353. Brown M, Wade J, Marshall J. Fundamental importance of arterial oxygen content in the regulation of cerebral blood flow in man. Brain 1985;108:83–91.
354. Aaslid R. Visually evoked dynamic blood flow response of the human cerebral circulation. Stroke 1987;18(4):771–5.
355. Siesjo BK. Cerebral circulation and metabolism. J Neurosurg 1984;60(5):883–908.
356. Paulson OB, Strandgaard S, Edvinsson L. Cerebral autoregulation. Cerebrovasc Brain Metab Rev 1990;2(2):161–92.
357. Kuchinsky W, Paulson O. Capillary circulation in the brain. Cerebrovasc Brain Metab Rev 1992;4:261–86.
358. LeDoux JE, Thompson ME, Iadecola C, et al. Local cerebral blood flow increases during auditory and emotional processing in the conscious rat. Science 1983;221(4610):576–8.
359. Born P, Leth H, Miranda MJ, et al. Visual activation in infants and young children studied by functional magnetic resonance imaging. Pediatr Res 1998;44(4):578–83.
360. Yamada H, Sadato N, Konishi Y, et al. A rapid brain metabolic change in infants detected by fMRI. Neuroreport 1997;8(17):3775–8.
361. Kato T, Kamei A, Takashima S, et al. Human visual cortical function during photic stimulation monitoring by means of near-infrared spectroscopy. J Cereb Blood Flow Metab 1993;13(3):516–20.
362. Meek JH, Firbank M, Elwell CE, et al. Regional hemodynamic responses to visual stimulation in awake infants. Pediatr Res 1998;43(6):840–3.
363. Sakatani K, Chen S, Lichty W, et al. Cerebral blood oxygenation changes induced by auditory stimulation in newborn infants measured by near infrared spectroscopy. Early Hum Dev 1999;55(3):229–36.
364. Bartocci M, Bergqvist LL, Lagercrantz H, et al. Pain activates cortical areas in the preterm newborn brain. Pain 2006;122(1–2):109–17.
365. Zaramella P, Freato F, Amigoni A, et al. Brain auditory activation measured by near-infrared spectroscopy (NIRS) in neonates. Pediatr Res 2001;49(2):213–9.
366. Bartocci M, Winberg J, Ruggiero C, et al. Activation of olfactory cortex in newborn infants after odor stimulation: a functional near-infrared spectroscopy study. Pediatr Res 2000;48(1):18–23.

367. Roche-Labarbe N, Wallois F, Ponchel E, et al. Coupled oxygenation oscillation measured by NIRS and intermittent cerebral activation on EEG in premature infants. Neuroimage 2007;36(3):718–27.
368. Mata M, Fink DJ, Gainer H, et al. Activity-dependent energy metabolism in rat posterior pituitary primarily reflects sodium pump activity. J Neurochem 1980; 34(1):213–5.
369. Paulson OB, Newman EA. Does the release of potassium from astrocyte endfeet regulate cerebral blood flow? Science 1987;237(4817):896–8.
370. Iadecola C. Regulation of the cerebral microcirculation during neural activity: is nitric oxide the missing link? Trends Neurosci 1993;16(6):206–14.
371. Caesar K, Akgoren N, Mathiesen C, et al. Modification of activity-dependent increases in cerebellar blood flow by extracellular potassium in anaesthetized rats. J Physiol (Lond) 1999;520(Pt 1):281–92.
372. McCarron JG, Halpern W. Potassium dilates rat cerebral arteries by two independent mechanisms. Am J Physiol 1990;259(3 Pt 2):H902–8.
373. Johnson TD, Marrelli SP, Steenberg ML, et al. Inward rectifier potassium channels in the rat middle cerebral artery. Am J Physiol 1998;274(2 Pt 2):R541–7.
374. Knot HJ, Zimmermann PA, Nelson MT. Extracellular K(+)-induced hyperpolarizations and dilatations of rat coronary and cerebral arteries involve inward rectifier K(+) channels. J Physiol (Lond) 1996;492(Pt 2):419–30.
375. Zaritsky JJ, Eckman DM, Wellman GC, et al. Targeted disruption of Kir2.1 and Kir2.2 genes reveals the essential role of the inwardly rectifying K(+) current in K(+)-mediated vasodilation [see comments]. Circ Res 2000;87(2):160–6.
376. Chrissobolis S, Ziogas J, Chu Y, et al. Role of inwardly rectifying K(+) channels in K(+)-induced cerebral vasodilatation in vivo [In Process Citation]. Am J Physiol Heart Circ Physiol 2000;279(6):H2704–12.
377. Astrup J, Heuser D, Lassen NA, et al. Evidence against H+ and K+ as main factors for the control of cerebral blood flow: a microelectrode study. Ciba Found Symp 1978;104(56):313–37.
378. O'Regan M. Adenosine and the regulation of cerebral blood flow. Neurol Res 2005;27(2):175–81.
379. Harder DR, Roman RJ, Gebremedhin D. Molecular mechanisms controlling nutritive blood flow: role of cytochrome P450 enzymes. Acta Physiol Scand 2000; 168(4):543–9.
380. Leniger-Follert E, Urbanics R, Lubbers W. Behavior of extracellular H+ and K+ activities during functional hyperemia of microcirculation in the brain cortex. Adv Neurol 1978;20(5):97–101.
381. Koehler RC, Gebremedhin D, Harder DR. Role of astrocytes in cerebrovascular regulation. J Appl Physiol 2006;100(1):307–17.
382. Zonta M, Angulo MC, Gobbo S, et al. Neuron-to-astrocyte signaling is central to the dynamic control of brain microcirculation. Nat Neurosci 2003;6(1):43–50.
383. Hossmann KA, Lechtape-Gruter H, Hossmann V. The role of cerebral blood flow for the recovery of the brain after prolonged ischemia. Z Neurol 1973;204(4):281–99.
384. Koch KA, Jackson DL, Schmiedl M, et al. Total cerebral ischemia: effect of alterations in arterial PCO2 on cerebral microcirculation. J Cereb Blood Flow Metab 1984;4(3):343–9.
385. Rosenberg A. Cerebral blood flow and O2 metabolism after asphyxia in neonatal lambs. Pediatr Res 1986;20:778–82.
386. Leffler CW, Busija DW, Beasley DG, et al. Postischemic cerebral microvascular responses to norepinephrine and hypotension in newborn pigs. Stroke 1989; 20(4):541–6.

387. Busija DW. Cerebral autoregulation. In: Phillis JW, editor. The regulation of cerebral blood flow. Boca Raton (FL): Chemical Rubber Company; 1993. p. 45–64.
388. Bari F, Louis TM, Meng W, et al. Global ischemia impairs ATP-sensitive K+ channel function in cerebral arterioles in piglets. Stroke 1996;27(10):1874–80 [discussion 80–1].
389. Kagstrom E, Smith ML, Siesjo B. Cerebral circulatory responses to hypercapnia and hypoxia in the recovery period following complete and incomplete cerebral ischemia in the rat. Acta Physiol Scand 1983;118:281–91.
390. Laptook A, Corbett R, Ruley J, et al. Blood flow and metabolism during and after repeated partial brain ischemia in neonatal piglets. Stroke 1992;23:380–7.
391. Conger J, Weil J. Abnormal vascular function following ischemia-reperfusion injury. J Investig Med 1995;43(5):431–2.
392. Mayhan W, Amundsen S, Faraci F, et al. Responses of cerebral arteries after ischemia and reperfusion in cats. Am J Physiol 1988;255:H879–84.
393. Rosenberg A. Regulation of cerebral blood flow after asphyxia in neonatal lambs. Stroke 1988;19:239–44.
394. Pryds O, Greisen G, Lou H, et al. Vasoparalysis associated with brain damage in asphyxiated term infants. J Pediatr 1990;117(1 Pt 1):119–25.
395. Lou HC. The "lost autoregulation hypothesis" and brain lesions in the newborn—an update. Brain Dev 1988;10(3):143–6.
396. Iadecola C, Zhang F, Casey R, et al. Inducible nitric oxide synthase gene expression in vascular cells after transient focal cerebral ischemia. Stroke 1996; 27:1373–80.
397. Leffler C, Beasley D, Busija D. Cerebral ischemia alters cerebral microvascular reactivity in newborn pigs. Am J Physiol 1989;257:H266–71.
398. Leffler CW, Mirro R, Armstead WM, et al. Prostanoid synthesis and vascular responses to exogenous arachidonic acid following cerebral ischemia in piglets. Prostaglandins 1990;40(3):241–8.
399. Leffler C, Mirro R, Armstead W, et al. Topical arachidonic acid restores pial arteriolar dilation to hypercapnea of postischemic newborn pig brain. Am J Physiol 1992;263:H746–51.
400. Lou HC. Autoregulation of cerebral blood flow and brain lesions in newborn infants. Lancet 1998;352(9138):1406.
401. Ingvar M. Cerebral blood flow and metabolic rate during seizures. Relationship to epileptic brain damage. Ann N Y Acad Sci 1986;462:194–206.
402. Boylan GB, Panerai RB, Rennie JM, et al. Cerebral blood flow velocity during neonatal seizures. Arch Dis Child Fetal Neonatal Ed 1999;80(2):F105–10.
403. Montecot C, Seylaz J, Pinard E. Carbon monoxide regulates cerebral blood flow in epileptic seizures but not in hypercapnia. Neuroreport 1998;9(10):2341–6.
404. Parfenova H, Carratu P, Tcheranova D, et al. Epileptic seizures cause extended postictal cerebral vascular dysfunction that is prevented by HO-1 overexpression. Am J Physiol Heart Circ Physiol 2005;288(6):H2843–50.
405. Carratu P, Pourcyrous M, Fedinec A, et al. Endogenous heme oxygenase prevents impairment of cerebral vascular functions caused by seizures. Am J Physiol Heart Circ Physiol 2003;285(3):H1148–57.
406. Montecot C, Borredon J, Seylaz J, et al. Nitric oxide of neuronal origin is involved in cerebral blood flow increase during seizures induced by kainate. J Cereb Blood Flow Metab 1997;17(1):94–9.
407. Busija DW, Leffler CW. Role of prostanoids in cerebrovascular responses during seizures in piglets. Am J Physiol 1989;256(1 Pt 2):H120–5.

Cytokines and Perinatal Brain Damage

Olaf Dammann, MD, SM[a], T. Michael O'Shea, MD, MPH[b,*]

KEYWORDS

- Cytokines • Developmental disability • Cerebral palsy
- Mental retardation • Periventricular leukomalacia
- Chorioamnionitis

Perinatal brain damage has been implicated in the pathogenesis of neurodevelopmental impairments and psychiatric illnesses. These conditions constitute an enormous source of human suffering and health care costs. For example, the average lifetime costs for mental retardation,[1] cerebral palsy,[1] and high-functioning autism exceed $1 million, and for individuals who have autism and mental retardation they exceed $5 million.[2]

The focus of this article is on specific aspects of the pathogenesis of perinatal brain damage in which cytokines and chemokines have been implicated. Epidemiologic studies indicate an association between maternal and neonatal infections and perinatal brain damage, even when the infection is distant from the brain. Experiments in animals indicate that the causal link between these two events probably involves cytokines and chemokines. Further, these inflammatory molecules are produced locally in the brain after exposure to various damage initiators, including experimental hypoxia-ischemia and infection/inflammation. Based on research completed in the past 2 decades, it seems plausible that interventions can be developed to prevent or attenuate brain damage attributable to the fetal or neonatal response to infection or some other initiator of inflammation.[3–5]

This article reviews evidence that infection outside of the brain can damage the brain and discusses specific cytokines and pathomechanisms that probably mediate the putative effect of remote infection on the developing brain. Events associated with increased circulating inflammatory cytokines, chemokines, and immune cells are described. Finally, studies of genetic variation in susceptibility to cytokine-related brain damage are reviewed. Possible neuroprotective intervention strategies for attenuating cytokine-mediated brain damage are discussed elsewhere in this issue.

[a] Division of Newborn Medicine, Floating Hospital for Children at Tufts Medical Center, 800 Washington Street, Box 854, Boston, MA 02111, USA
[b] Wake Forest University School of Medicine, Winston-Salem, NC 27157, USA
* Corresponding author.
E-mail address: moshea@wfubmc.edu (T.M. O'Shea).

Clin Perinatol 35 (2008) 643–663
doi:10.1016/j.clp.2008.07.011 perinatology.theclinics.com

INFECTION DISTANT FROM THE BRAIN CAN DAMAGE THE DEVELOPING BRAIN

In a study completed more than 40 years ago, infants who had bacteria recovered from their cardiac blood at postmortem examination were estimated to be 34 times more likely to have histologic white matter damage than infants whose cardiac blood was sterile.[6] No bacteria were found in the brain of any infant who had cerebral white matter damage. These observations led to the hypothesis that a circulating, noninfectious product of inflammation could lead to brain damage. The investigators tested their hypothesis by injecting sterile endotoxin into the peritoneal cavity of newborn kittens,[7,8] monkeys, and rabbits[8] and found white matter damage. At about the same time, others had shown that the offspring of rats given endotoxin in the days before delivery had reduced white matter volume.[9] Further epidemiologic support was provided by the Collaborative Perinatal Project (CPP), a study of about 54,000 pregnancies occurring between 1959 and 1966. In that study, chorionitis (ie, marked neutrophil infiltration of the chorion) was associated with an increased risk for cerebral palsy.[10] Further, among the 560 newborns in the CPP cohort who were born alive, died within the first 28 days, and had postmortem examination of the brain, the occurrence of maternal urinary tract infection with fever was associated with a more than 400-fold increase in the risk for white matter damage, and definite or suspect septicemia with a more than 40-fold increase.[11]

Over the past 30 years, a large body of epidemiologic studies in humans[12] and experimental studies in animals[13] has been added in support of the concept that infection distant from the brain can damage the developing brain,[14] that endotoxin initiates a brain-damaging process,[15,16] and that inflammatory proteins play a role in mediating the damage.[17,18]

In 2000, a meta-analysis of 19 studies concluded that clinical chorioamnionitis is associated with cerebral palsy and cystic periventricular leukomalacia (ie, cerebral white matter damage on neuroimaging studies).[19] It is estimated that about 11% of all cases of cerebral palsy in term and near-term infants are attributable to chorioamnionitis, assuming that it is a causal factor.[20] Studies of neonatal encephalopathy also are relevant, because term neonates who have encephalopathy have a risk for cerebral palsy that is 100 times that of neonates who do not have encephalopathy. In a population-based study, infants who had encephalopathy accounted for 24% of all cases of cerebral palsy in term infants.[21] Maternal pyrexia[22,23] has been associated with a threefold to fourfold, and chorioamnionitis with a fivefold,[23] increase in the odds of neonatal encephalopathy.

Maternal infection, including that evidenced only by neutrophil infiltration of the placenta,[24] is a frequent antecedent of preterm delivery, resulting from either preterm labor or preterm rupture of the fetal membranes.[25] Among preterm infants, maternal chorioamnionitis is associated not only with evidence of brain damage on cranial ultrasound examination but also with cerebral palsy.[19] These observations lead to the hypothesis that the link between prematurity and cerebral palsy is attributable, at least in part, to their being causally related to maternal infection.[26,27]

It would seem that prenatal and postnatal infections are potentially harmful to the developing brain. Postnatal sepsis was associated with white matter damage at autopsy.[6] In a large cohort of extremely low birth weight infants, sepsis and sepsis with necrotizing enterocolitis were associated with an increased risk for delayed mental development at 18 months adjusted age, even when adjusting for 18 potential confounders.[28]

Although the larger body of research relates maternal infection to white matter injury, inflammatory processes may present a hazard also to the cerebral cortex. In an autopsy study, polymicrogyria was found in 78% of infants who had evidence of infection of the placenta but in none of those who did not have this finding.[29] Maternal influenza infection during the second trimester has been associated with an increased risk for schizophrenia.[30] Among very low birth weight infants, maternal fever at birth was associated with an almost fourfold increase in the risk for nonverbal intelligence at 9 years of age in a cohort of very low birth weight infants.[31]

WHICH CYTOKINES MIGHT BE INVOLVED?

Cytokines, chemokines, and growth factors are ubiquitous signaling molecules that help orchestrate almost all bodily functions of growth and development and acute responses, such as fever and inflammation. An important aspect of cytokine biology is the high degree of overlap in source, target cell, and function. This redundancy makes it difficult to identify individual cytokines as "most important" in specific settings. In addition, some cytokines can have apparently contradicting functions. For example, interleukin (IL)-6 is considered both a pro- and anti-inflammatory cytokine (see the sections on pro- and anti-inflammatory cytokines below).

Which cytokines, chemokines, and growth factors might be involved in the process of perinatal brain damage and repair is context specific. Three context levels, among others, are of utmost importance when considering the role of cytokines in brain-damaging processes.

First, fetal and neonatal inflammatory responses to the various perinatal challenges are likely to occur at multiple levels. At the systemic level, the so-called "acute phase response"[32] involves molecules synthesized mainly in the liver (eg, CRP, IL-6), by white blood cells and the endothelium. At the local (brain) level, the neuroinflammatory response is of crucial importance.

Second, the relative importance of individual molecules is likely to vary by level and characteristics of the insult. Obviously, most research on the roles for cytokines in perinatal brain damage that focuses on one or a few individual molecules in the setting of defined insults comes from bench science groups, most of which focus on hypoxia-ischemia, inflammation, and excitotoxicity,[33] or on combinations of multiple challenges.[34,35]

Third, timing of the insults during brain development is certainly an effect modifier. Although the well-known differences between term and preterm infants could be attributable to different challenges (exposure to intrauterine infection in preterm and perinatal energy failure in term infants), at least part of the neuropathologic differences between the two groups of newborns is likely to be because of their different developmental stages.

In what follows, we highlight a few examples of molecules that have been investigated over the past years. For the purpose of structure, we have deliberately chosen to present these data in functional groups. We are fully aware, however, that some molecules overlap in function or belong to multiple groups. For example, IL-6 is considered both anti- and proinflammatory, and IL-2 is both a cytokine and a growth factor.

Proinflammatory Cytokines

Proinflammatory cytokines have been at the forefront of clinical and laboratory investigations of fetal and neonatal brain damage in the past decade. Initial suggestions were that proinflammatory cytokines, such as tumor necrosis factor (TNF)–α, can affect the developing brain and blood-brain barrier[36] and that intrauterine

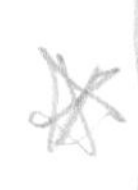

infection and a proinflammatory cytokine response are involved in the pathogenesis of preterm brain white matter damage.[26,27] Since then, the theory has come of age[14,37,38] and is now close to reaching the status of "received knowledge."[13,16,39–45] At the center of the paradigm is the notion that fetal exposure to a strong proinflammatory challenge (intrauterine infection) elicits a fetal inflammatory response that contributes to preterm delivery[46] and brain damage in the preterm newborn,[38] without leading to brain infection.[14]

TNF-α, interferon (IFN)–gamma, IL-1, IL-6, and IL-18[47] are the proinflammatory cytokines that have been studied frequently in term,[48–54] preterm,[55–64] and mixed populations.[65] Most, but not all, of these studies have found elevated levels of these mediators in newborns who had evidence of perinatal brain damage compared with controls. A role for the proinflammatory cytokines is further suggested by reports[66–68] supporting the hypothesis[69] of an association between single-nucleotide polymorphisms (SNPs) in the genes that encode for such cytokines and brain damage.

The major role for experimental studies in attempts to prevent or attenuate perinatal brain injury by interfering with the cytokine cascade is in the realm of blocking individual cytokines. For example, in one study, coadministration of lipopolysaccharide (LPS) with IL-1 receptor antagonist, but not with TNF-α antibody, significantly attenuated LPS-induced white matter injury.[70]

Anti-Inflammatory Cytokines

Cytokines that function as immunomodulatory regulators by antagonizing proinflammatory responses are sometimes called anti-inflammatory cytokines. Soluble receptors for proinflammatory cytokines can have similar function. Major anti-inflammatory cytokines include IL-1 receptor antagonist, IL-4, IL-6, IL-10, IL-11, and IL-13, and transforming growth factor (TGF)–β.[71]

Only a few of these anti-inflammatory/immunomodulatory cytokines have been studied clinically in relation to perinatal brain damage. Probably the best studied is IL-10, which has protective properties in microglial culture studies after a proinflammatory insult[72] and in rat pups born to *Escherichia coli*–infected dams.[73] In newborn mice subjected to intracerebral injection of the excitotoxic stimulus ibotenate (which by itself induces white matter lesions similar to those seen in periventricular leukomalacia), pretreatment with intraperitoneal IL-10 alone had no detectable effect, whereas IL-10 co-administered with IL-1β reduced the toxic effects of IL-1β, suggesting that exogenous IL-10 might be neuroprotective mainly in inflammatory contexts.[74] This result is in keeping with our clinical observation that infants homozygous for the high IL-10 producer −1082 G allele were significantly less likely to develop ultrasound-defined periventricular echodensities.[75]

TGF-β3 was found expressed in the brains of neonatal rats that had posthemorrhagic hydrocephalus[76] and in cerebrospinal fluid of preterm infants who had this condition.[77] If TGF-β turns out to be part of an endogenous protection factor derived from astrocytes,[78] it might reduce damage (eg, by blocking IL-1–induced activation of microglia cells).[79] In an excitotoxicity context, TGF-β seems to help orchestrate IL-9/mast cell interactions that lead to exacerbation of excitotoxic brain damage by increased extracellular histamine concentrations.[80] In the adult rat, cerebroventricular administration of TGF-β improves only short-term, but not long-term, neuropathology and neurologic function.[81]

Chemokines

The central role for chemokines in immunity is to help orchestrate leukocyte trafficking, thereby "engendering the adaptive immune response."[82] Chemokine biology offers various linkage points for intervention in neurologic diseases,[83] including those with a neuroinflammatory component.[84]

The chemokine nomenclature recently underwent revision.[85] In our subsequent discussion of examples for chemokine functions in perinatal brain injury, we use the new and old chemokine names side by side.

The "oldest" and probably best studied chemokine is CXCL8 (IL-8), well known to neonatologists as one of the serum biomarkers of neonatal sepsis.[86] In term newborns, serum levels of CXCL8 (IL-8) are elevated among those who have MRI-defined neuroabnormalities and adverse neurologic outcome.[87] It is also associated with intraventricular hemorrhage in preterm infants,[64] with levels being comparatively higher in cerebrospinal fluid than in serum,[88] which might indicate its production inside the CNS, where microglial cells are one potential production site of CXCL8 (IL-8).[89] Indeed, the crucial role of microglia cells in the neuroinflammatory process leading to developmental disability is now widely acknowledged.[90]

Chemokines are up-regulated in immature rat brain after hypoxic-ischemic challenge[91] and in mature rodents after a systemic bolus of LPS.[92] This up-regulation was followed by a transient neutrophil invasion of the infarct region and an activation of microglia/macrophages, CD4 lymphocytes, and astroglia for up to at least 42 days of postnatal age implicating a chronic component of immunoinflammatory activation in the immature animals.[91] These findings support our suggestion that white cell invasion might be part of the pathogenesis of perinatal white matter damage.[93]

Growth Factors

A vast variety of growth factors are implicated in brain development and damage/repair mechanisms. For the sake of brevity, we focus on only four in this section.

IL-2 is the major cytokine/growth factor for T lymphocytes by stimulating their clonal expansion. We have previously argued[94] that its toxicity to oligodendrocytes and myelin[95] and that the observation IL-2 and its receptor have been identified in areas of cerebral white matter damage in human newborns in the absence of lymphocytes[96] raises the possibility that the IL-2 originated outside the brain.

In adult models of stroke, vascular endothelial growth factor (VEGF) has neuroprotective properties as a reducer of apoptosis (programmed cell death) and initiation of neurogenesis and maturation of heterologous newborn neurons in adult rat brains after stroke.[97] VEGF is expressed in hypoxic neonatal rodent white matter[98] and reduces excitotoxic brain lesions in the developing mouse.[99] This finding supports the hypothesis that VEGF is part of an endogenous protection response.[3]

Inflammation at birth seems to be associated with a systemic up-regulation of insulinlike growth factor (IGF) and a down-regulation of its binding proteins.[100] Because IGF improves oligodendrocyte survival after hypoxic insult[101] and reduces hypoxia/ischemia-induced brain damage in fetal sheep[102] and newborn rats,[103] it would be interesting to know whether IGF might also be part of the developing organism's anti-inflammatory response geared toward brain protection in experimental models using LPS challenge.

One most interesting growth factor involved in multiple developmental processes is neuregulin (NRG). Our recent proposal that NRG is a potential endogenous protector of the perinatal brain[104] is based on its role in brain development,[105] particularly in oligodendrocyte development,[106] its neuroprotective effects in the setting of ischemia,[107–110] and its involvement in the pathogenesis of neuropsychiatric disorders, such as schizophrenia,[111] which shares with perinatal brain injury an antenatal infection/inflammation-related etiology.[112]

PROPOSED MECHANISMS

Just as context is important for which cytokines are involved in perinatal brain damage causation, it is also important for how they might be involved. By this we refer to the experimental paradigm used to study cytokine actions in animal experiments of perinatal brain damage causation.

The following are examples of intricacies that should be kept in mind. First, the cytokine cascade in experimentally induced ischemia might differ in quality and in quantity from the cytokine response to intracerebrally injected LPS. Second, responses might differ between paradigms of direct cerebral LPS exposure and remote systemic/transplacental exposure,[13] which does not even implicate the presence of LPS in the brain. On the other hand, different paradigms might have some central aspects in common, such as microglia activation as one key pathomechanisms and the premyelinating oligodendrocyte as the major cellular target in white matter damage.[45] Third, differences in species, timing, dosage, and definition of experimental study endpoint are clearly nontrivial. Finally, some general issues of causal inference[113] deserve consideration when integrating experimental results with other sources of evidence.

Cytokine Upregulation

Both hypoxia-ischemia and exposure to infection/LPS[13] are followed by a prominent neuroinflammatory response in the immature brain. Inhibition of such neuroinflammatory cascades might help reduce brain injury.[5] For example, intravenous melatonin reduces microglial activation and apoptotic cell death in a fetal ovine umbilical cord occlusion model.[114] Similarly, administration of glycine 2-methyl proline glutamate leads to reduced IL-6 expression and reduced brain damage in a neonatal rat model of hypoxia-ischemia with treatment starting 2 hours after the insult.[115] The immunomodulatory cytokine IL-10 reduces the inflammatory response of microglial cells after LPS challenge[72] and is neuroprotective in a mouse model using intracerebral ibotenate injection.[74] Although it does not reduce damage in the developing piglet brain if administered after the onset of inflammation,[116] it seems to be protective when administered concomitantly.[116]

Proinflammatory cytokines directly exert deleterious effects in the developing brain. For example, injection of IL-1 leads to neuronal death and delayed myelination in neonatal rats.[117] TNF-α induces cell death in mature oligodendrocytes, probably by apoptosis-inducing factor (AIF).[118] In developing oligodendrocytes, exposure to TNF seems to be associated with increased apoptosis[119] and reduced staining for myelin basic protein (MBP),[120] which helps explain the reduced myelination that is considered a hallmark of inflammation-associated diffuse white matter damage in fetal rodents[121] and preterm infants.[122]

Extracerebral Exposure to Lipopolysaccharide

Our conceptual model of remote infection as a damage initiator[14] assumes that the fetus (and its brain) are not directly exposed to bacterial antigen. Indeed, much of our proposal that cytokines are involved in neonatal brain damage after exposure to intrauterine infection was based on the assumption that damage can develop in the absence of bacterial antigen in the brain, with cytokines playing the role of the "dangerous messenger," being both a secondary proinflammatory signal in the brain and a direct cause of cell death and delayed myelination.[37] This scenario has been modeled in animal studies that have shown that exposure of the dam to intraperitoneal LPS leads to up-regulation of IL-1,[123,124] TNF,[123,125–127] and neurotrophic factors brain-derived neurotrophic factor (BDNF) and NGF[128] in neonatal rat brain. In some of these and closely related models in fetal sheep,[129] rabbits,[130,131] and guinea pigs[132] the remote infection results in fetal brain damage. In mice, the remote infection paradigm of maternal intraperitoneal LPS exposure leads to up-regulation of chemokine CCL2 (MCP-1), IL-6 and IL-1β, and growth factor VEGF, among other growth and differentiation factors, and the down-regulation of genes involved in axon guidance and neurogenesis.[133] It also leads to long-term memory changes[134] and behavioral changes in the adult offspring of mice exposed to intraperitoneal LPS challenge, such as increased anxiety and reduced aggression.[135] Recent studies suggest a potential role for oxidative stress in brain damage induced by antenatal remote infection scenarios.[136–138] In sum, these observations support the hypothesis that intrauterine exposure to an extracerebral inflammatory stimulus can lead to brain damage in the immature animal without bacterial antigen gaining access to the brain. The finding that antenatal exposure to inflammation might not only affect brain well-being but also suppresses the neonatal inflammatory response[139] adds an interesting level of complexity to the recently developed multiple-hit models,[34,35] which in themselves offer intriguing opportunities for future studies of cytokine patterns in dual paradigm scenarios.

Intracerebral Endotoxin Binding and Microglial Activation

What if LPS does gain access to the fetal/neonatal brain? Although we still lack evidence that this is actually the case in human perinatal brain damage, some experimentalists have already modeled this interesting scenario.

When injected into the rat brain at postnatal day 5, LPS induces white matter rarefaction and necrosis, ventricular enlargement, and a prominent neuroinflammatory response.[140] Microglial cells seem to be the only brain cells that possess LPS-binding TLR4 receptors and seem to be necessary for LPS-induced oligodendrocyte death[141] and neurodegeneration.[142] TLR-dependent pathways involving intracellular heat shock protein signaling of microglia activation might help explain the bidirectional relationship between brain damage and neuroinflammation in multiple inflammatory contexts.[143] Minocycline, an inhibitor of microglia activation, reduces inflammatory response and brain damage after intracerebral LPS challenge.[144] Similar effects were observed in experiments that used hypoxia-ischemia as the damage inducer,[145] indicating that microglial activation might be an important mediator of damage induction in LPS- and energy failure–related paradigms.

White Cell Tissue Migration

A few years ago, we proposed that recruitment of white blood cells might play a role in perinatal white matter damage.[93] Multiple intraperitoneal LPS injections over the first 8 postnatal days induce an acute inflammatory response, a prominent breakdown of the blood-brain barrier for proteins in the white matter, and white matter paucity.[146] Even short-term disruption of blood-brain barrier integrity can contribute to LPS-induced inflammatory brain damage in 35-day-old rats.[147] Indeed, macrophage-like cells appear in the close vicinity of blood vessels in the white matter of fetal sheep after a single, low-dose intravenous LPS challenge.[148] It will be interesting to learn from future research whether blocking blood-brain transfer of white cells can attenuate neuroinflammation and brain damage in the remote infection paradigm.

Sustained Activation

Along the lines of white cell involvement, we further propose that an interplay between the innate and adaptive components of immunity is highly likely to be part of white matter damage pathogenesis.[94] This argument is based on the multiple linkage points between the two systems, created by crosstalk between dendritic cells, natural killer cells, and monocytes/macrophages on the innate side, and T cells on the adaptive side of immunity. (We further expand on the importance of T cells in the next section.) One exciting potential implication for intervention designers might be the window of opportunity opened by prolonged and possibly persistent inflammation generated by such innate–adaptive immune interactions.[149]

TWO FACES OF NEUROINFLAMMATION

What has recently been called the "dual role of inflammation in CNS disease"[150] incorporates aspects of what we refer to as the interplay between proinflammatory challenge and endogenous protection responses.[3] Multiple aspects of neuroimmune responses in the brain might help explain the purported ambivalent role of inflammation in the CNS, which is still not unanimously accepted in the neuroimmunology community.[151] First, it is increasingly recognized that the immune system and the CNS overlap in expression of inflammatory cytokines and neurotrophic factors. Indeed, BDNF and glial cell–derived neurotrophic factor are produced not only in the CNS but also by immune cells.[150] Conversely, B-cell activating factor not only is a product of white blood cells but also is produced by astrocytes and seems to play a role in multiple sclerosis.[152] Second, classic proinflammatory neurotoxic signals, such as TNF, also seem to elicit potentially protective effects. For example, TNF-receptor knockout mice sustain greater damage after focal ischemia than wild-type animals.[153] Moreover, TNF stimulation of astrocytes leads to BDNF production by these cells.[154] Third, T cells specific to MBP seem to contribute to damage limitation after initial damage.[155] Such a "protective neuroimmunity" mechanism is likely to involve microglial cells,[156] which were suspected more than a decade ago to exert not only potentially damaging but also beneficial effects.[157] The possibility to enhance protective neuroimmune responses by way of T cell–based vaccination in neurodegenerative disorders is tempting.[158] Fourth, immune signals are involved in adult hippocampal neurogenesis.[159] In essence, T cells seem to be necessary for spatial learning and the production of BDNF in the adult brain.[160] It will be interesting to learn from groups who will pursue such studies in the developing brain. What follows from the above points is that links between the innate and adaptive immune systems might not only contribute to perinatal brain damage[94] but also offer target points for the design of neuroprotective intervention.

POTENTIAL INITIATORS OF INFLAMMATION IN FETUSES AND NEONATES

Some of the earliest experiments linking infection and cerebral white matter damage involved exposure of immature animals to endotoxin, or LPS. LPS binding to specific toll-like receptors (TLR) constitutes an early molecular event leading from endotoxin exposure to inflammation. The binding of endotoxin to TLR activates signal-transduction pathways that induce the expression of genes coding for various immune-response proteins, such as inflammatory cytokines. TLR and other pattern recognition receptors may be secreted or located on the surface of phagocytes and serve to recognize molecules produced by microbial pathogens.[161] Organisms recognized by TLR include group B *Streptococcus*, *Listeria monocytogenes*, *Mycoplasma hominis*, *Candida albicans*, cytomegalovirus, and *Enterobactericeae*.[162] Based on the frequency with which these organisms are implicated as pathogens in neonates, it is not surprising that multiple antecedents have been identified that could induce the production of effectors of innate immunity. Clinical events associated with a fetal inflammatory response include chorioamnionitis,[52,163–165] whereas those associated with a neonatal inflammatory response include sepsis,[166–170] necrotizing enterocolitis (NEC),[171] and pulmonary infections.

Compared with uninfected controls, very preterm neonates who have either confirmed or suspected sepsis have higher umbilical cord blood levels of Il-6, but not TNF-α. Infants born to mothers who have more severe grades of chorioamnionitis and infants who have funisitis have higher umbilical cord blood levels of IL-6[164,165] and CXCL8 (IL-8)[165] than those who do not have these histologic findings. Infants born to women from whose placenta *Ureaplasma urealyticum* was cultured were more likely to have this organism in their blood cultures and were three times more likely to have elevated levels of IL-6.[172] Histologic chorioamnionitis also has been associated with increased levels of CXCL8 (IL-8) in blood[52] and tracheal aspirates,[163] and increased levels of the chemokine CCL5 (RANTES) in blood.[52] In a study of infants suspected of having early-onset sepsis, levels of IL-6, CXCL8 (IL-8), and TNF-α were elevated at the time when sepsis was initially suspected (<48 hours of age). Twenty-four hours later, CXCL8 (IL-8) and TNF-α levels were similar to uninfected controls, but IL-6 remained elevated.[166] In a study of very low birth weight infants suspected of having late-onset sepsis, the levels of multiple chemokines, IL-6, IL-10, IL-12p70, and TNF-α were higher among infants who had confirmed infections. All of the chemokines as well as IL-6 and IL-10 remained elevated 24 hours later.[167] Also elevated in late-onset systemic infections are anti-inflammatory cytokines, such as IL-4 and IL-10.[168]

In a study of infants who had necrotizing enterocolitis, those who had the most severe disease (stage 3) had higher levels of CXCL8 (IL-8) than either infants who had milder NEC or controls who did not have NEC, and the level of CXCL8 (IL-8) continued to increase over the 72 hours when serial measurements were made.[171] Differences were not found when comparing infants who had sepsis and NEC and infants who had NEC only. IL-10, an anti-inflammatory cytokine, also was higher in infants who had stage 3 NEC when compared with controls and with infants who had milder NEC. Significant group differences were not found for either IL-1β or the anti-inflammatory protein IL-1ra.

Among term infants, elevated blood levels of inflammatory cytokines have been associated with indicators of perinatal asphyxia, infection, and encephalopathy. In a group of 20 infants who had fetal acidemia, respiratory depression, and low Apgar scores, cerebrospinal fluid levels of IL-6 were higher among those infants who had more severe neonatal encephalopathy.[48] This elevation in IL-6 could be attributable to brain damage manifesting as neonatal encephalopathy or to antecedents of encephalopathy, which include chorioamnionitis.[173] Blood levels of IL-6, along with IL-1β,[54,87] TNF-α,[54] CXCL8 (IL-8),[87] and IL-12,[87] also are elevated in infants who have encephalopathy. This association was found even among infants born to mothers who were not diagnosed with chorioamnionitis.[87] Antecedents of neonatal encephalopathy other than chorioamnionitis (eg, hypoxia-ischemia) thus might lead to elevated levels of inflammatory cytokines in the blood. Higher levels of IL-1β, IL-6, TNF-α, and CXCL8 (IL-8), in the blood of neonates who have encephalopathy have been associated with increased anaerobic brain metabolism, as assessed with magnetic resonance spectroscopy, and with abnormal neurodevelopmental outcome.[87]

Lung injury, which occurs in many critically ill neonates, and even in otherwise healthy premature infants, has been consistently associated with elevations in inflammatory cytokine and chemokine levels in respiratory tract secretions. CXCL8 (IL-8) and IL-6 are found in tracheal aspirates of preterm infants treated with mechanical ventilation for respiratory distress syndrome, and as early as the first day of life levels of CXCL8 (IL-8) are higher among those who eventually develop bronchopulmonary dysplasia.[174] These infants have, by the second day of life, higher levels of TNF-α,[175,176] IL-6,[176] and IL-β,[175,176] and macrophage inhibitory protein–1α (MIP-1α)–activated macrophages.[175] That mechanical ventilation may be an inducer of inflammation is suggested by the finding that within hours after birth, preterm infants who required mechanical ventilation had significantly higher numbers of activated phagocytes in their blood as compared with preterm nonventilated controls[177] (and no difference was found comparing umbilical cord blood specimens from these two groups). Although not studied in vivo, increased pressure in lung venular capillaries, as would be expected when a patent ductus arteriosus leads to excessive pulmonary blood flow, has been found in vitro to cause proinflammatory responses in endothelial cells (eg, expression of P-selectin).[178]

GENETIC SUSCEPTIBILITY TO INFLAMMATION-RELATED BRAIN DAMAGE

There is increasing evidence that inherited cytokine or chemokine polymorphisms influence the risk for pre- and perinatal brain damage.[179] Included are polymorphisms of genes regulating expression of proinflammatory cytokines and chemokines along with anti-inflammatory cytokines. Increased production of TNF-α is associated with an SNP at position −308 in the promoter region of the TNF-α gene. Patients who have this SNP have a sevenfold increase in the risk for central nervous system malaria[180] and for preterm delivery.[181] In a study of 27 infants born before 32 weeks' gestation, the TNF-α promoter −308 was associated with severe intraventricular hemorrhage (Papile grade 3 or 4),[182] although the association was statistically significant only among males.[68] In a study of 119 very low birth weight infants, TNF-α promoter −308 was associated with an almost twofold increase in the risk for all grades of intraventricular hemorrhage.[183] Although in one study of children born before 32 weeks' gestation, those who had cerebral palsy were not more likely to have the TNF-α promoter −308 gene,[184] this association was found in a much larger study (443 cases and 883 controls).[185] In analyses stratified by gestational age and clinical type of cerebral palsy, the association with TNF-α promoter −308 was strongest among children who had quadriplegia who were born at term and those who had hemiplegia born before 32 weeks. Further, an SNP in the gene for mannose-binding lectin (which is involved in complement activation) was associated with an increased risk for diplegia.[185]

An SNP in the IL-6 gene promoter at position −174 (CC genotype) has been associated with enhanced production in LPS-stimulated monocytes of neonates, but not adults. Among infants born before 32 weeks' gestation, this polymorphism has been associated with an increased risk for periventricular hemorrhage and cerebral white matter damage on cranial ultrasound, although no association was found with developmental scores at 2 and 5 years of age.[186] In another study of very preterm infants, another polymorphism associated with higher IL-6 synthesis (−572 C allele) found no difference in the frequency of cranial ultrasound abnormalities but worse cognitive development.[67]

Further (albeit indirect) evidence that genetic variation influences the risk for brain damage related to inflammation comes from studies of genetic variation in apolipoprotein E, a lipid transport protein that also plays a role in repair after cell injury. The three common alleles of this protein differ only of the basis of one or two amino acids. Among infants who underwent cardiopulmonary bypass for repair of congenital heart disease, the ϵ2 allele of apolipoprotein E was associated with lower scores on a standardized measure of psychomotor development at 1 year of age.[187] In another study, early cognitive functioning at 2 years of age was worse among infants who had the ϵ2 or ϵ3 allele.[188]

Finally, a polymorphism that results in increased production of the anti-inflammatory cytokine IL-10 has been associated with a marked decrease in the risk for cerebral white matter damage. In a study of 39 very low birth weight infants[189] and another study of 15 very preterm infants[75] who had the GG allele for IL-10(−1082) genotype, none had cerebral white matter damage, as compared with 10% (30/313) of infants who had the GA or AA allele. Of 15 infants who had the GG allele for whom developmental follow-up data were available, none had cerebral palsy, as compared with the expected 10% of those children who did not have this allele.[75]

SUMMARY

More than 30 years ago, evidence from epidemiologic studies and experiments in animals indicated that infection remote from the brain is a potential cause of cerebral white matter damage in human neonates. Since that time, a large body of evidence has accumulated suggesting that the link between infection and brain damage involves various mediators of inflammation, including cytokines, chemokines, and immune cells. Inflammatory mediators also are involved in brain-damaging processes that follow energy deprivation, as may occur with intrapartum asphyxia. Equally important is the role of cytokines in modulation of inflammation and repair after inflammation-related brain damage. Genetic polymorphisms in genes coding for inflammatory mediators could explain, at least in part, genetic susceptibility to pre- and perinatal brain damage. Strategies to reduce the frequency and extent of pre- and perinatal brain damage may derive from therapeutic interventions that either enhance the production or activity of certain "damage protectors" (eg, anti-inflammatory cytokines) or inhibit the production or activity of specific "damage mediators" (eg, inflammatory cytokines).

REFERENCES

1. Honeycutt A, Dunlap L, Chen H, et al. Economic costs associated with mental retardation, cerebral palsy, hearing loss, and vision impairment—United States, 2003. MMWR Morb Mortal Wkly Rep 2004;53(3):57–9.
2. Jarbrink K, Knapp M. The economic impact of autism in Britain. Autism 2001; 5(1):7–22.
3. Dammann O, Leviton A. Brain damage in preterm newborns: might enhancement of developmentally-regulated endogenous protection open a door for prevention? Pediatrics 1999;104:541–50.
4. Dammann O, Cesario A, Hallen M. NEOBRAIN—an EU-funded project committed to protect the newborn brain. Neonatology 2007;92(4):217–8.
5. Wolfberg AJ, Dammann O, Gressens P. Anti-inflammatory and immunomodulatory strategies to protect the perinatal brain. Semin Fetal Neonatal Med 2007; 12(4):296–302.
6. Leviton A, Gilles F, Neff R, et al. Multivariate analysis of risk of perinatal telencephalic leukoencephalopathy. Am J Epidemiol 1976;104:621–6.
7. Gilles FH, Leviton A, Kerr CS. Endotoxin leukoencephalopathy in the telencephalon of the newborn kitten. J Neurol Sci 1976;27:183–91.
8. Gilles FH, Averill DR, Kerr CS. Neonatal endotoxin encephalopathy. Ann Neurol 1977;2(1):49–56.

9. Ornoy A, Altshuler G. Maternal endotoxemia, fetal anomalies, and central nervous-system damage—rat model of a human problem. Am J Obstet Gynecol 1976;124(2):196–204.
10. Nelson KB, Ellenberg JH. Predictors of low and very low birth-weight and the relation of these to cerebral-palsy. JAMA 1985;254(11):1473–9.
11. Leviton A, Gilles FH. Acquired perinatal leukoencephalopathy. Ann Neurol 1984; 16(1):1–8.
12. Wu YW. Systematic review of chorioamnionitis and cerebral palsy. Ment Retard Dev Disabil Res Rev 2002;8(1):25–9.
13. Wang XY, Rousset CI, Hagberg H, et al. Lipopolysaccharide-induced inflammation and perinatal brain injury. Semin Fetal Neonatal Med 2006;11(5): 343–53.
14. Dammann O, Leviton A. Infection remote from the brain, neonatal white matter damage, and cerebral palsy in the preterm infant. Semin Pediatr Neurol 1998; 5:190–201.
15. Hagberg H, Mallard C. Effect of inflammation on central nervous system development and vulnerability. Curr Opin Neurol 2005;18(2):117–23.
16. Dammann O, Leviton A. Inflammatory brain damage in preterm newborns—dry numbers, wet lab, and causal inferences. Early Hum Dev 2004;79(1):1–15.
17. Silverstein FS, Barks JD, Hagan P, et al. Cytokines and perinatal brain injury. Neurochem Int 1997;30(4–5):375–83.
18. Dammann O, Leviton A. Intrauterine infection, cytokines, and brain damage in the preterm newborn. Pediatr Res 1997;42(1):1–8.
19. Wu YW, Colford JM. Chorioamnionitis as a risk factor for cerebral palsy—a meta-analysis. JAMA 2000;284(11):1417–24.
20. Wu YW, Escobar GJ, Grether JK, et al. Chorioamnionitis and cerebral palsy in term and near-term infants. JAMA 2003;290(20):2677–84.
21. Badawi N, Felix JF, Kurinczuk JJ, et al. Cerebral palsy following term newborn encephalopathy: a population-based study. Dev Med Child Neurol 2005;47(5): 293–8.
22. Badawi N, Kurinczuk JJ, Keogh JM, et al. Intrapartum risk factors for newborn encephalopathy: the Western Australian case-control study. Br Med J 1998; 317(7172):1554–8.
23. Blume HK, Li CI, Loch CM, et al. Intrapartum fever and chorioamnionitis as risks for encephalopathy in term newborns: a case-control study. Dev Med Child Neurol 2008;50(1):19–24.
24. Holzman C, Lin XM, Senagore P, et al. Histologic chorioamnionitis and preterm delivery. Am J Epidemiol 2007;166(7):786–94.
25. Romero R, Gomez R, Chaiworapongsa T, et al. The role of infection in preterm labour and delivery. Paediatr Perinat Epidemiol 2001;15:41–56.
26. Leviton A. Preterm birth and cerebral-palsy—is tumor-necrosis-factor the missing link. Dev Med Child Neurol 1993;35(6):553–6.
27. Adinolfi M. Infectious-diseases in pregnancy, cytokines and neurological impairment—an hypothesis. Dev Med Child Neurol 1993;35(6):549–53.
28. Stoll BJ, Hansen NI, Adams-Chapman I, et al. Neurodevelopmental and growth impairment among extremely low-birth-weight infants with neonatal infection. JAMA 2004;292(19):2357–65.
29. Toti P, De Felice C, Palmeri ML, et al. Inflammatory pathogenesis of cortical polymicrogyria: an autopsy study. Pediatr Res 1998;44(3):291–6.
30. Brown AS, Susser ES. In utero infection and adult schizophrenia. Ment Retard Dev Disabil Res Rev 2002;8(1):51–7.

31. Dammann O, Drescher J, Veelken N. Maternal fever at birth and non-verbal intelligence at age 9 years in preterm infants. Dev Med Child Neurol 2003; 45(3):148–51.
32. Gabay C, Kushner I. Mechanisms of disease—acute-phase proteins and other systemic responses to inflammation. N Engl J Med 1999;340:448–54.
33. Hagberg H, Peebles D, Mallard C. Models of white matter injury: comparison of infectious, hypoxic-ischemic, and excitotoxic insults. Ment Retard Dev Disabil Res Rev 2002;8(1):30–8.
34. Hagberg H, Dammann O, Mallard C, et al. Preconditioning and the developing brain. Semin Perinatol 2004;28(6):389–95.
35. Mallard C, Hagberg H. Inflammation-induced preconditioning in the immature brain. Semin Fetal Neonatal Med 2007;12(4):280–6.
36. Megyeri P, Abraham CS, Temesvari P, et al. Recombinant human tumor-necrosis-factor-alpha constricts pial arterioles and increases blood-brain-barrier permeability in newborn piglets. Neurosci Lett 1992;148(1–2):137–40.
37. Dammann O, Leviton A. Maternal intrauterine infection, cytokines, and brain damage in the preterm newborn. Pediatr Res 1997;42:1–8.
38. Dammann O, Leviton A. The role of the fetus in perinatal infection and neonatal brain injury. Curr Opin Pediatr 2000;12:99–104.
39. Patrick LA, Smith GN. Proinflammatory cytokines: a link between chorioamnionitis and fetal brain injury. J Obstet Gynaecol Can 2002;24(9):705–9.
40. Cornette L. Fetal and neonatal inflammatory response and adverse outcome. Semin Fetal Neonatal Med 2004;9(6):459–70.
41. Edwards AD, Tan S. Perinatal infections, prematurity and brain injury. Curr Opin Pediatr 2006;18(2):119–24.
42. Back SA. Perinatal white matter injury: the changing spectrum of pathology and emerging insights into pathogenetic mechanisms. Ment Retard Dev Disabil Res Rev 2006;12(2):129–40.
43. Adams-Chapman I. Neonatal infection and long-term neurodevelopmental outcome in the preterm infant. Curr Opin Infect Dis 2006;19(3):290–7.
44. Murthy V, Kennea NL. Antenatal infection/inflammation and fetal tissue injury. Best Pract Res Clin Obstet Gynaecol 2007;21(3):479–89.
45. Khwaja O, Volpe JJ. Pathogenesis of cerebral white matter injury of prematurity. Arch Dis Child Fetal Neonatal Ed 2008;93(2):F152–161.
46. Romero R, Espinoza J, Goncalves LF, et al. The role of inflammation and infection in preterm birth. Semin Reprod Med 2007;25(1):21–39.
47. Felderhoff-Mueser U, Schmidt OI, Oberholzer A, et al. IL-18: a key player in neuroinflammation and neurodegeneration? Trends Neurosci 2005;28(9):487–93.
48. MartinAncel A, GarciaAlix A, PascualSalcedo D, et al. Interleukin-6 in the cerebrospinal fluid after perinatal asphyxia is related to early and late neurological manifestations. Pediatrics 1997;100(5):789–94.
49. Nelson KB, Dambrosia JM, Grether JK, et al. Neonatal cytokines and coagulation factors in children with cerebral palsy. Ann Neurol 1998;44:665–75.
50. Grether JK, Nelson KB, Dambrosia JM, et al. Interferons and cerebral palsy. J Pediatr 1999;134(3):324–32.
51. Oygur N, Sonmez O, Saka O, et al. Predictive value of plasma and cerebrospinal fluid tumour necrosis factor-alpha and interleukin-1 beta concentrations on outcome of full term infants with hypoxic-ischaemic encephalopathy. Arch Dis Child 1998;79(3):F190–3.
52. Shalak LF, Laptook AR, Jafri HS, et al. Clinical chorioamnionitis, elevated cytokines, and brain injury in term infants. Pediatrics 2002;110(4):673–80.

53. Silveira RC, Procianoy RS. Interleukin-6 and tumor necrosis factor-alpha levels in plasma and cerebrospinal fluid of term newborn infants with hypoxic-ischemic encephalopathy. J Pediatr 2003;143(5):625–9.
54. Aly H, Khashaba MT, El Ayouty M, et al. IL-6 and TNF-alpha and outcomes of neonatal hypoxic ischemic encephalopathy. Brain Dev 2006;28(3):178–82.
55. Yoon BH, Romero R, Yang SH. Interleukin-6 concentrations in umbilical cord plasma are elevated in neonates with white matter lesions associated with periventricular leukomalacia. Am J Obstet Gynecol 1996;174:1433–40.
56. Yoon BH, Jun JK, Romero R, et al. Amniotic fluid inflammatory cytokines (interleukin-6, interleukin-1beta, and tumor necrosis factor-alpha), neonatal brain white matter lesions, and cerebral palsy. Am J Obstet Gynecol 1997;177(1):19–26.
57. Yoon BH, Romero R, Kim CJ, et al. High expression of tumor necrosis factor-alpha and interleukin-6 in periventricular leukomalacia. Am J Obstet Gynecol 1997;177(2):406–11.
58. Duggan PJ, Maalouf EF, Watts TL, et al. Intrauterine T-cell activation and increased proinflammatory cytokine concentrations in preterm infants with cerebral lesions. Lancet 2001;358(9294):1699–700.
59. Yanowitz TD, Jordan JA, Gilmour CH, et al. Hemodynamic disturbances in premature infants born after chorioamnionitis: association with cord blood cytokine concentrations. Pediatr Res 2002;51(3):310–6.
60. Minagawa K, Tsuji Y, Ueda H, et al. Possible correlation between high levels of IL-18 in the cord blood of pre-term infants and neonatal development of periventricular leukomalacia and cerebral palsy. Cytokine 2002;17(3):164–70.
61. Nelson KB, Grether JK, Dambrosia JM, et al. Neonatal cytokines and cerebral palsy in very preterm infants. Pediatr Res 2003;53(4):600–7.
62. Heep A, Behrendt D, Nitsch P, et al. Increased serum levels of interleukin 6 are associated with severe intraventricular haemorrhage in extremely premature infants. Arch Dis Child 2003;88(6):F501–4.
63. Viscardi RM, Muhumuza CK, Rodriguez A, et al. Inflammatory markers in intrauterine and fetal blood and cerebrospinal fluid compartments are associated with adverse pulmonary and neurologic outcomes in preterm infants. Pediatr Res 2004;55(6):1009–17.
64. Hansen-Pupp I, Harling S, Berg AC, et al. Circulating interferon-gamma and white matter brain damage in preterm infants. Pediatr Res 2005;58(5):946–52.
65. Kaukola T, Satyaraj E, Patel DD, et al. Cerebral palsy is characterized by protein mediators in cord serum. Ann Neurol 2004;55(2):186–94.
66. Harding D, Dhamrait S, Millar A, et al. Is interleukin-6-174 genotype associated with the development of septicemia in preterm infants? Pediatrics 2003;112(4):800–3.
67. Harding D, Brull D, Humphries SE, et al. Variation in the interleukin-6 gene is associated with impaired cognitive development in children born prematurely: a preliminary study. Pediatr Res 2005;58(1):117–20.
68. Heep A, Schueller AC, Kattner E, et al. Association of two tumour necrosis factor gene polymorphisms with the incidence of severe intraventricular haemorrhage in preterm infants. J Med Genet 2005;42(7):604–8.
69. Dammann O, Durum SK, Leviton A. Modification of the infection-associated risks of preterm birth and white matter damage in the preterm newborn by polymorphisms in the tumor necrosis factor-locus? Pathogenesis 1998;2:1–7.
70. Cai ZW, Pang Y, Lin SY, et al. Differential roles of tumor necrosis factor-alpha and interleukin-1 beta in lipopolysaccharide-induced brain injury in the neonatal rat. Brain Res 2003;975(1–2):37–47.

71. Opal SM, Depalo VA. Anti-inflammatory cytokines. Chest 2000;117(4):1162–72.
72. Kremlev SG, Palmer C. Interleukin-10 inhibits endotoxin-induced pro-inflammatory cytokines in microglial cell cultures. J Neuroimmunol 2005; 162(1–2):71–80.
73. Rodts-Palenik S, Wyatt-Ashmead J, Pang Y, et al. Maternal infection-induced white matter injury is reduced by treatment with interleukin-10. Am J Obstet Gynecol 2004;191(4):1387–92.
74. Mesples B, Plaisant F, Gressens P. Effects of interleukin-10 on neonatal excitotoxic brain lesions in mice. Brain Res Dev Brain Res 2003;141(1–2):25–32.
75. Dordelmann M, Kerk J, Dressler F, et al. Interleukin-10 high producer allele and ultrasound-defined periventricular white matter abnormalities in preterm infants: a preliminary study. Neuropediatrics 2006;37(3):130–6.
76. Cherian S, Thoresen M, Silver IA, et al. Transforming growth factor-beta s in a rat model of neonatal posthaemorrhagic hydrocephalus. Neuropathol Appl Neurobiol 2004;30(6):585–600.
77. Heep A, Stoffel-Wagner B, Bartmann P, et al. Vascular endothelial growth factor and transforming growth factor-beta 1 are highly expressed in the cerebrospinal fluid of premature infants with posthemorrhagic hydrocephalus. Pediatr Res 2004;56(5):768–74.
78. Lin CH, Cheng FC, Lu YZ, et al. Protection of ischemic brain cells is dependent on astrocyte-derived growth factors and their receptors. Exp Neurol 2006; 201(1):225–33.
79. Basu A, Krady JK, Enterline JR, et al. Transforming growth factor beta 1 prevents IL-1 beta-induced microglial activation, whereas TNF alpha- and IL-6-stimulated activation are not antagonized. Glia 2002;40(1):109–20.
80. Mesples B, Fontaine RH, Lelievre V, et al. Neuronal TGF-beta(1) mediates IL-9/mast cell interaction and exacerbates excitotoxicity in newborn mice. Neurobiol Dis 2005;18(1):193–205.
81. Guan J, Miller OT, Waugh KM, et al. TGF beta-I and neurological function after hypoxia-ischemia in adult rats. Neuroreport 2004;15(6):961–4.
82. Charo IF, Ransohoff RM. Mechanisms of disease—the many roles of chemokines and chemokine receptors in inflammation. N Engl J Med 2006;354(6):610–21.
83. Savarin-Vuaillat C, Ransohof RM. Chemokines and chemokine receptors in neurological disease: raise, retain, or reduce? Neurotherapeutics 2007;4(4): 590–601.
84. Ubogu EE, Cossoy MB, Ransohoff RM. The expression and function of chemokines involved in CNS inflammation. Trends Pharmacol Sci 2006;27(1):48–55.
85. Bacon K, Baggiolini M, Broxmeyer H, et al. Chemokine/chemokine receptor nomenclature. J Interferon Cytokine Res 2002;22(10):1067–8.
86. Ng PC, Lam HS. Diagnostic markers for neonatal sepsis. Curr Opin Pediatr 2006;18(2):125–31.
87. Bartha AI, Foster-Barber A, Miller SP, et al. Neonatal encephalopathy: association of cytokines with MR spectroscopy and outcome. Pediatr Res 2004;56(6): 960–6.
88. Ellison VJ, Mocatta TJ, Winterbourn CC, et al. The relationship of CSF and plasma cytokine levels to cerebral white matter injury in the premature newborn. Pediatr Res 2005;57(2):282–6.
89. Ehrlich LC, Hu SX, Sheng WS, et al. Cytokine regulation of human microglial cell IL-8 production. J Immunol 1998;160(4):1944–8.
90. Chew LJ, Takanohashi A, Bell M. Microglia and inflammation: impact on developmental brain injuries. Ment Retard Dev Disabil Res Rev 2006;12(2):105–12.

91. Bona E, Andersson AL, Blomgren K, et al. Chemokine and inflammatory cell response to hypoxia-ischemia in immature rats. Pediatr Res 1999;45(4):500–9.
92. Thibeault I, Laflamme N, Rivest S. Regulation of the gene encoding the monocyte chemoattractant protein 1 (MCP-1) in the mouse and rat brain in response to circulating LPS and proinflammatory cytokines. J Comp Neurol 2001;434(4): 461–77.
93. Dammann O, Durum S, Leviton A. Do white cells matter in white matter damage? Trends Neurosci 2001;24(6):320–4.
94. Leviton A, Dammann O, Durum SK. The adaptive immune response in neonatal cerebral white matter damage. Ann Neurol 2005;58(6):821–8.
95. Curatolo L, Valsasina B, Caccia C, et al. Recombinant human IL-2 is cytotoxic to oligodendrocytes after in vitro self aggregation. Cytokine 1997;9(10):734–9.
96. Kadhim H, Tabarki B, De Prez C, et al. Interleukin-2 in the pathogenesis of perinatal white matter damage. Neurology 2002;58(7):1125–8.
97. Sun FY, Guo X. Molecular and cellular mechanisms of neuroprotection by vascular endothelial growth factor. J Neurosci Res 2005;79(1–2):180–4.
98. Kaur C, Sivakumar V, Ang LS, et al. Hypoxic damage to the periventricular white matter in neonatal brain: role of vascular endothelial growth factor, nitric oxide and excitotoxicity. J Neurochem 2006;98(4):1200–16.
99. Laudenbach V, Fontaine RH, Medja F, et al. Neonatal hypoxic preconditioning involves vascular endothelial growth factor. Neurobiol Dis 2007;26(1):243–52.
100. Hansen-Pupp I, Hellstrom-Westas L, Cilio CM, et al. Inflammation at birth and the insulin-like growth factor system in very preterm infants. Acta Paediatr 2007;96(6):830–6.
101. Wood TL, Loladze V, Altieri S, et al. Delayed IGF-1 administration rescues oligodendrocyte progenitors from glutamate-induced cell death and hypoxic-ischemic brain damage. Dev Neurosci 2007;29(4–5):302–10.
102. Guan J, Bennet L, George S, et al. Insulin-like growth factor-1 reduces postischemic white matter injury in fetal sheep. J Cereb Blood Flow Metab 2001;21(5):493–502.
103. Brywe KG, Mallard C, Gustavsson M, et al. IGF-I neuroprotection in the immature brain after hypoxia-ischemia, involvement of Akt and GSK3 beta? Eur J Neurosci 2005;21(6):1489–502.
104. Dammann O, Bueter W, Leviton A, et al. Neuregulin-1: a potential endogenous protector in perinatal brain white matter damage. Neonatology 2008;93(3): 182–7.
105. Bernstein HG, Lendeckel U, Bertram I, et al. Localization of neuregulin-1 alpha (heregulin-alpha) and one of its receptors, ErbB-4 tyrosine kinase, in developing and adult human brain. Brain Res Bull 2006;69(5):546–59.
106. Vartanian T, Fischbach G, Miller R. Failure of spinal cord oligodendrocyte development in mice lacking neuregulin. Proc Natl Acad Sci U S A 1999; 96(2):731–5.
107. Xu ZF, Jiang J, Ford G, et al. Neuregulin-1 is neuroprotective and attenuates inflammatory responses induced by ischemic stroke. Biochem Biophys Res Commun 2004;322(2):440–6.
108. Xu ZF, Croslan DR, Harris AE, et al. Extended therapeutic window and functional recovery after intraarterial administration of neuregulin-1 after focal ischemic stroke. J Cereb Blood Flow Metab 2006;26(4):527–35.
109. Xu ZF, Ford GD, Croslan DR, et al. Neuroprotection by neuregulin-1 following focal stroke is associated with the attenuation of ischemia-induced pro-inflammatory and stress gene expression. Neurobiol Dis 2005;19(3):461–70.

110. Li YG, Xu ZF, Ford GD, et al. Neuroprotection by neuregulin-1 in a rat model of permanent focal cerebral ischemia. Brain Res 2007;1184:277–83.
111. Corfas G, Roy K, Buxbaum J. Neuregulin 1-erbB signaling and the molecular/cellular basis of schizophrenia. Nat Neurosci 2004;7(6):575–80.
112. Brown AS. Prenatal infection as a risk factor for schizophrenia. Schizophr Bull 2006;32(2):200–2.
113. Dammann O, Leviton A. Perinatal brain damage causation. Dev Neurosci 2007;29(4–5):280–8.
114. Welin AK, Svedin P, Lapatto R, et al. Melatonin reduces inflammation and cell death in white matter in the mid-gestation fetal sheep following umbilical cord occlusion. Pediatr Res 2007;61(2):153–8.
115. Svedin P, Guan J, Mathai S, et al. Delayed peripheral administration of a GPE analogue induces astrogliosis and angiogenesis and reduces inflammation and brain injury following hypoxia-ischemia in the neonatal rat. Dev Neurosci 2007;29(4–5):393–402.
116. Lyng K, Munkeby BH, Saugstad OD, et al. Effect of interleukin-10 on newborn piglet brain following hypoxia-ischemia and endotoxin-induced inflammation. Biol Neonate 2005;87(3):207–16.
117. Cai ZW, Lin SY, Pang Y, et al. Brain injury induced by intracerebral injection of interleukin-1beta and tumor necrosis factor-alpha in the neonatal rat. Pediatr Res 2004;56(3):377–84.
118. Jurewicz A, Matysiak M, Tybor K, et al. Tumour necrosis factor-induced death of adult human oligodendrocytes is mediated by apoptosis inducing factor. Brain 2005;128:2675–88.
119. Pang Y, Cai ZW, Rhodes PG. Effect of tumor necrosis factor-alpha on developing optic nerve oligodendrocytes in culture. J Neurosci Res 2005;80(2):226–34.
120. Cammer W, Zhang H. Maturation of oligodendrocytes is more sensitive to TNF alpha than is survival of precursors and immature oligodendrocytes. J Neuroimmunol 1999;97(1–2):37–42.
121. Wang XY, Hagberg H, Zhu CL, et al. Effects of intrauterine inflammation on the developing mouse brain. Brain Res 2007;1144:180–5.
122. Inder TE, Wells SJ, Mogridge NB, et al. Defining the nature of the cerebral abnormalities in the premature infant: a qualitative magnetic resonance imaging study. J Pediatr 2003;143(2):171–9.
123. Cai ZW, Pan ZL, Pang Y, et al. Cytokine induction in fetal rat brains and brain injury in neonatal rats after maternal lipopolysaccharide administration. Pediatr Res 2000;47(1):64–72.
124. Rousset CI, Chalon S, Cantagrel S, et al. Maternal exposure to LPS induces hypomyelination in the internal capsule and programmed cell death in the deep gray matter in newborn rats. Pediatr Res 2006;59(3):428–33.
125. Urakubo A, Jarskog LF, Lieberman JA, et al. Prenatal exposure to maternal infection alters cytokine expression in the placenta, amniotic fluid, and fetal brain. Schizophr Res 2001;47(1):27–36.
126. Ling ZD, Gayle DA, Ma SY, et al. In utero bacterial endotoxin exposure causes loss of tyrosine hydroxylase neurons in the postnatal rat midbrain. Mov Disord 2002;17(1):116–24.
127. Bell MJ, Hallenbeck JM. Effects of intrauterine inflammation on developing rat brain. J Neurosci Res 2002;70(4):570–9.
128. Gilmore JH, Jarskog LF, Vadlamudi S. Maternal infection regulates BDNF and NGF expression in fetal and neonatal brain and maternal-fetal unit of the rat. J Neuroimmunol 2003;138(1–2):49–55.

129. Duncan JR, Cock ML, Scheerlinck JP, et al. White matter injury after repeated endotoxin exposure in the preterm ovine fetus. Pediatr Res 2002;52(6):941–9.
130. Debillon T, Gras-Leguen C, Verielle V, et al. Intrauterine infection induces programmed cell death in rabbit periventricular white matter. Pediatr Res 2000; 47(6):736–42.
131. Debillon T, Gras-Leguen C, Leroy S, et al. Patterns of cerebral inflammatory response in a rabbit model of intrauterine infection-mediated brain lesion. Brain Res Dev Brain Res 2003;145(1):39–48.
132. Harnett EL, Dickinson MA, Smith GN. Dose-dependent lipopolysaccharide-induced fetal brain injury in the guinea pig. Am J Obstet Gynecol 2007;197(2): e1–7.
133. Liverman CS, Kaftan HA, Cui L, et al. Altered expression of pro-inflammatory and developmental genes in the fetal brain in a mouse model of maternal infection. Neurosci Lett 2006;399(3):220–5.
134. Golan HM, Lev V, Hallak M, et al. Specific neurodevelopmental damage in mice offspring following maternal inflammation during pregnancy. Neuropharmacology 2005;48(6):903–17.
135. Hava G, Vered L, Yael M, et al. Alternations in behaviour in adults offspring mice following maternal inflammation during pregnancy. Dev Psychobiol 2006;48(2): 162–8.
136. Paintlia MK, Paintlia AS, Contreras MA, et al. Lipopolysaccharide-induced peroxisomal dysfunction exacerbates cerebral white matter injury: attenuation by N-acetyl cysteine. Exp Neurol 2008;210:560–76.
137. Lante F, Meunier J, Guiramand J, et al. Neurodevelopmental damage after prenatal infection: role of oxidative stress in the fetal brain. Free Radic Biol Med 2007;42(8):1231–45.
138. Lante F, Meunier J, Guiramand J, et al. Late N-acetylcysteine treatment prevents the deficits induced in the offspring of dams exposed to an immune stress during gestation. Hippocampus 2008;18(6):602–9.
139. Lasala N, Zhou HP. Effects of maternal exposure to LPS on the inflammatory response in the offspring. J Neuroimmunol 2007;189(1–2):95–101.
140. Pang Y, Cai ZW, Rhodes PG. Disturbance of oligodendrocyte development, hypomyelination and white matter injury in the neonatal rat brain after intracerebral injection of lipopolysaccharide. Brain Res Dev Brain Res 2003; 140(2):205–14.
141. Lehnardt S, Lachance C, Patrizi S, et al. The toll-like receptor TLR4 is necessary for lipopolysaccharide-induced oligodendrocyte injury in the CNS. J Neurosci 2002;22(7):2478–86.
142. Lehnardt S, Massillon L, Follett P, et al. Activation of innate immunity in the CNS triggers neurodegeneration through a toll-like receptor 4-dependent pathway. Proc Natl Acad Sci U S A 2003;100(14):8514–9.
143. Lehnardt S, Schott E, Trimbuch T, et al. A vicious cycle involving release of heat shock protein 60 from injured cells and activation of toll-like receptor 4 mediates neurodegeneration in the CNS. J Neurosci 2008;28(10):2320–31.
144. Fan LW, Pang Y, Lin S, et al. Minocycline attenuates lipopolysaccharide-induced white matter injury in the neonatal rat brain. Neuroscience 2005; 133(1):159–68.
145. Cai Z, Lin S, Fan LW, et al. Minocycline alleviates hypoxic-ischemic injury to developing oligodendrocytes in the neonatal rat brain. Neuroscience 2006; 137(2):425–35.

146. Stolp HB, Dziegielewska KM, Ek CJ, et al. Long-term changes in blood-brain barrier permeability and white matter following prolonged systemic inflammation in early development in the rat. Eur J Neurosci 2005;22(11):2805–16.
147. Stolp HB, Ek CJ, Johansson PA, et al. Effect of minocycline on inflammation-induced damage to the blood-brain barrier and white matter during development. Eur J Neurosci 2007;26(12):3465–74.
148. Yan EW, Castillo-Melendez M, Nicholls T, et al. Cerebrovascular responses in the fetal sheep brain to low-dose endotoxin. Pediatr Res 2004;55(5):855–63.
149. Dammann O. Persistent neuro-inflammation in cerebral palsy: a therapeutic window of opportunity? Acta Paediatr 2007;96(1):6–7.
150. Hohlfeld R, Kerschensteiner M, Meinl E. Dual role of inflammation in CNS disease. Neurology 2007;68:S58–63.
151. Crutcher KA, Gendelman HE, Kipnis J, et al. Debate: "is increasing neuroinflammation beneficial for neural repair?". J Neuroimmune Pharmacol 2006;1(3):195–211.
152. Krumbholz M, Theil D, Derfuss T, et al. BAFF is produced by astrocytes and up-regulated in multiple sclerosis lesions and primary central nervous system lymphoma. J Exp Med 2005;201(2):195–200.
153. Bruce AJ, Boling W, Kindy MS, et al. Altered neuronal and microglial responses to excitotoxic and ischemic brain injury in mice lacking TNF receptors. Nat Med 1996;2(7):788–94.
154. Saha RN, Liu A, Pahan K. Up-regulation of BDNF in astrocytes by TNF-alpha: a case for the neuroprotective role of cytokine. J Neuroimmune Pharmacol 2006;1(2):212–22.
155. Moalem G, Leibowitz-Amit R, Yoles E, et al. Autoimmune T cells protect neurons from secondary degeneration after central nervous system axotomy. Nat Med 1999;5(1):49–55.
156. Schwartz M, Butovsky O, Bruck W, et al. Microglial phenotype: is the commitment reversible? Trends Neurosci 2006;29(2):68–74.
157. Banati RB, Graeber MB. Surveillance. Intervention and cytotoxicity—is there a protective role of microglia. Dev Neurosci 1994;16(3–4):114–27.
158. Schwartz M, Kipnis J. Therapeutic T cell-based vaccination for neurodegenerative disorders—the role of CD4(+) CD25(+) regulatory T cells. Ann NY Acad Sci 2005;1051:701–8.
159. Ziv Y, Schwartz M. Immune-based regulation of adult neurogenesis: implications for learning and memory. Brain Behav Immun 2008;22(2):167–76.
160. Ziv Y, Ron N, Butovsky O, et al. Immune cells contribute to the maintenance of neurogenesis and spatial learning abilities in adulthood. Nat Neurosci 2006;9(2):268–75.
161. Medzhitov R, Janeway C. Innate immune recognition: mechanisms and pathways. Immunol Rev 2000;173:89–97.
162. Levy O. Innate immunity of the newborn: basic mechanisms and clinical correlates. Nat Rev Immunol 2007;7(5):379–90.
163. De Dooy J, Colpaert C, Schuerwegh A, et al. Relationship between histologic chorioamnionitis and early inflammatory variables in blood, tracheal aspirates, and endotracheal colonization in preterm infants. Pediatr Res 2003;54(1):113–9.
164. Kashlan F, Smulian J, Shen-Schwarz S, et al. Umbilical vein interleukin 6 and tumor necrosis factor alpha plasma concentrations in the very preterm infant. Pediatr Infect Dis J 2000;19(3):238–43.

165. Kaukola T, Herva R, Perhomaa M, et al. Population cohort associating chorioamnionitis, cord inflammatory cytokines and neurologic outcome in very preterm, extremely low birth weight infants. Pediatr Res 2006;59(3):478–83.
166. Martin H, Olander B, Norman M. Reactive hyperemia and interleukin 6, interleukin 8, and tumor necrosis factor-alpha in the diagnosis of early-onset neonatal sepsis. Pediatrics 2001;108(4):E61.
167. Ng PC, Li K, Chui KM, et al. IP-10 is an early diagnostic marker for identification of late-onset bacterial infection in preterm infants. Pediatr Res 2007;61(1):93–8.
168. Ng PC, Li K, Wong RP, et al. Proinflammatory and anti-inflammatory cytokine responses in preterm infants with systemic infections. Arch Dis Child 2003;88(3): 209–13.
169. Franz AR, Bauer K, Schalk A, et al. Measurement of interleukin 8 in combination with C-reactive protein reduced unnecessary antibiotic therapy in newborn infants: a multicenter, randomized, controlled trial. Pediatrics 2004; 114(1):1–8.
170. Verboon-Maciolek MA, Thijsen SF, Hemels MA, et al. Inflammatory mediators for the diagnosis and treatment of sepsis in early infancy. Pediatr Res 2006;59(3): 457–61.
171. Edelson MB, Bagwell CE, Rozycki HJ. Circulating pro- and counterinflammatory cytokine levels and severity in necrotizing enterocolitis. Pediatrics 1999;103(4): 766–71.
172. Goldenberg RL, Andrews WW, Goepfert AR, et al. The Alabama preterm birth study: umbilical cord blood Ureaplasma urealyticum and mycoplasma hominis cultures in very preterm newborn infants. Am J Obstet Gynecol 2008;198(1): e1–5.
173. Whitaker AH, Feldman JF, VanRossem R, et al. Neonatal cranial ultrasound abnormalities in low birth weight infants: relation to cognitive outcomes at six years of age. Pediatrics 1996;98(4):719–29.
174. Munshi UK, Niu JO, Siddiq MM, et al. Elevation of interleukin-8 and interleukin-6 precedes the influx of neutrophils in tracheal aspirates from preterm infants who develop bronchopulmonary dysplasia. Pediatr Pulmonol 1997;24(5):331–6.
175. Murch SH, Costeloe K, Klein NJ, et al. Early production of macrophage inflammatory protein-1 alpha occurs in respiratory distress syndrome and is associated with poor outcome. Pediatr Res 1996;40(3):490–7.
176. Jonsson B, Tullus K, Brauner A, et al. Early increase of TNF alpha and IL-6 in tracheobronchial aspirate fluid indicator of subsequent chronic lung disease in preterm infants. Arch Dis Child 1997;77(3):F198–201.
177. Turunen R, Nupponen I, Siitonen S, et al. Onset of mechanical ventilation is associated with rapid activation of circulating phagocytes in preterm infants. Pediatrics 2006;117(2):448–54.
178. Kuebler WM, Ying XY, Singh B, et al. Pressure is proinflammatory in lung venular capillaries. J Clin Invest 1999;104(4):495–502.
179. Baier RJ. Genetics of perinatal brain injury in the preterm infant. Front Biosci 2006;11:1371–87.
180. Mcguire W, Hill AV, Allsopp CE, et al. Variation in the TNF-alpha promoter region associated with susceptibility to cerebral malaria. Nature 1994;371(6497): 508–11.
181. Aidoo M, Mcelroy PD, Kolczak MS, et al. Tumor necrosis factor-alpha promoter variant 2 (TNF2) is associated with pre-term delivery, infant mortality, and

malaria morbidity in western Kenya: Asenibo Bay Cohort project IX. Genet Epidemiol 2001;21(3):201–11.
182. Papile LA, Munsickbruno G, Schaefer A. Relationship of cerebral intraventricular hemorrhage and early-childhood neurologic handicaps. J Pediatr 1983;103(2): 273–7.
183. Adcock K, Hedberg C, Loggins J, et al. MCP-1-2518 and TGF-beta(1) +915 polymorphisms are not associated with the development of chronic lung disease in very low birth weight infants. Genes Immun 2003;4(6):420–6.
184. Nelson KB, Dambrosia JM, Iovannisci DM, et al. Genetic polymorphisms and cerebral palsy in very preterm infants. Pediatr Res 2005;57(4):494–9.
185. Gibson CS, MacLennan AH, Goldwater PN, et al. The association between inherited cytokine polymorphisms and cerebral palsy. Am J Obstet Gynecol 2006;194(3):674–80.
186. Harding DR, Dhamrait S, Whitelaw A, et al. Does interleukin-6 genotype influence cerebral injury or developmental progress after preterm birth? Pediatrics 2004;114(4):941–7.
187. Gaynor JW, Gerdes M, Zackai EH, et al. Apolipoprotein E genotype and neurodevelopmental sequelae of infant cardiac surgery. J Thorac Cardiovasc Surg 2003;126(6):1736–45.
188. Wright RO, Hu H, Silverman EK, et al. Apolipoprotein E genotype predicts 24-month Bayley Scales Infant Development score. Pediatr Res 2003;54(6):819–25.
189. Yanamandra K, Boggs P, Loggins J, et al. Interleukin-10-1082 G/A polymorphism and risk of death or bronchopulmonary dysplasia in ventilated very low birth weight infants. Pediatr Pulmonol 2005;39(5):426–32.

The Use of Amplitude Integrated Electroencephalography for Assessing Neonatal Neurologic Injury

Mona C. Toet, MD, PhD*, Linda G.M. van Rooij, MD,
Linda S. de Vries, MD, PhD

KEYWORDS

- Amplitude-integrated electroencephalography
- Cerebral function monitor • Hypoxia-ischemia
- Asphyxia • Neonatal seizures
- Neurodevelopmental outcome

Amplitude-integrated electroencephalography (aEEG), or the cerebral function monitor (CFM), was originally designed by Maynard[1] in the late 1960s to perform continuous electrocortical monitoring. Prior[2,3] developed the clinical application, mainly in adult patients during anesthesia and intensive care, after cardiac arrest, during status epilepticus, and after heart surgery. The first studies performed in newborns are from the early 1980s.[4–6] During the first 2 decades, aEEG was recorded with the analog CFM. Initial studies focused on maturation of the background pattern in low-risk preterm infants.[5–7] It quickly became clear, however, that long-term recordings in high-risk full-term infants with neonatal encephalopathy (NE) was the main contribution of this technique.[4,8–10]

The term *amplitude-integrated electroencephalography* is currently preferred to denote a method for encephalographic monitoring, because CFM is used to refer to specific equipment. The electroencephalography (EEG) signal for analog single-channel aEEG was initially recorded from one pair of parietally placed electrodes (corresponding to P3 and P4, according to the international EEG 10-20 classification, ground F_z). With the introduction of several digital machines, recording of more than just the single

Dr. de Vries and Dr. Toet have been involved in the development or testing of the instruments from which records are shown in this article. They do not have an economic interest in the production or sales of these instruments.

Department of Neonatology, University Medical Center, Wilhelmina Children's Hospital, KE 04.123.1, PO Box 85090, 3508 AB Utrecht, The Netherlands
* Corresponding author.
E-mail address: m.toet@umcutrecht.nl (M.C. Toet).

Clin Perinatol 35 (2008) 665–678
doi:10.1016/j.clp.2008.07.017 perinatology.theclinics.com

channel has also become possible. Using two channels (F3–P3 and F4–P4 or C3–P3 and C3–P4, ground F_Z),[11,12] according to the international EEG 10-20 classification, provides information about hemispheric asymmetry, which may be especially helpful in children with a unilateral brain lesion. The signal is amplified and passed through an asymmetric band-pass filter that strongly prefers higher frequencies over lower ones and suppresses activity less than 2 Hz and greater than 15 Hz to minimize artifacts from such external sources as sweating, movement, muscle activity, and electrical interference.

Additional processing includes semilogarithmic amplitude presentation, rectification, smoothing, and considerable time compression (**Fig. 1**). The signal is displayed on a semilogarithmic scale at slow speed (6 cm/h) at the cot side. A second tracing continuously displays the original EEG from one or more channels. The electrode impedance is continuously recorded but not necessarily displayed; however, there is an alarm when there is high impedance, often attributable to a loose electrode. The band width in the output reflects variations in minimum and maximum EEG amplitude, both of which depend on the maturity and severity of illness of the newborn. Because of the semilogarithmic scale used to plot the output, changes in background activity of extremely low amplitude (<5 μV) are enhanced. The information in the aEEG trace can be enhanced by modifying the gray scale so that a particular intensity represents the amount of time the signal spends at that amplitude. This feature is useful when defining the lower border of the trace (**Fig. 2**C) and analyzing changes caused by ictal periods.

ASSESSMENT OF AMPLITUDE-INTEGRATED ELECTROENCEPHALOGRAPHY BACKGROUND PATTERN

The aEEG traces are assessed visually based on pattern recognition and classified into the five following categories in full-term infants (see **Fig. 2**):[13]

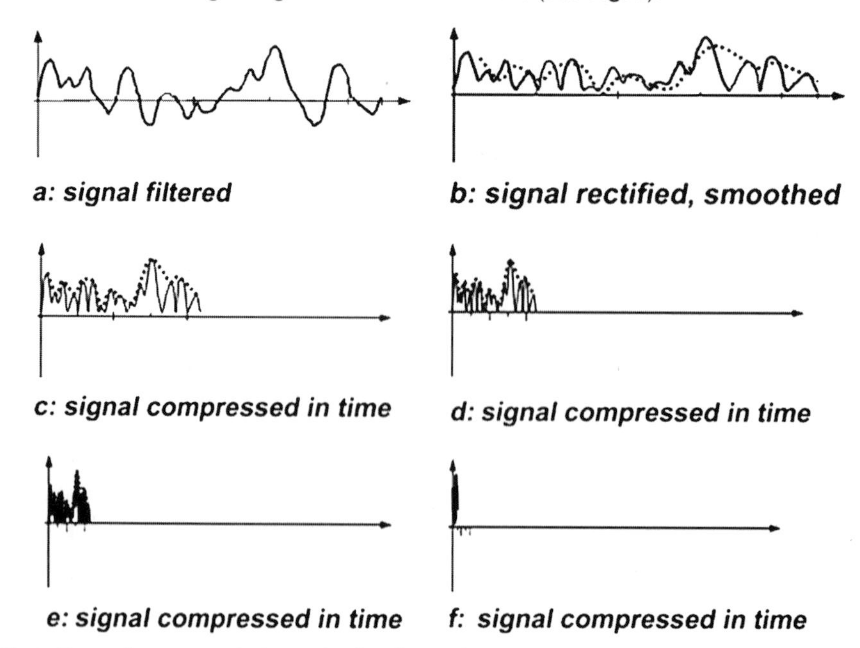

Fig. 1. From electroencephalography (EEG) signal to aEEG signal.

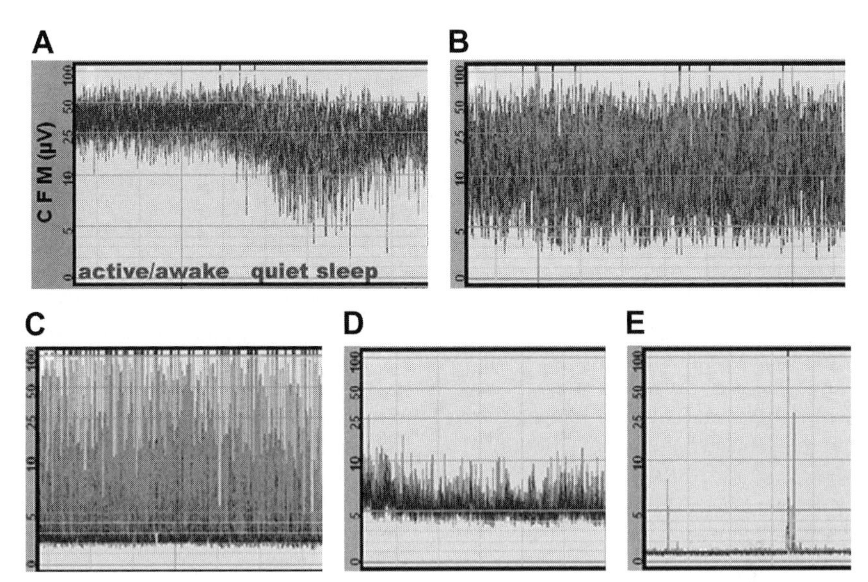

Fig. 2. Different background patterns: continuous normal voltage (CNV) (*A*), discontinuous normal voltage (DNV) (*B*), burst suppression (BS) (*C*), continuous low voltage (CLV) (*D*), and flat trace (FT) (*E*).

1. Continuous normal voltage pattern (CNV): continuous activity with lower (minimum) amplitude around (5) to 7 to 10 µV and maximum amplitude around 10 to 25 (to 50) µV (see **Fig. 2**A)
2. Discontinuous normal voltage pattern (DNV): discontinuous background, with variable minimum amplitude, but less than 5 µV and maximum amplitude greater than 10 µV (see **Fig. 2**B)
3. Burst suppression (BS): discontinuous background with minimum amplitude without variability at 0 to 1 (2) µV and bursts with amplitude greater than 25 µV (see **Fig. 2**C)
4. Continuous low voltage (CLV): continuous background pattern of extremely low voltage (around or less than 5 µV) (see **Fig. 2**D)
5. Inactive flat trace (FT): mainly inactive (isoelectric tracing) background less than 5 µV (see **Fig. 2**E)

During longer recordings a sleep-wake cycling (SWC) pattern should be present, seen as continuous activity with regularly cycling patterns: intervals of continuous activity (awake, active sleep) intermixed with periods of slightly lower voltage (for term infant, broadest bandwidth: minimum of 6–8 µV, maximum of 15–20 µV; narrowest bandwidth: minimum of 6–8 µV, maximum of 9–15 µV; see **Fig. 2**A).

AMPLITUDE-INTEGRATED ELECTROENCEPHALOGRAPHY IN NEONATAL ENCEPHALOPATHY

The value of the background pattern in the prediction of neurodevelopmental outcome was already well established with the use of standard EEG.[14] A poor background pattern, which persists beyond the first 12 to 24 hours after birth (BS, CLV, and FT) is well known to carry a poor prognosis. The interburst interval (IBI) can be calculated, and it was shown, using standard EEG, that a predominant IBI duration of more than 30 seconds correlated with the occurrence of an unfavorable neurologic outcome and subsequent epilepsy ($P = .04$ and $P = .033$, respectively).[15] Continuous calculation of the IBI is now also available on- and off-line in some of the digital devices. Over the years, several groups have studied the relation between the background pattern recorded within 3 to 12 hours after birth and subsequent neurodevelopmental outcome (**Table 1**).

The first studies assessed aEEG during the first 12 to 24 hours, but with recent interest in early intervention strategies, aEEG has also been assessed as early as 3 to 6 hours after birth to see whether it could play a role in selection of infants at risk for developing NE.[9,10,16–20] The predictive value of the presence of a poor background pattern (BS, CLV, or FT) for subsequent poor neurodevelopmental outcome at 18 to 24 months was assessed in these different studies. The predictive values obtained by different groups were similar. Positive and negative predictive values were slightly lower when aEEG was assessed at 3 instead of 6 hours after birth, but they were still considered sufficiently high to use this technique for early selection in hypothermia or other intervention studies.[21] Combining a neurological examination with aEEG performed less than 12 hours after birth further increased predictive accuracy from 75% to 85%.[20] In the meta-analysis of eight studies described by Spitzmiller and colleagues,[22] a sensitivity of 91% (confidence interval [CI]: 87%–95%) and a negative likelihood ratio of 0.09 for aEEG tracings was found to predict poor outcome accurately.

A negative relation was recently reported between aEEG amplitude measures, Sarnat grades, and MRI abnormality scores. The relation was strongest for the minimum amplitude measures in both hemispheres. A minimum amplitude of less than 4 μV was useful in predicting severe MRI abnormalities.[11]

The use of aEEG should not be restricted to full-term infants with NE associated with problems around the time of delivery. Other conditions presenting with NE or seizures in the neonatal period are indications to use this technique (eg, meningoencephalitis, metabolic disorders, congenital malformations, use of muscle paralysis, after open-heart surgery, extracorporeal membrane oxygenation [ECMO]).[23,24]

The usefulness of aEEG in predicting outcome after cardiac arrest and induced hypothermia has also been described in adults.[25]

Table 1
Predictive values of abnormal background patterns (burst suppression, continuous low voltage, flat trace) during the first 3, 6, and 12 hours of life to predict adverse outcomes (death or handicap)

	Sensitivity (%)	Specificity (%)	Positive Predictive Value (%)	Negative Predictive Value (%)
6 hours: Hellström-Westas et al (n = 47)	95	89	86	96
6 hours: Eken et al (n = 34)	94	79	84	92
6 hours: Toet et al (n = 68)	91	86	86	96
3 hours: Toet et al (n = 68)	85	77	78	84
6 hours: al Naqeeb et al (n = 56)	93	70	77	90
12 hours: Shalak et al (n = 15)	79	89	73	91
6 hours: vanRooij et al (n = 161)	83	85	88	91
6 hours: Shany et al (n = 39)	100	87	69	100

Data modified from references.

RECOVERY OF THE BACKGROUND PATTERN

In a large study of 160 full-term infants admitted and recorded with aEEG within 6 hours after birth, 65 had an initial FT or CLV pattern and 25 had an initial BS pattern. The background pattern recovered to a CNV pattern within 24 hours in only 6 (9%) of the 65 infants in the FT/CLV group, and 5 of them were normal at follow-up. In the BS group, the background pattern improved to normal voltage in 12 (48%) of the 25 infants within 24 hours. Of these infants, 2 survived with mild disability and 4 were normal. The patients who did not recover died in the neonatal period or survived with a severe disability. Although the actual number of infants with background recovery within 24 hours was small (9%), more than half of these infants (61%) had a normal or mildly abnormal outcome.[26] The difference in outcome for these two background pattern groups is of interest. The insult around the time of delivery in the FT/CLV group was almost invariably acute and severe but presumably of shorter duration than in those with a persistent FT/CLV background pattern and in those with a BS pattern. aEEG by itself was apparently not sufficient to make an accurate prediction in the BS group. The authors therefore have a policy to perform additional neurophysiologic (visual and somatosensory evoked potentials) and neuroimaging studies (ultrasound and MRI). This study stressed the importance of continuing aEEG registration beyond the first 12 to 24 hours after birth. None of the infants in this cohort had been treated with hypothermia.

Data about a possible effect of hypothermia on aEEG voltage are scarce.[27] In one study, there was no effect of mild hypothermia on aEEG voltage in neonates receiving ECMO.[27] There are no data about a possible effect of mild hypothermia on the rate of recovery of a depressed background pattern. When morphine is used for sedation during hypothermia, care should be taken to interpret the background, because it was recently shown that morphine clearance is reduced during hypothermia and potentially toxic serum concentrations of morphine may occur with moderate hypothermia and infusion rates greater than 10 μg/kg/h, which may affect recovery of the background pattern.[28]

A longer registration should also allow assessment of the presence, quality, and time of onset of SWC (see **Fig. 2**A). The authors have shown that the presence, time of onset, and quality of SWC reflects the severity of the hypoxic-ischemic insult to which newborns have been exposed.[29] The time of onset of SWC was shown to predict neurodevelopmental outcome based on whether SWC returns before 36 hours (good outcome) or after 36 hours (bad outcome).

Using this method, an accurate prediction was made in 82% of the 171 newborns with different degrees of encephalopathy. These data are in agreement with those of two other reports.[19,30] Although the infants who were treated with antiepileptic drugs for seizures had a significantly later onset of SWC, no significant effect on time of onset of SWC was seen with two or fewer antiepileptic drugs. This was confirmed by another study in which aEEG recordings were compared with MRI abnormalities. The investigators found little effect of antiepileptic drugs on the relation between aEEG amplitude and cerebral injury as assessed by their MRI assessment score.[11]

Timing of the insult is an important issue in infants with hypoxic-ischemic encephalopathy (HIE). Often, it is not immediately clear whether there is a prelabor insult, a peripartum insult, or both. Timing has an effect on aEEG and also on the subsequent effect of neuroprotective strategies, such as cooling. It also affects the time of onset of seizures after birth, which was shown in a study by Filan and colleagues.[31] They showed that with a prelabor insult, the first seizures occur before 12 hours after birth, whereas in infants with a peripartum insult, the onset of seizures is generally after 18 to 20 hours after birth.

CORRELATION BETWEEN AMPLITUDE-INTEGRATED ELECTROENCEPHALOGRAPHY AND STANDARD ELECTROENCEPHALOGRAPHY

There have been several studies in which aEEG and standard EEG were performed simultaneously to compare the two techniques. Overall, there seemed to be a good correlation between the aEEG and EEG background patterns in the full-term infant with moderate to severe NE.[32,33]

Detection of Epileptic Seizure Activity

Seizure burden is known to be high in encephalopathic neonates.[34] A recent video-conventional EEG study by Murray and colleagues[34] shows that only one third of neonatal EEG seizures display clinical signs on simultaneous video recordings. Two thirds of these clinical manifestations are unrecognized or misinterpreted by experienced neonatal staff. Clinical diagnosis is therefore not sufficient for the recognition and management of neonatal seizures.

A rapid increase in the lower and upper margins of the aEEG tracing is suggestive of an ictal discharge (**Fig. 3**A). Seizures can be recognized as single seizures, repetitive seizures, or status epilepticus (see **Figs. 3**B, **3**C). The latter usually looks like a "saw-tooth" pattern. Correct interpretation is greatly improved by simultaneous raw EEG recordings available on the digital devices, and the gray-scale software available on some of the newer machines also helps to make the correct diagnosis (see **Fig. 3**C).[35]

Since the increased use of continuous monitoring, it has become apparent that subclinical seizures are common and frequently continue after administration of the first antiepileptic drug.[36,37] This so-called "uncoupling" or "electroclinical dissociation" has recently been reported by several groups and was found in 50% to 60% of the children studied. aEEG can play an important role in the detection of these subclinical seizures. Being aware of this phenomenon has highlighted the poor therapeutic effect of most of the commonly used antiepileptic drugs. Drugs that were considered to have a good therapeutic effect in the past often only suppress the clinical symptoms. Continuous EEG or aEEG recording, preferably with simultaneous video recording, is therefore required to assess the therapeutic effect of antiepileptic drugs.

Even status epilepticus is not uncommon and occurred in 18% of 56 full-term infants admitted with neonatal seizures.[38] The duration of status epilepticus may influence prognosis as well. In a group of 48 infants with HIE and aEEG-detected status epilepticus, there was a significant difference in the background pattern and in the duration of the status epilepticus in infants with a poor outcome compared with those with a good outcome. The background pattern at the onset of status epilepticus was the main predictor of outcome in all neonates with status epilepticus.[38]

Using a single channel or even two channels does not allow detection of all seizures. Because of the nature of the technique, it is not surprising that brief seizure activity and focal seizure activity may be missed.[33,39] This was recently also shown by Shellhaas and colleagues[40] in a large data set of 125 conventional EEG recordings with 851 neonatal seizures. Ninety-four percent of the conventional EEG recordings detected one or more seizures on the C3-to-C4 channel, and 81% of the neonatal seizures originated from central-temporal or midline vertex electrodes.[41] The C3-to-C4–derived aEEG recordings were evaluated by six neonatologists who did not have access to the "raw" EEG recordings. Detection of individual seizures seemed to be difficult (12%–38%) without access to the raw EEG recordings, especially when the seizures

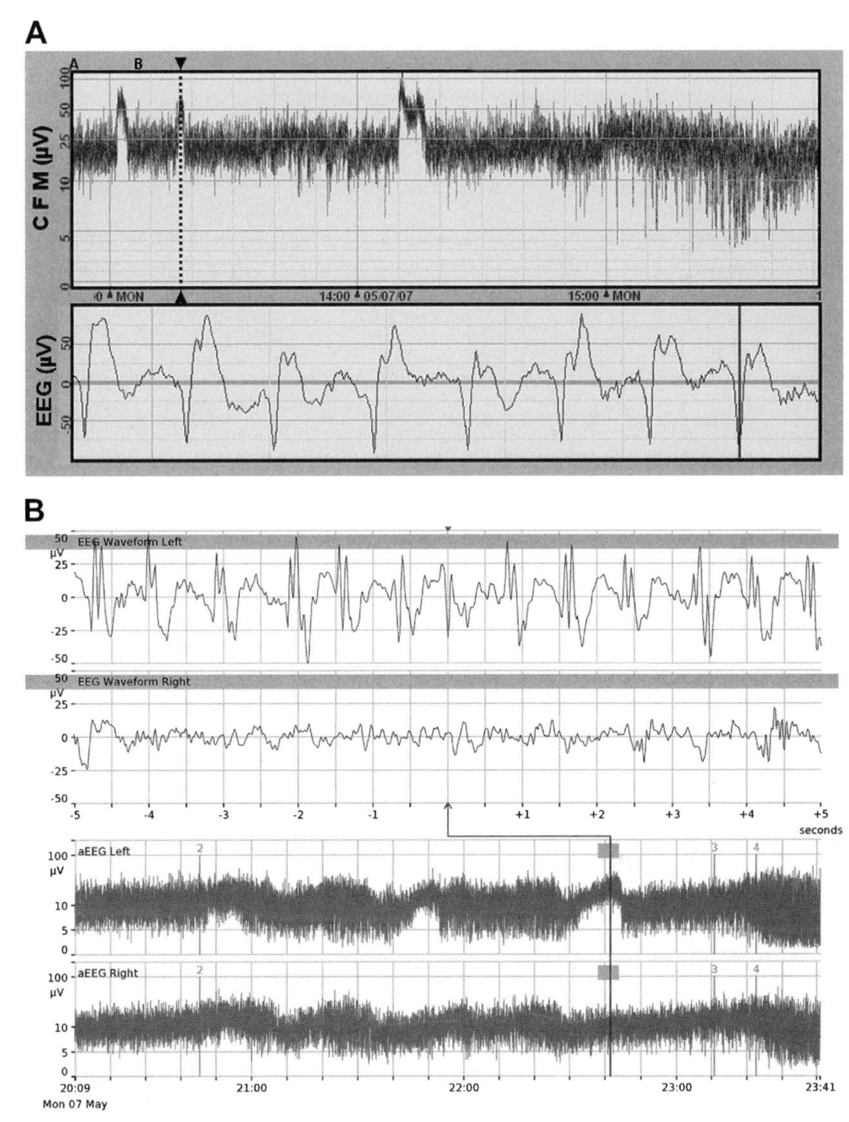

Fig. 3. (*A*) Three seizures on a good background pattern, with the raw electroencephalographic data taken during the second seizure. (*B*) Subsequent bilateral recording of the same child shows a left-sided ictal discharge. MRI later showed a left-sided middle cerebral artery infarct. (*C*) Status epilepticus and repetitive seizures. The seizure detection marker is presented as blocks in orange above the recording.

were infrequent, brief, or of low amplitude. There were no false-positive results among 19 control records. Infants who have focal seizures, however, tend to develop more widespread ictal discharges during the continuous registration, which can be identified.[33] Some therefore say that the long duration of the aEEG registration seems to outweigh the limitations of obtaining detailed information during a much shorter 30-minute standard EEG registration.

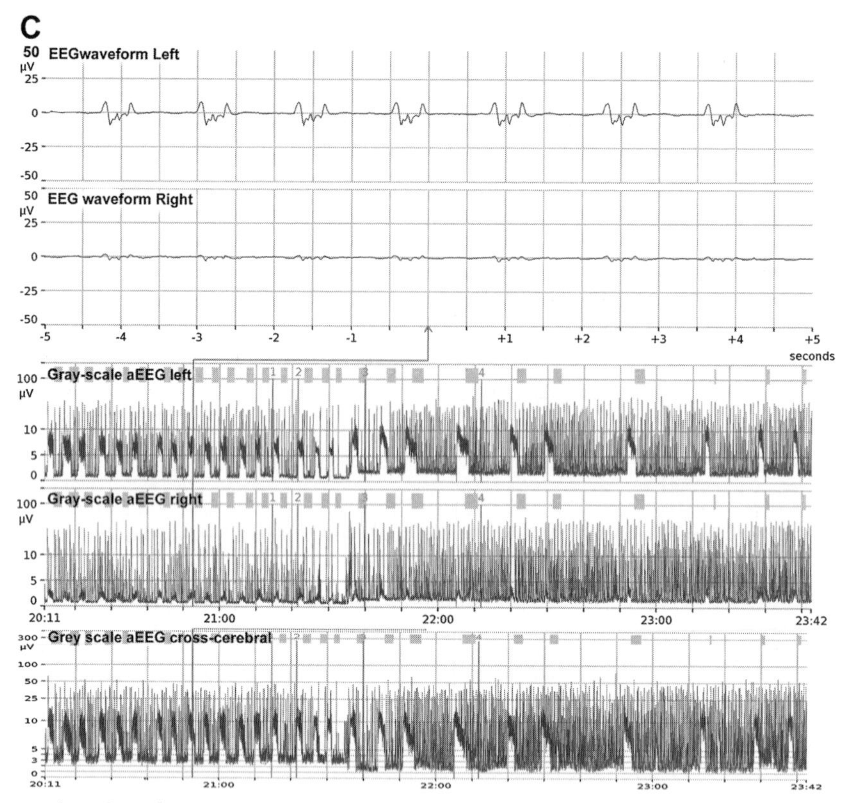

Fig. 3. (*continued*)

Whether the use of two channels (or more) is indicated in all infants is still under debate. In the authors' own population of 222 full-term infants admitted between 2002 and 2006 with NE or seizures, 21% had a predominantly unilateral lesion.

Using a two-channel recording, it was noted that some ictal discharges arose from the affected hemisphere, but these discharges could usually be recognized on the cross-cerebral recording (see **Fig. 3**B) (L.G.M. van Rooij, unpublished data, 2008). Comparing the two-channel data with the crossover recording, there was good agreement with regard to classification of the background pattern with only small differences in amplitudes. Seeing an asymmetry in background pattern or seizures occurring predominantly in one hemisphere can suggest a unilateral lesion, often before the diagnosis is made with neuroimaging.

ROLE OF AMPLITUDE-INTEGRATED ELECTROENCEPHALOGRAPHY IN NEUROPROTECTIVE STRATEGIES

Immediate access to aEEG monitoring in full-term infants with NE, often admitted at night or during the weekend, is one of many advantages of this technique. It is easy to learn by senior and junior doctors and the nursing staff and can immediately provide information about the background activity and presence of seizures within hours after birth. In one study, this information was required as soon as possible after birth for selection of patients for neuroprotective intervention.[21]

PITFALLS AND ARTIFACTS

One can use a classification system based on pattern recognition[9,16] or look at actual values of lower and upper margins of activity.[17] Although one would be inclined to prefer values rather than patterns, values may be misleading, because the voltage may be affected by scalp edema and interelectrode distance.[11] In the study of Shah and colleagues[11] with two-channel recordings, cutoff values of 4 and 9 μV were used instead of cutoff values of 5 and 10 μV from the criteria of al Naqeeb and colleagues[17] in the one-channel recording because of a smaller distance between the central and parietal electrodes (C3–P3 and C4–P4 with an electrode distance of 2.5 cm) in the two-channel recording compared with the one-channel electrode distance.

The lower margin may be elevated because of extracranial activity (e.g. electrocardiographic [ECG] interference or interference from a high-frequency ventilator). This so-called "drift of the baseline" is especially seen in infants with a severely depressed background pattern (**Fig. 4**).[42]

The simultaneous recording of the real EEG, present on the newer digital devices, may help in the identification of artifacts,[43] which are quite common during long-term recordings. Hagmann and colleagues[42] show that 12% of their 200 hours of recording was affected by artifacts. This was attributable to electrical interference in 55% of instances, which could be ECG artifact (39%) or fast activity (>50 Hz, 61%), and was attributable to movement artifact in the remaining 45%. They state that the dual facility (aEEG with simultaneous raw EEG) is crucial for the correct interpretation of the aEEG data. Inappropriate electrode position can also lead to aEEG recordings with artifact or drift of the baseline.

In a recent study by Sarkar and colleagues,[44] 54 infants with moderate or severe HIE were evaluated with aEEG for selection for hypothermic neuroprotection. Seven encephalopathic infants with "normal" aEEG recordings were not cooled but were subsequently shown to have abnormalities on MRI. These investigators concluded that

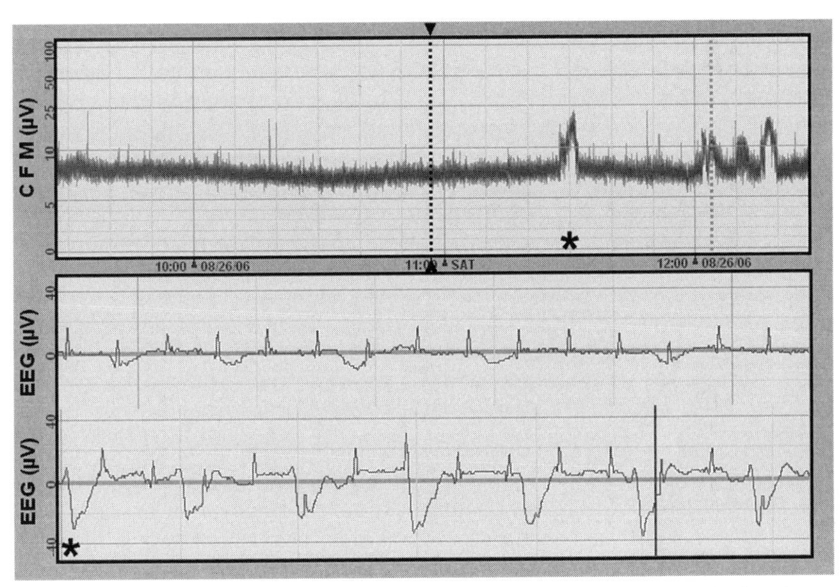

Fig. 4. FT with "drift of the baseline" attributable to an ECG artifact. The original EEG recording is shown by the dotted line and during seizure activity (*).

there was a poor correlation between early aEEG recordings and short-term adverse outcome, with a sensitivity of 54.8% and a negative predictive value of only 44%. All these normal aEEG recordings, however, had ECG artifacts, which could explain the drift of the baseline (J.D. Barks, personal communication, 2008). Retrospectively, these patients would have been eligible for the cooling study on the basis of their background pattern.

Medication can also affect the background pattern, as was mentioned previously. Antiepileptic drugs can give a temporary decrease in amplitude on the aEEG recording, although this did not influence prognosis.[11,29] Other drugs can also have this effect, as was shown by a recent case report concerning an overdose of morphine.[45]

The authors therefore recommend the use of pattern recognition, taking the values of upper and lower margins into account as well. Hellström-Westas and colleagues[9,13] classified aEEG from asphyxiated full-term infants as CNV, DNV, BS, CLV, and FT.

SEIZURE-LIKE ARTIFACTS

Any movement or handling of the baby, with a sudden increase in the baseline of the aEEG recording, can also mimic seizure activity on aEEG. The simultaneous recorded single-channel raw EEG signal can help to interpret aEEG traces more accurately.[43] In addition, marking events on the aEEG recording by nursing staff is important.

DISCUSSION

Experience with continuous aEEG is increasing, and many neonatal intensive care units would now find it hard to imagine treating a full-term infant with NE without the use of this monitoring device.

The three main features that are provided with aEEG are the background pattern on admission, the rate of recovery seen during the first 24 to 48 hours after birth, the presence or absence of SWC, and the presence of electrographic discharges and the effect of treatment with antiepileptic drugs. It is not yet known whether hypothermia has an effect on the rate of recovery of a depressed background pattern.

Having access to the raw EEG recording on the new digital machines has helped the authors to read the aEEG recording better, especially with regard to the diagnosis of electrographic discharges and distinction from artifacts. Recognition of the drift of the baseline is especially important. Correct interpretation of background patterns is vital in children with HIE eligible for interventions, such as hypothermia.

New software has become available, enabling calculation of the IBI and the number of bursts per hour on-line, which has been shown to be of predictive value using standard EEG.[15] Interpretation of the different background patterns has become more reliable using the new gray scale (see **Fig. 3**C).

It should be stressed, however, that aEEG is a monitoring device and does not replace standard EEG. Especially in the more intermediate discontinuous background pattern, correct interpretation may be difficult and ictal discharges may be especially difficult to identify with this background pattern. After introduction of aEEG, one usually finds an increase in the number of standard EEG requests rather than a decrease. With some of the digital machines, it is possible to be connected to the network, and on-line access in the neurophysiology department or even from home may be possible.

With the increased use of aEEG, physicians have become more aware of the limited effect of the commonly used antiepileptic drugs, such as phenobarbitone and phenytoin.[46] Other antiepileptic drugs, such as lidocaine and midazolam, have been used as second-line drugs.[47–50] There is uncertainty whether treatment of electrographic discharges is in the best interest of the infant. A potential beneficial effect of treating clinical and subclinical seizures was suggested by finding a relatively lower incidence of postneonatal epilepsy in two groups of infants who were treated for clinical and subclinical seizures (8%–9%), compared with previous reports in the literature in infants who only received treatment of EEG-confirmed clinical seizures.[51–54] This was further supported by data of other groups.[55,56] The first randomized study of treatment of subclinical seizures (SuSeQue) is underway, with 11 neonatal units participating in The Netherlands and Belgium.

Data obtained in animal experiments suggested a possible apoptotic neurodegenerative effect of commonly used antiepileptic drugs at concentrations relevant for seizure control in humans.[57] There are several case reports using new drugs, such as levetiracetam and lamotrigine, which also may have a neuroprotective effect. Randomized controlled trials using these drugs are likely to be performed in the near future.[58,59]

In conclusion, the authors have become increasingly aware of the importance of continuous monitoring of electrocortical activity. Although aEEG may provide limited information when it comes to seizure detection, it is reliable in recognizing background abnormalities, which have been shown to be strongly predictive of neurodevelopmental outcome. Recognition of artifacts influencing background patterns is especially important in those infants eligible for interventions, such as hypothermia. Although not supported by all, the authors only consider neonatal intensive care of the infant with NE or seizures to be optimal when a continuous aEEG monitor is used.[60]

REFERENCES

1. Maynard DE. EEG analysis using an analogue frequency analyser and a digital computer. Electroencephalogr Clin Neurophysiol 1967;23(5):487.
2. Prior PF. EEG monitoring and evoked potentials in brain ischaemia. Br J Anaesth 1985;57(1):63–81.
3. Prior PF, Maynard DE. Monitoring cerebral function. Long-term recordings of cerebral electrical activity and evoked potentials. Amsterdam: Elsevier; 1986. p. 1–441.
4. Bjerre I, Hellström-Westas L, Rosen I, et al. Monitoring of cerebral function after severe birth asphyxia in infancy. Arch Dis Child 1983;58:997–1002.
5. Verma UL, Archbald F, Tejani NA, et al. Cerebral function monitor in the neonate. I: normal patterns. Dev Med Child Neurol 1984;26:154–61.
6. Viniker DA, Maynard DE, Scott DF. Cerebral function studies in neonates. Clin Electroencephalogr 1984;15:185–92.
7. Thornberg E, Thiringer K. Normal pattern of the cerebral function monitor trace in term and preterm neonates. Acta Paediatr Scand 1990;79:20–5.
8. Hellström-Westas L, Rosen I, Svenningsen NW. Silent seizures in sick infants in early life. Acta Paediatr Scand 1985;74:741–8.
9. Hellström-Westas L, Rosen I, Svenningsen NW. Predictive value of early continuous amplitude integrated EEG recordings on outcome after severe birth asphyxia in full term infants. Arch Dis Child Fetal Neonatal Ed 1995;72:F34–8.
10. Eken P, Toet MC, Groenendaal F, et al. Predictive value of early neuroimaging, pulsed Doppler and neurophysiology in fullterm infants with hypoxic-ischemic encephalopathy. Arch Dis Child 1995;73:F75–80.
11. Shah DK, Lavery S, Doyle LW, et al. Use of 2-channel bedside electroencephalogram monitoring in term-born encephalopathic infants related to cerebral injury defined by magnetic resonance imaging. Pediatrics 2006;118(1):47–55.

12. Lavery S, Shah DK, Hunt RW, et al. Single versus bihemispheric amplitude-integrated electroencephalography in relation to cerebral injury and outcome in the term encephalopathic infant. J Paediatr Child Health 2008;44:285–90.
13. Hellström-Westas L, Rosén I, de Vries LS, et al. Amplitude-integrated EEG classification and interpretation in preterm and term infants. Neonatal Review 2006; 7(2):e76–86.
14. Holmes GL, Lombroso CT. Prognostic value of background patterns in the neonatal EEG. J Clin Neurophysiol 1993;10(3):323–52.
15. Menache CC, Bourgeois BF, Volpe JJ. Prognostic value of neonatal discontinuous EEG. Pediatr Neurol 2002;27(2):93–101.
16. Toet MC, Hellström-Westas L, Groenendaal F, et al. Amplitude integrated EEG 3 and 6 hours after birth in full term neonates with hypoxic-ischaemic encephalopathy. Arch Dis Child Fetal Neonatal Ed 1999;81(1):F19–23.
17. Al Naqeeb N, Edwards AD, Cowan F, et al. Assessment of neonatal encephalopathy by amplitude integrated electroencephalography. Pediatrics 1999;103:1263–71.
18. Thornberg E, Ekstrom-Jodal B. Cerebral function monitoring: a method of predicting outcome in term neonates after severe perinatal asphyxia. Acta Paediatr 1994;83(6):596–601.
19. Ter Horst HJ, Sommer C, Bergman KA, et al. Prognostic significance of amplitude-integrated EEG during the first 72 hours after birth in severely asphyxiated neonates. Pediatr Res 2004;55(6):1026–33.
20. Shalak LF, Laptook AR, Velaphi SC, et al. Amplitude-integrated electroencephalography coupled with an early neurologic examination enhances prediction of term infants at risk for persistent encephalopathy. Pediatrics 2003;111(2):351–7.
21. Gluckman PD, Wyatt JS, Azzopardi D, et al. Selective head cooling with mild systemic hypothermia after neonatal encephalopathy: multicentre randomised trial. Lancet 2005;365(9460):663–70.
22. Spitzmiller E, Phillips T, Meinzen-Derr J, et al. Amplitude-integrated EEG is useful in predicting neurodevelopmental outcome in full-term infants with hypoxic-ischaemic encephalopathy: a meta-analysis. J Child Neurol 2007;22(9):1069–78.
23. Toet MC, Flinterman A, Laar I, et al. Cerebral oxygen saturation and electrical brain activity before, during, and up to 36 hours after arterial switch procedure in neonates without pre-existing brain damage: its relationship to neurodevelopmental outcome. Exp Brain Res 2005;165(3):343–50.
24. Pappas A, Shankaran S, Stockmann PT, et al. Changes in amplitude-integrated electroencephalography in neonates treated with extracorporeal membrane oxygenation: a pilot study. J Pediatr 2006;148(1):125–7.
25. Rundgren M, Rosén I, Friberg H. Amplitude-integrated EEG predicts outcome after cardiac arrest and induced hypothermia. Intensive Care Med 2006;32(6):836–42.
26. van Rooij LGM, Toet MC, Osredkar D, et al. Recovery of amplitude integrated electroencephalographic background patterns within 24 hours of perinatal asphyxia. Arch Dis Child Fetal Neonatal Ed 2005;90(3):F245–51.
27. Horan M, Azzopardi D, Edwards D, et al. Lack of influence of mild hypothermia on amplitude integrated-electroencephalography in neonates receiving extracorporeal membrane oxygenation. Early Hum Dev 2007;83:69–75.
28. Róka Anikó, Tamas Melinda Kis, Vásárhelyi Barna, et al. Elevated morphine concentrations in neonates treated with morphine and prolonged hypothermia for hypoxic ischemic encephalopathy. Pediatrics 2008;121:e844–9.
29. Osredkar D, Toet MC, van Rooij LGM, et al. Sleep-wake cycling on amplitude-integrated EEG in full-term newborns with hypoxic-ischemic encephalopathy. Pediatrics 2005;115(2):327–32.

30. Thorngren-Jerneck K, Hellström-Westas L, Ryding E, et al. Cerebral glucose metabolism and early EEG/aEEG in term newborn infants with hypoxic-ischemic encephalopathy. Pediatr Res 2003;54(6):854–60.
31. Filan P, Boylan GB, Chorley G, et al. The relationship between the onset of electrographic seizure activity after birth and time of cerebral injury in utero. BJOB 2004;111:1–4.
32. Hellstrőm-Westas L. Comparison between tape-recorded and amplitude integrated EEG monitoring sick newborn infants. Acta Paediatr Scand 1992;81(10): 812–9.
33. Toet MC, van der Meij W, de Vries LS, et al. Comparison between simultaneously recorded amplitude integrated EEG (cerebral function monitor) and standard EEG in neonates. Pediatrics 2002;109(5):772–9.
34. Murray DM, Boylan GB, Ali I, et al. Defining the gap between electrographic seizure burden, clinical expression, and staff recognition of neonatal seizures. Arch Dis Child Fetal Neonatal Ed 2008;93:F187–91.
35. Shah DK, Mackay MT, Lavery S, et al. The accuracy of bedside EEG monitoring as compared with simultaneous continuous conventional EEG for seizure detection in term infants. Pediatrics 2008;121(6):1146–54.
36. Boylan GB, Rennie JM, Pressler RM, et al. Phenobarbitone, neonatal seizures, and video-EEG. Arch Dis Child Fetal Neonatal Ed 2002;86(3):F165–70.
37. Scher MS, Alvin J, Gaus L, et al. Uncoupling of EEG-clinical neonatal seizures after antiepileptic drug use. Pediatr Neurol 2003;28(4):277–80.
38. van Rooij LGM, de Vries LS, Handryastuti S, et al. Neurodevelopmental outcome in term infants with status epilepticus detected with amplitude-integrated electroencephalography. Pediatrics 2007;120(2):e354–63.
39. Rennie JM, Chorley G, Boylan GB, et al. Non-expert use of the cerebral function monitor for neonatal seizure detection. Arch Dis Child Fetal Neonatal Ed 2004; 89(1):F37–40.
40. Shellhaas RA, Soaita AI, Clancy R, et al. Sensitivity of amplitude-integrated electroencephalography for neonatal seizure detection. Pediatrics 2007;120(4):770–7.
41. Shellhaas RA, Clncy RR. Characterization of neonatal seizures by conventional EEG and single-channel EEG. Clin Neurophysiol 2007;118(10):2156–61.
42. Hagmann CF, Robertson NJ, Azzopardi D. Artifacts on electroencephalograms may influence amplitude-integrated EEG classification: a qualitative analysis in neonatal encephalopathy. Pediatrics 2006;118:2552–4.
43. de Vries NK, ter Horst HJ, Bos AF. The added value of simultaneous EEG and amplitude-integrated EEG recordings in three newborn infants. Neonatology 2007; 91:212–6.
44. Sarkar S, Barks JD, Donn SM. Should amplitude-integrated electroencephalography be used to identify infants suitable for hypothermic neuroprotection? J Perinatol 2008;28(2):117–22.
45. Niemarkt NJ, Halbertsma FJ, Andriessen P, et al. Amplitude-integrated electroencephalographic changes in a newborn induced by overdose of morphine and corrected with naloxone. Acta Paediatr 2008;97:127–34.
46. Painter MJ, Scher MS, Stein AD, et al. Phenobarbital compared with phenytoin for the treatment of neonatal seizures. N Engl J Med 1999;341(7):485–9.
47. Boylan GB, Rennie JM, Chorley G, et al. Second-line anticonvulsant treatment of neonatal seizures. Neurology 2004;62(3):486–8.
48. Hellström-Westas L, Svenningsen NW, Westgren U, et al. Lidocaine for treatment of severe seizures in newborn infants. II. Blood concentrations of lidocaine and metabolites during intravenous infusion. Acta Paediatr 1992;81(10):35–9.

49. Malingre M, van Rooij LGM, Rademaker CM, et al. Development of an optimal lidocaine infusion strategy in neonatal seizures. Eur J Pediatr 2006;165(9):598–604.
50. van Leuven K, Groenendaal F, Toet MC, et al. Midazolam and amplitude integrated EEG in asphyxiated full-term neonates. Acta Paediatr 2004;93(9):1221–7.
51. Hellström-Westas L, Blennow G, Lindroth M, et al. Low risk of seizure recurrence after early withdrawal of anti-epileptic treatment in the neonatal period. Arch Dis Child 1995;72(1):F97–101.
52. Toet MC, Groenendaal F, Osredkar D, et al. Postneonatal epilepsy following amplitude-integrated EEG-detected neonatal seizures. Pediatr Neurol 2005;32(4):241–7.
53. Clancy RR, Legido A. Postnatal epilepsy after EEG-confirmed neonatal seizures. Epilepsia 1991;32(1):69–76.
54. Brunquell PJ, Glennon CS, Dimario FJ, et al. Prediction of outcome based on clinical seizure type in newborn infants. J Pediatr 2002;140(6):707–12.
55. Miller SP, Weiss J, Barnwell A, et al. Seizure-associated brain injury in term newborns with perinatal asphyxia. Neurology 2002;58(4):542–8.
56. Oliveira AJ, Nunes M, Haertel LM, et al. Duration of rhythmic EEG patterns in neonates: new evidence for clinical and prognostic significance of brief rhythmic discharges. Clin Neurophysiol 2000;111(9):1646–53.
57. Bittigau P, Sifringer M, Genz K, et al. Antiepileptic drugs and apoptosis in the developing brain. Proc Natl Acad Sci USA 2002;99(23):15089–94.
58. Barr PA, Buettiker VE, Antony JH. Efficacy of lamotrigine in refractory neonatal seizures. Pediatr Neurol 1999;20(2):161–3.
59. Shoemaker MT, Rotenberg JS. Levetiracetam for the treatment of neonatal seizures. J Child Neurol 2007;22(1):95–8.
60. Freeman JM. The use of amplitude-integrated electroencephalography: beware of its unintended consequences. Pediatrics 2007;119(3):615–7.

Anatomic Changes and Imaging in Assessing Brain Injury in the Term Infant

Russell K. Lawrence, MD[a], Terrie E. Inder, MD[a,b,*]

KEYWORDS

- Term encephalopathy • Neuroimaging • Cerebral injury

Neonatal encephalopathy occurs in from three to five per 1000 live births[1] and presents many challenges to clinicians. Hypoxic-ischemic encephalopathy (HIE), the most common cause (1 per 1000 live births), continues to have significant morbidity and mortality despite advances in neonatal intensive care. As many as 10% to 60% infants die in the newborn period, and up to 25% of survivors go on to develop poor long-term neurodevelopmental outcome. This population accounts for 15% to 28% of children who develop cerebral palsy,[2] often with a more severe form than those who do not have a history of encephalopathy.[3] MRI has proved value in evaluating infants who have perinatal asphyxia.[4,5] The construction of a time frame for a potential injury has critical importance from medical and legal perspectives. Although some references state that only 8% to 15% of term infants who have encephalopathy or seizures have evidence of perinatal asphyxia,[6,7] other sources state that 90% of these infants have evidence by MRI and histology of perinatal acquired injuries.[8] Conventional MRI along with diffusion and spectroscopic MRI provides information on the nature of the injury, clues on the timing, and the later prognosis in term encephalopathic neonates. This article addresses optimization of MRI in newborns along with the common patterns of cerebral injury in asphyxiated term newborns.

WHY UNDERTAKE NEUROIMAGING AND WHICH MODALITY SHOULD BE USED?

History and physical examination are not sufficient to determine the nature and extent of brain injury and have variable prognostic value. Although cranial ultrasound is

[a] Department of Pediatrics, St. Louis Children's Hospital, Washington University, One Children's Place, St. Louis, MO 63110, USA
[b] Department of Neurology and Radiology, Washington University, St. Louis, MO, USA
* Corresponding author. Department of Pediatrics, St. Louis Children's Hospital, Washington University, One Children's Place, St. Louis, MO 63110.
E-mail address: inder_t@kids.wustl.edu (T.E. Inder).

Clin Perinatol 35 (2008) 679–693
doi:10.1016/j.clp.2008.07.013
perinatology.theclinics.com

frequently used in term infants who have encephalopathy, it rarely discloses the true nature of the cerebral pathology. Cranial ultrasound provides poor contrast for lesions of the brain parenchyma. Acute stroke, for example, can be difficult to detect compared with CT and MRI.[9] In addition, because ultrasound images typically are obtained through the anterior fontanel, there is a limited field of view that does not "see" the cerebral convexities where cortical neuronal injury occurs. Furthermore, image detail in the posterior fossa, which is far from the transducer, often is poor.

CT has been available for approximately 30 years and continues to be widely used for term encephalopathic infants because of its speed and ease of acquisition. CT provides excellent views of bone and also is very sensitive for the detection of hemorrhage, which appears bright. It allows differentiation of white and gray matter, although the contrast between these two types of tissue is low in comparison with MRI. CT scans usually require that infants be removed from an ICU, which is a disadvantage compared with cranial ultrasound. Alternatively, the scan time is shorter than that of a typical MRI study. Further, infants are more readily accessible while in a scanner, in the event of an emergency, than for an MRI scan, although there is a trend in MRI magnet design toward more open magnet configurations, which provide better patient access.

A further issue for CT is the exposure of the infant brain to ionizing radiation. There are two main areas of concern related to this exposure—first, the risk for future malignancy and second, cognitive impairment. Recently, Hall and colleagues[10] suggested that even low doses of ionizing radiation, similar to those delivered by CT scans, may affect brain and cognitive development adversely. Currently, it is unclear what long-term effects, if any, low doses of cranial irradiation, such as those delivered during a cranial CT scan, may have when administered during infancy, a phase of rapid brain development. Until such data are available, it is reasonable to restrict the use of this neuroimaging technique to selected settings in which the information obtained from the imaging study is of clear benefit to a patient.

In contrast, there have been no concerns over safety with MRI. MRI provides the best delineation of the pattern of injury and is the strongest predictor of neurodevelopmental outcome in term encephalopathic newborns. Although the American Academy of Neurology recommended the use of MRI as the neuroimaging method of choice for term encephalopathy nearly a decade ago, it has not been universally adopted because of limited availability and access to MRI for sick infants.

HOW TO UNDERTAKE MRI IN A NEWBORN

MRI in encephalopathic newborns is challenging because of the severity of illness and the limited experience by MRI technologists and neuroradiologists. All infants require a thorough search for any metallic objects that would interfere with the magnet. All MRI-compatible monitoring devices are placed before wrapping an infant. These include some form of cardiorespiratory monitoring along with pulse oximetry. MRI-compatible intravenous pumps, ventilators, and incubators are commercially available and may be necessary for critically ill infants.

To maximize signal-to-noise ratio, a dedicated neonatal head coil is ideal, but if not available, an adult knee coil can be used as a substitute. Specialized sequences are essential because of the high water content of the neonatal brain. The majority of centers use a 1-T or 1.5-T magnet, but there is an increasing use of 3-T magnets in clinical research. Used correctly, 3-T magnets can acquire images with shorter acquisition time and greater anatomic resolution.[11,12]

To maximize the study and avoid motion artifact, infants must remain still. An organized approach can avoid wasting time on inadequate images. Feeding and bundling an infant approximately half an hour before the study often results in deep sleep with little movement, avoiding the need for sedation. Equipment, such as vacuum papooses, can be helpful. Because of the noise from certain MRI sequences, ear protection is recommended. The authors use neonatal earmuffs (Natus MiniMuffs, Natus Medical, San Carlos, California), but other options, such as moldable ear putty or shielding with gauze, are acceptable. If these techniques fail to keep an infant still, sedation can be used. Common agents used are midazolam hydrochloride (0.1 mg/kg), lorazepam (0.1 mg/kg), or oral chloral hydrate (30–75 mg/kg).[5,13–15] These medications always should be administered under the watchful eye of a physician experienced in sedating newborns.

THE MAJOR PATTERNS OF BRAIN INJURY IN THE ENCEPHALOPATHIC TERM INFANT

The patterns of injury in term newborns have been delineated on MRI and neuropathology. For MRI, the common classification schemes separate lesions into focal, multifocal, or diffuse injury.[16] This article reviews a neuropathologic classification proposed by Volpe[1] and well visualized on MRI. The injury types discussed include selective neuronal necrosis, parasagittal cerebral injury, periventricular leukomalacia, and, lastly, focal and multifocal ischemic brain necrosis. Although these lesions are discussed as separate discrete entities, overlap is common.

Selective Neuronal Necrosis

After exposure to ischemic injury, there often is necrosis of the neurons in a characteristic, often widespread pattern. This is the most common form of injury in term hypoxic-ischemic infants with common overlap with other patterns of injury. Unlike parasagittal cerebral injury (discussed later), these lesions are not solely from hypotension. The high-energy demand within neurons may account for their selective vulnerability.[17] Four different patterns of neuronal necrosis commonly are seen. These patterns vary depending on the severity and timing of the initial insult.

The first form of selective neuronal necrosis that is seen is that of diffuse neuronal injury affecting the cerebral cortex, basal ganglia, hippocampus, brainstem, and cerebellum (**Fig. 1**). Injury of this magnitude results forms a severe, prolonged perinatal insult, such as total placental abruption, cord prolapse, or some form of vascular interruption. In term infants, the involvement of the cerebrum includes the perirolandic cortex, border zones in the cerebral cortex, the depths of the sulci, the hippocampus, and all regions of deep nuclear gray matter and thalamus. Other areas of involvement include brainstem, cerebellum (most commonly Purkinje's cells), and, less commonly, the anterior horn cells of the spinal cord. Not surprisingly, these diffuse lesions carry a poor prognosis.

The second form of selective neuronal injury is the cerebral–deep nuclear neuronal injury, which combines neuronal damage in the deep nuclear gray matter with injury in the cerebral cortex, usually the parasagittal areas of the perirolandic cortex (**Fig. 2**). Affected areas of the deep nuclear gray matter that are more vulnerable include the putamen and the ventrolateral thalamus. This pattern accounts for 35% to 65% of term infants after hypoxic-ischemic insults.[18–20] Insults are described as a "prolonged, partial insult," meaning that a moderate to severe vascular insult evolved in a more gradual manner. Like diffuse neuronal injury, these lesions carry with them a poor long-term prognosis.

The third form is deep nuclear gray matter–brainstem, which often results from an abrupt-severe insult. This pattern of neuronal injury seems to affect only the deep gray matter without cerebral involvement. Affected areas include the basal ganglia,

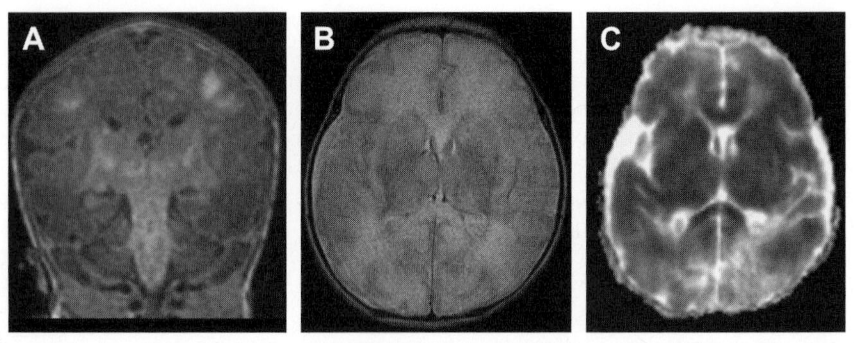

Fig. 1. Diffuse neuronal injury in a term infant who had a history of severe hypoxic-ischemic injury. Images were acquired at 7 days of life. (*A*) Coronal T1W image shows interruption of the posterior limbs bilaterally with diffuse hyperintensities in the watershed regions of the gyri in a parasagittal distribution. In addition, the high signal in the deep nuclear gray matter can be visualized. (*B*) Axial T2W image shows injury throughout the deep nuclear gray matter with diffuse white matter hyperintensity and loss of differentiation between white matter and the cortical ribbon. (*C*) Axial DWI where restricted diffusion from injury (decreased ADC) is represented by dark lesions. This image shows diffuse diffusion restriction in the deep nuclear gray matter, white matter, and cortex bilaterally still apparent at day 7.

the thalamus, and the tegmentum of the brainstem. Only with the increased use of MRI has the frequency of this pattern been appreciated. Long-term prognosis, like the other forms of deep nuclear gray matter injury, is poor, although the severity of the brainstem lesion influences mortality.

The final form of selective neuronal necrosis is pontosubicular necrosis with injury to the neurons of the ventral pons and the subiculum of the hippocampi.[21] Causes of this injury include hypoxia, acute ischemia, hypocapnia, hyperoxemia, and hypoglycemia.[22–25] The least common form of neuronal necrosis in term infants, this pattern is more recognized in premature infants, often associated with periventricular leukomalacia. Recent studies of by Bruck and colleagues[26] indicate that in pontosubicular neuronal cell death is apoptotic in nature on pathologic examination.

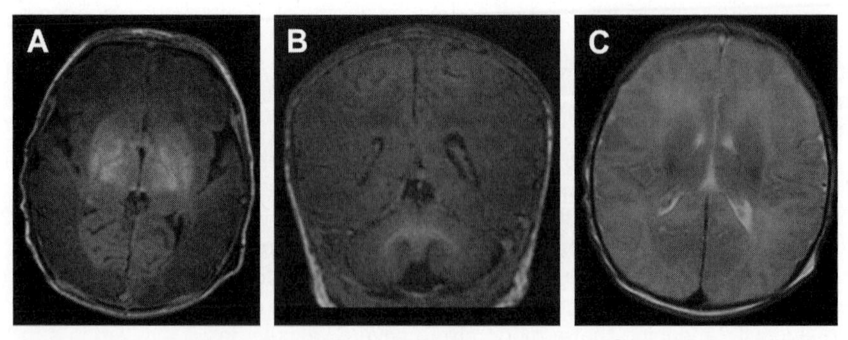

Fig. 2. Deep nuclear gray matter with cortical injury in a term infant who had a history of severe hypoxic-ischemic injury. (*A*) Axial T1W image shows hyperintense severe injury throughout the deep nuclear gray matter. (*B*) Coronal T1W image shows the extension of this hyperintense injury from the deep nuclear gray matter up into the parasagittal region of the cortex. (*C*) Axial T2W image demonstrates low intensity extending from the deep nuclear gray matter into the parasagittal cortex bilaterally.

Parasagittal Cerebral Injury

Parasagittal cerebral injury is unique to term infants, occurring over the cerebral cortex and the underlying subcortical white matter of the parasagittal regions. Parietal-occipital regions are affected most commonly. Injury usually is bilateral in distribution and results from mild to moderate hypotension in this watershed region between the anterior, middle, and posterior cerebral circulation. This lesion is referred to as a "watershed injury" in many MRI publications. The neuropathology is not well established in humans, as most affected infants survive. As isolated lesions, parasagittal cerebral injury in term neonates progresses to mild to moderate neurodevelopmental delay (motor and cognitive). This pattern results in a significantly better prognosis than deep nuclear gray matter injury. In a recent MRI study of 78 term HIE infants, 45% (the largest subgroup) had watershed injury as the predominant pattern and had better neurodevelopmental outcome than those who have deep nuclear gray matter involvement.[27]

Periventricular Leukomalacia

Necrotic damage to the white matter dorsal and lateral to the external angles of the lateral ventricle (PVL) has been well described in premature infants but also is seen (less commonly) in term infants after hypoxic-ischemic injury (**Fig. 3**). Diffuse and cystic PVL, especially in preterm infants, relates to an increased risk for adverse neurodevelopmental outcome.[28]

Ischemic Perinatal Stroke

The incidence of ischemic perinatal stroke ranges from 1 per 2300 to 1 per 5000 live births[29–32] and is recognized as the second most common cause of term

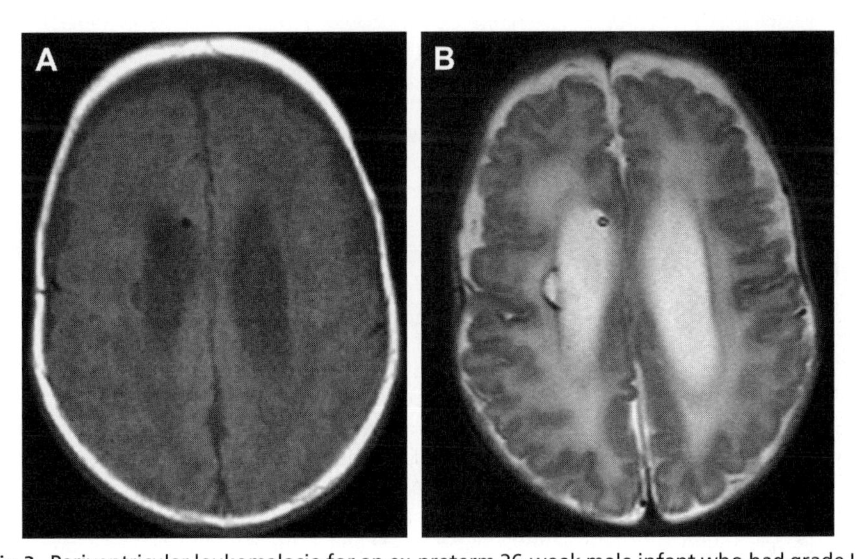

Fig. 3. Periventricular leukomalacia for an ex-preterm 26-week male infant who had grade III intraventricular hemorrhage and post-hemorrhagic hydrocephalus requiring a shunt. Images were acquired at term equivalent. (*A*) Axial T1W image shows a focal cystic hypointensity along the right periventricular region. (*B*) Axial T2W image shows this injury as a hyperintense lesion again along the right periventricular area. Furthermore, there is diffuse hyperintensity of the white matter bilaterally consistent with diffuse and focal periventricular leukomalacia.

encephalopathy. Arterial lesions, usually unilateral, most commonly involve the middle cerebral artery, with the left cerebral hemisphere affected more frequently than the right. Venous thrombosis most commonly affects the superior sagittal sinus.

MRI METHODS

The diagnosis of the nature and timing of cerebral injury in encephalopathic infants requires the optimal application of MRI. In this section the most common MRI modalities, including conventional images (T1-weighted [T1W] and T2-weighted [T2W]), diffusion-weighted imaging (DWI), diffusion tensor imaging, magnetic resonance spectroscopy (MRS), and magnetic resonance angiogram and venogram, are discussed.

Conventional Images

Conventional images include T1W (short repetition and short echo times) and T2W images (long repetition times and long echo times). These sequences offer superiority in differentiating cortical gray matter from cerebral white matter and myelinated from unmyelinated white matter compared with ultrasound and CT. Injury appears hypointense on T1W and hyperintense in T2W in the acute phase, then hyperintense on T1W and hypointense on T2W later within the first week. Although useful in the clinical setting, conventional images alone can overlook damage in the acute phase (<4 days).

Diffusion-Weighted Imaging

DWI measures the random self-diffusion of water through the brain tissue. This self-diffusion of water in tissue is referred to as apparent diffusion; thus, the term, *apparent diffusion coefficient* (*ADC*), the quantitative measure of tissue diffusivity. Brain tissue after ischemic injury experiences a decrease in water diffusion compared with healthy adjacent tissue. After neonatal ischemic brain injury, ADC values can decrease slowly as compared with adult stroke, with up to 30% of infants having normal-appearing DWI in the first 12 to 24 hours (**Fig. 4**).[33] DWI imaging progresses with pseudonormalization of the ADC occurring by 7 to 10 days, a time when injury should be apparent on conventional MRI. Secondary alterations in cerebral regions, such as wallerian degeneration in axonal pathways after a primary neuronal injury, can frame shift these acute changes. For example, restriction in the posterior limb of the internal capsule (PLIC) or corpus callosum may become noticeable on days 6 to 10.[34] Thus, care must be taken in interpretation of the timing of the insult based solely on restriction in ADC but the pattern of restriction should be considered.

Magnetic Resonance Spectroscopy

MRS is based on the ability of the same nuclei in various molecules to demonstrate different resonant frequencies due to different electron densities. The most commonly applied nucleus for this use is the 1H proton. The signal is expressed in parts per million (ppm) and can detect N-acetylasparate (NAA), creatine + phosphocreatine (Cr), choline (Cho), myoinositol, glutamine, glutamate, glucose, taurine, and lactate. NAA (a free amino acid) is present in large quantities in the developing brain in neuronal tissue and developing oligodendrocytes, making it a great indicator of intact central nervous tissue.[35] Several studies have used NAA ratios (NAA/Cr and NAA/Cho) to assess the degree of brain injury in animal models and human infants.[36–38] ^{1}H-MRS also detects this presence of lactate, a doublet peak at 1.3 ppm that is upright at 288 ms echo time and inverted at 144 ms echo time (**Fig. 5**), and is a useful marker for tissue injury.

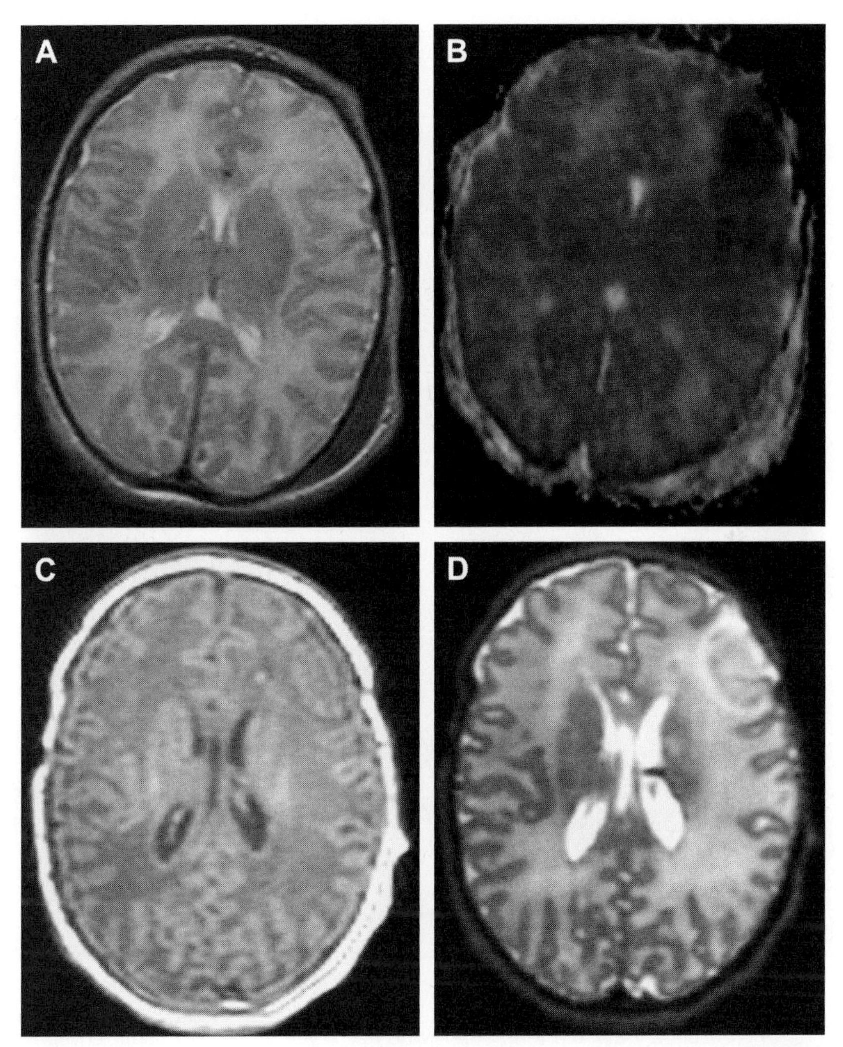

Fig. 4. Left frontal cortical stroke in a term infant who was imaged twice during the first week of life. The first two images (*A, B*) were obtained at 48 to 72 hours of life and images (*C, D*) were done at 7 days of life. Axial T2W image (*A*) shows no obvious cortical injury whereas in the DWI (*B*) there is restricted diffusion over the left frontal cortex. At 7 days, axial T1W (*C*) and T2W (*D*) show evidence of injury to the right frontal cortex.

Magnetic Resonance Angiography/Magnetic Resonance Venography

Magnetic resonance angiography and venography are noninvasive techniques used to delineate arterial and venous supply and topography while avoiding catheterization and contrast administration.[39–41] In newborns, however, there are limitations with small caliber vessels and slow cerebral flow compared with children and adults, making flow voids more frequent.[42] Care in interpretation is critical.

THE CLINICAL INTERPRETATION OF MRI IN THE TERM ENCEPHALOPATHIC INFANT

The aim in undertaking neurologic imaging of sick term infants who have suspected brain injury is to aid the history and examination in answering, What is the nature

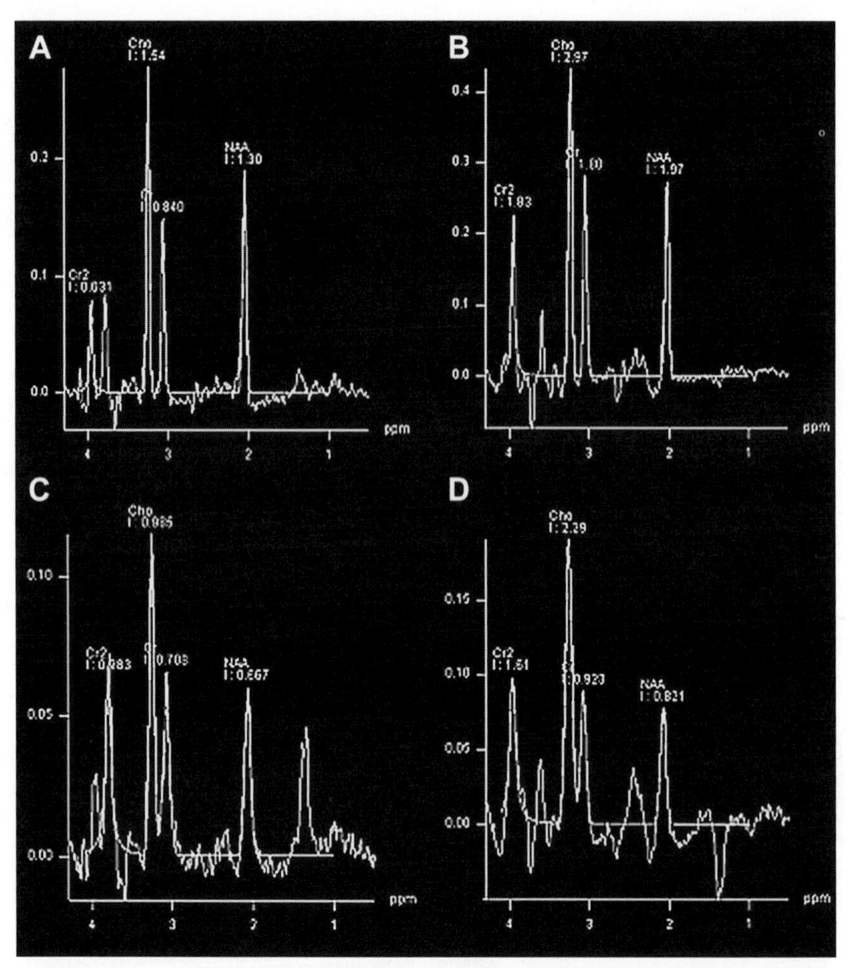

Fig. 5. MRS in two different term infants. The first (*A, B*) are from a term infant who had seizures on day of life 4 without evidence of hypoxic-ischemic encephalopathy. The second data (*C, D*) are from a 1-day-old term infant who had severe hypoxic-ischemic encephalopathy. (*A, B*) Both 288 and 144 echo times show a normal NAA peak without evidence of a lactate doublet peak at 1.3 ppm. (*C*) The 288 echo time shows a decreased NAA peak along with a doublet peak at 1.3 ppm suspicious for lactate. (*D*) The 144 echo time helps confirm the doublet as a lactate peak and not artifact from lipid. Lactate, unlike lipid, inverts downward during the shorter echo time. These (*C, D*) are consistent with severe neuronal injury and poor prognosis.

and extent of brain injury? What was the likely cause of the injury? When did the injury occur? Are there ways to intervene other than supportive care that could have an impact on outcome? and What is the prognosis for the patient? The final section of this review addresses these questions using MRI.

Conventional Imaging

In the first 48 hours after injury there may be no visible changes on conventional MRI. If MRI abnormalities are present at this time, T1W images appear hypointense whereas

T2W images appear hyperintense. The hyperintensity in affected areas on T2W images evolves into hypointensity by 6 to 10 days of life.[16] Acutely affected infants may only demonstrate diffuse edema of the cortical tissue on conventional images. This increase in water content of the brain tissue causes the cortex to become isointense with adjacent white matter, making differentiation of the border between the two tissues difficult. Areas of involvement vary according to the nature and severity of the insult. Mild hypoxic-ischemic injuries commonly involve the bilateral putamen, the ventrolateral nucleus of the thalamus, the parasagittal cortex, and the underlying subcortical white matter overlying the vascular boundary zone. More severe injuries also include diffuse areas of the deep and superficial gray matter along with diffuse white matter involvement. Chronically, this pattern evolves into a picture of multicystic encephalopathy (**Fig. 6**).

An area to pay particular attention to is the PLIC. In images of healthy neonates, the internal capsule appears hyperintense on T1W imaging and hypointense on T2W images compared with adjacent structures. If injured, the PLIC appears hypointense on T1 images relative to the thalamus and putamen by 5 days after injury. Abnormal signal intensity in the posterior limb is a powerful prognostic indicator for poor neurodevelopmental outcome,[15] correctly predicting outcome in 92% of infants who have stage II HIE.[5]

The pattern of injury on conventional imaging carries important prognostic value. Several studies have divided patterns of injury into watershed predominant or deep nuclear gray matter predominant with long-term follow-up. Deep nuclear gray matter (basal ganglia or thalamus) predominance is associated with more intensive need for resuscitation, more severe encephalopathy, increased seizure burden, and worse neurodevelopmental outcome as far out as 5 years of age.[19,27,43]

Conventional images provide a robust measure of the nature and severity of injury when done after a week from the initial insult, correlating well with neurodevelopmental outcome.[4,5,15,44] Conventional MRI in the first 4 days often is limited, however, in delineating injury.

Diffusion-Weighted Imaging/Diffusion Tensor Imaging

In contrast to conventional MRI, diffusion imaging is sensitive to acute cerebral injury. By 2 to 3 days, restriction in the ADC is clearly visible with brain injury, although it may

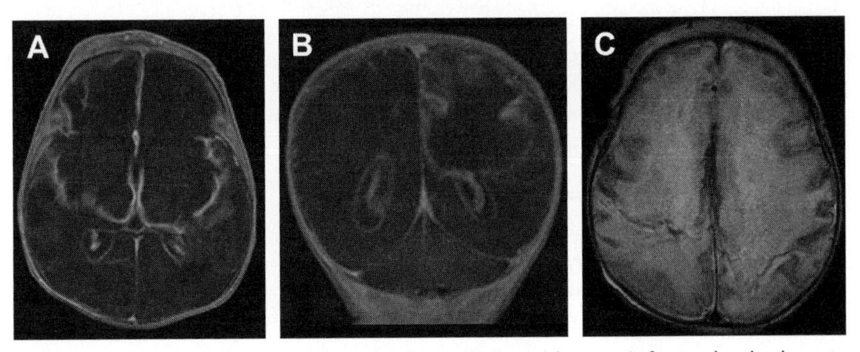

Fig. 6. Severe multicystic encephalopathy in a 12-day-old term infant who had proteus meningitis. The first group of images (*A, B*) are T1W axial (*A*) and coronal (*B*) images showing severe white and gray matter loss in the frontal, parietal, and temporal lobes. This tissue loss is replaced largely by fluid. (*C*) T2W axial image also shows diffuse injury with necrosis of white and gray matter.

underestimate the full extent[13] or be difficult to visualize with moderate injury.[14] The evolution in diffusion over time in HIE infants has been described with basal ganglia injury in the early postnatal period.[45] In the first 12 to 24 hours there may be no visible changes in diffusion imaging.[33] The pattern of the early predominance of the ventrolateral nucleus of the thalami (first 48 hours) becomes more evident in the putamen, corticospinal tracts, and the perirolandic cortex by 3 to 5 days of life. Subcortical white matter and white matter pathways, such as the corpus callosum and the cingulum, show involvement by 6 to 7 days after injury. Clues to the timing and extent of brain injury, therefore, can be elucidated by DWI within the first 4 days of life. Although changes in diffusion can be detected as early as 6 hours after injury, the most significant change in diffusion occurs between 2 to 4 days after the insult.[33,46] These changes in diffusion correlate not only with later conventional imaging but also with neurodevelopmental outcome.[47] If DWI shows involvement of the PLIC with an ADC of 0.74 or less, poor neurodevelopmental outcome is highly likely.[48] The presence of wallerian degeneration in the PLIC on DWI also is a strong predictor for hemiplegia.[49]

Measuring anisotropy (relative anisotropy or fractional anisotropy [FA]) with diffusion tensor imaging gives additional information. Anisotropy decreases with severe and moderate white matter and deep nuclear gray matter injury during the first week of life, whereas ADC decreases only with severe injury. Anisotropy (FA) values continue to decrease during the second week of life and do not undergo pseudonormalization like ADC values. Thus, the pairing of FA values with ADC can add information on severity and timing of injury. In a mild and moderate HIE population, FA correlated with short-term neurodevelopmental outcome.[50]

Magnetic Resonance Spectroscopy

The in vivo assessment of metabolites was first described in neonates by Groendaal and colleagues, who observed higher lactate and lower NAA values in the basal ganglia in infants with poor outcome at 3 months after postasphyxial encephalopathy.[36] Since this observation, studies have looked at metabolite ratios (lactate/Cho, lactate/Cr, NAA/Cho) and absolute levels (lactate and NAA) and correlated them with outcome. The abnormal rise in lactate and fall in NAA are most significant within the first week after injury, with lactate detected within 24 hours after injury whereas NAA starts to decrease after 48 hours.[38,45] An elevated lactate/Cho ratio has been shown to be most predictive for neurodevelopmental outcome.[51–57] These metabolite levels can remain abnormal for long periods of time. Elevated lactate levels are seen for months after injury, thus do not indicate acute injury. Persistence of lactate signifies a worse prognosis.[53] When MRS of the basal ganglia and parasagittal cortex (watershed area) has been compared with DWI in the acute postnatal period, MRS appeared superior in predicting poor outcome.[58]

Putting it all Together

Modern MRI techniques offer ways to answer the fundamental questions on etiology, timing, and prognosis in term encephalopathic infants. The information garnered from an MRI always must be placed into the context of the clinical picture of the infant. The combination of imaging done at approximately 48 hours, followed by a second scan between 7 and 10 days, seems to offer the most robust amount of information. For example, an acute perinatal injury may reveal no injury on conventional images on the first scan but show obvious changes on diffusion, anisotropy, or abnormalities on spectroscopy. A second scan then would confirm the injury with visible changes on conventional images by days 7 to 10. Alternatively, if an early scan at 2 days demonstrates clear changes on conventional imaging, this may indicate that the initial injury occurred in utero. Spectroscopy and diffusion images can help support or contradict this assumption based on their appearance. If ADC values on the first MRI scan in the primary area of involvement already have begun to pseudonormalize or increase in value, this supports that the injury occurred greater than 5 days ago. Anisotropy measures, as discussed previously, remain decreased for a longer period of time than diffusion and are more sensitive to moderate injury. Caution should be taken when attempting to interpret scans done between 4 and 5 days of age. If an injury is perinatal, diffusion changes may be commencing pseudonormalization, whereas the conventional imaging may not yet display clear changes. This "normal" scan can lead to false reassurance for families and physicians.

Causes may be teased out once the pattern and the timing of the initial insult are established. Combining this observation with the clinical history provides clues to possible mechanisms. For example, the pattern of diffuse neuronal injury with acute diffuse abnormalities on day 2 along with elevated lactate (MRS) and minimal conventional changes is consistent with an acute perinatal event, such as placental abruption, cord prolapse, or maternal shock. Such sentinel acute perinatal events occur in fewer than 25% of term encephalopathic infants (Vermont Oxford Network Encephalopathy Registry, J. Horbar, personal communication, June 2008). In contrast, a pattern of abnormal T1/T2 imaging with less pronounced diffusion findings and reduced NAA (MRS) on day 2 may be found with a history of intrauterine growth restriction or maternal diabetes, suggesting a much earlier timing that labor/delivery with fetal vulnerability. Again, there can be overlap with chronic and acute changes co-existing.

Interventions that can alter the course of hypoxic-ischemic injury in neonates mainly are still hypothetical and not yet fully integrated into clinical practice. One exception is hypothermia (systemic or selective head cooling), which is gaining acceptance among the neonatal community. Several large prospective randomized studies have shown promising results.[59,60] How hypothermia affects pattern, severity, and evolution of injury by MRI are not yet well established. Preliminary observations, all on small groups of infants, have found that mild hypothermia reduced the severity of basal ganglia, thalamic, and cortical lesions, likely mirroring improved clinical outcome on neurodevelopmental follow-up.[61–63] Concern has been raised about the potential of hypothermia to alter the extent and timing of injury but more systematic data are required.

The capacity of MRI to aid in prognosis based on the pattern of injury is well established. Although conventional imaging, spectroscopy, DWI, and diffusion tensor imaging have all shown prognostic value on their own, using them in combination holds the most potential.[64] Injury documented by conventional changes or abnormalities of diffusion or spectroscopy, involving the deep nuclear gray matter, carries a poor prognosis.[4,19,20,27,51,58,65] Most significant of the structures in the deep nuclear gray matter is the internal capsule, carrying crucial motor and sensory pathways from the cortex to the spinal cord and thalamus. Injury involving the white matter without deep nuclear gray matter or cerebral involvement has an overall more favorable prognosis. Focal and diffuse white matter injury in the absence of gray matter involvement, however, predicts long-term morbidity, many times presenting in the early school years as learning and behavioral issues.[43] Stage I-II HIE often presents with normal conventional imaging and only with measures of diffusion and anisotropy can these abnormalities of white matter be detected.[50] More data on long-term neurodevelopmental outcomes in school age from milder forms of injury are required.

SUMMARY

MRI offers a powerful tool in assessing encephalopathic term infants. Understanding the classical patterns of brain injury and the clinical scenarios can aid physicians in interpretation of the imaging findings for answering crucial questions, such as timing, possible cause, and long-term prognosis of infants. Finally, as future neuroprotective strategies become standard of care in the neonatal intensive care, MRI will provide a powerful tool for evaluating the impact of such interventions.

REFERENCES

1. Volpe J, editor. Neurology of the newborn. 4th edition. Philadelphia: Saunders; 2001.
2. Himmelmann K, Hagberg G, Beckung E, et al. The changing panorama of cerebral palsy in Sweden. IX. Prevalence and origin in the birth-year period 1995–1998. Acta Paediatr 2005;94(3):287–94.
3. Gaffney G, Flavell V, Johnson A, et al. Cerebral palsy and neonatal encephalopathy. Arch Dis Child Fetal Neonatal Ed 1994;70(3):F195–200.
4. Biagioni E, Mercuri E, Rutherford M, et al. Combined use of electroencephalogram and magnetic resonance imaging in full-term neonates with acute encephalopathy. Pediatrics 2001;107(3):461–8 [see comment].
5. Rutherford MA, Pennock JM, Counsell SR, et al. Abnormal magnetic resonance signal in the internal capsule predicts poor neurodevelopmental outcome in infants with hypoxic-ischemic encephalopahty. Pediatrics 1998;102(2):323–8.
6. Nelson KB, Leviton A. How much of neonatal encephalopathy is due to birth asphyxia? Am J Dis Child 1991;145(11):1325–31.
7. Blair E, Stanley FJ. Intrapartum asphyxia: a rare cause of cerebral palsy. J Pediatr 1988;112(4):515–9 [see comment] [erratum appears in J Pediatr 1988 Aug;113(2):420].
8. Cowan F, Rutherford M, Groenendaal F, et al. Origin and timing of brain lesions in term infants with neonatal encephalopathy. Lancet 2003;361(9359):736–42 [see comment].
9. Golomb MR, Dick PT, MacGregor DL, et al. Cranial ultrasonography has a low sensitivity for detecting arterial ischemic stroke in term neonates. J Child Neurol 2003;18(2):98–103.
10. Hall P, Adami HO, Trichopoulos D, et al. Effect of low doses of ionising radiation in infancy on cognitive function in adulthood: Swedish population based cohort study. BMJ 2004;328(7430):19.
11. Schmitt F, Grosu D, Mohr C, et al. [3 Tesla MRI: successful results with higher field strengths]. Radiologe 2004;44(1):31–47 [in German].
12. Frayne R, Goodyear BG, Dickhoff P, et al. Magnetic resonance imaging at 3.0 Tesla: challenges and advantages in clinical neurological imaging. Invest Radiol 2003;38(7):385–402.
13. Robertson RL, Ben-Sira L, Barnes PD, et al. MR line-scan diffusion-weighted imaging of term neonates with perinatal brain ischemia. AJNR Am J Neuroradiol 1999;20(9):1658–70 [see comment].
14. Rutherford M, Counsell S, Allsop J, et al. Diffusion-weighted magnetic resonance imaging in term perinatal brain injury: a comparison with site of lesion and time from birth. Pediatrics 2004;114(4):1004–14.
15. Jyoti R, O'Neil R, Jyoti R, et al. Predicting outcome in term neonates with hypoxic-ischaemic encephalopathy using simplified MR criteria. Pediatr Radiol 2006; 36(1):38–42.

16. Triulzi F, Parazzini C, Righini A, et al. Patterns of damage in the mature neonatal brain. Pediatr Radiol 2006;36(7):608–20.
17. Chugani HT, Phelps ME, Mazziotta JC. Positron emission tomography study of human brain functional development. Ann Neurol 1987;22(4):487–97.
18. Martin E, Barkovich AJ. Magnetic resonance imaging in perinatal asphyxia. Arch Dis Child Fetal Neonatal Ed 1995;72(1):F62–70.
19. Kuenzle C, Baenziger O, Martin E, et al. Prognostic value of early MR imaging in term infants with severe perinatal asphyxia. Neuropediatrics 1994;25(4): 191–200.
20. Rutherford M, Pennock J, Schwieso J, et al. Hypoxic-ischaemic encephalopathy: early and late magnetic resonance imaging findings in relation to outcome. Arch Dis Child Fetal Neonatal Ed 1996;75(3):F145–51 [see comment].
21. Friede R, editor. Developmental nuropathology. 2nd edition. Berlin: Springer Verlag; 1989.
22. Mito T, Kamei A, Takashima S, et al. Clinicopathological study of pontosubicular necrosis. Neuropediatrics 1993;24(4):204–7.
23. Friede RL. Ponto-subicular lesions in perinatal anoxia. Arch Pathol Lab Med 1972; 94(4):343–54.
24. Hashimoto K, Takeuchi Y, Takashima S. Hypocarbia as a pathogenic factor in pontosubicular necrosis. Brain Dev 1991;13(3):155–7.
25. Ahdab-Barmada M, Moossy J, Painter M. Pontosubicular necrosis and hyperoxemia. Pediatrics 1980;66(6):840–7.
26. Bruck Y, Bruck W, Kretzschmar HA, et al. Evidence for neuronal apoptosis in pontosubicular neuron necrosis. Neuropathol Appl Neurobiol 1996;22(1):23–9.
27. Miller SP, Ramaswamy V, Michelson D, et al. Patterns of brain injury in term neonatal encephalopathy. J Pediatr 2005;146(4):453–60.
28. Woodward LJ, Anderson PJ, Austin NC, et al. Neonatal MRI to predict neurodevelopmental outcomes in preterm infants. N Engl J Med 2006;355(7):685–94.
29. Schulzke S, Weber P, Luetschg J, et al. Incidence and diagnosis of unilateral arterial cerebral infarction in newborn infants. J Perinat Med 2005;33(2):170–5.
30. Lynch JK, Hirtz DG, DeVeber G, et al. Report of the national institute of neurological disorders and stroke workshop on perinatal and childhood stroke. Pediatrics 2002;109(1):116–23.
31. Hunt RW, Inder TE. Perinatal and neonatal ischaemic stroke: a review. Thromb Res 2006;118(1):39–48.
32. Nelson KB, Lynch JK. Stroke in newborn infants. Lancet Neurol 2004;3(3):150–8.
33. McKinstry RC, Miller JH, Snyder AZ, et al. A prospective, longitudinal diffusion tensor imaging study of brain injury in newborns. Neurology 2002;59(6):824–33 [see comment].
34. Neil JJ, Inder TE. Detection of wallerian degeneration in a newborn by diffusion magnetic resonance imaging (MRI). J Child Neurol 2006;21(2):115–8.
35. Bhakoo KK, Pearce D. In vitro expression of N-acetyl aspartate by oligodendrocytes: implications for proton magnetic resonance spectroscopy signal in vivo. J Neurochem 2000;74(1):254–62.
36. Groenendaal F, Veenhoven RH, van der Grond J, et al. Cerebral lactate and N-acetyl-aspartate/choline ratios in asphyxiated full-term neonates demonstrated in vivo using proton magnetic resonance spectroscopy. Pediatr Res 1994;35(2): 148–51.
37. Penrice J, Lorek A, Cady EB, et al. Proton magnetic resonance spectroscopy of the brain during acute hypoxia-ischemia and delayed cerebral energy failure in the newborn piglet. Pediatr Res 1997;41(6):795–802.

38. Barkovich AJ, Baranski K, Vigneron D, et al. Proton MR spectroscopy for the evaluation of brain injury in asphyxiated, term neonates. AJNR Am J Neuroradiol 1999;20(8):1399–405.
39. Koelfen W, Wentz U, Freund M, et al. Magnetic resonance angiography in 140 neuropediatric patients. Pediatr Neurol 1995;12(1):31–8.
40. Koelfen W, Freund M, Konig S, et al. Results of parenchymal and angiographic magnetic resonance imaging and neuropsychological testing of children after stroke as neonates. Eur J Pediatr 1993;152(12):1030–5.
41. Ayanzen RH, Bird CR, Keller PJ, et al. Cerebral MR venography: normal anatomy and potential diagnostic pitfalls. AJNR Am J Neuroradiol 2000;21(1):74–8.
42. Widjaja E, Shroff M, Blaser S, et al. 2D time-of-flight MR venography in neonates: anatomy and pitfalls. AJNR Am J Neuroradiol 2006;27(9):1913–8.
43. Barnett A, Mercuri E, Rutherford M, et al. Neurological and perceptual-motor outcome at 5-6 years of age in children with neonatal encephalopathy: relationship with neonatal brain MRI. Neuropediatrics 2002;33(5):242–8.
44. Barkovich AJ, Hajnal BL, Vigneron D, et al. Prediction of neuromotor outcome in perinatal asphyxia: evaluation of MR scoring systems. AJNR Am J Neuroradiol 1998;19(1):143–9.
45. Barkovich AJ, Miller SP, Bartha A, et al. MR imaging, MR spectroscopy, and diffusion tensor imaging of sequential studies in neonates with encephalopathy. AJNR Am J Neuroradiol 2006;27(3):533–47.
46. Soul JS, Robertson RL, Tzika AA, et al. Time course of changes in diffusion-weighted magnetic resonance imaging in a case of neonatal encephalopathy with defined onset and duration of hypoxic-ischemic insult. Pediatrics 2001; 108(5):1211–4.
47. Johnson AJ, Lee BC, Lin W. Echoplanar diffusion-weighted imaging in neonates and infants with suspected hypoxic-ischemic injury: correlation with patient outcome. AJR Am J Roentgenol 1999;172(1):219–26.
48. Hunt RW, Neil JJ, Coleman LT, et al. Apparent diffusion coefficient in the posterior limb of the internal capsule predicts outcome after perinatal asphyxia. Pediatrics 2004;114(4):999–1003.
49. De Vries LS, Van der Grond J, Van Haastert IC, et al. Prediction of outcome in new-born infants with arterial ischaemic stroke using diffusion-weighted magnetic resonance imaging. Neuropediatrics 2005;36(1):12–20.
50. Malik GK, Trivedi R, Gupta RK, et al. Serial quantitative diffusion tensor MRI of the term neonates with hypoxic-ischemic encephalopathy (HIE). Neuropediatrics 2006;37(6):337–43.
51. Boichot C, Walker PM, Durand C, et al. Term neonate prognoses after perinatal asphyxia: contributions of MR imaging, MR spectroscopy, relaxation times, and apparent diffusion coefficients. Radiology 2006;239(3):839–48.
52. Miller SP, Newton N, Ferriero DM, et al. Predictors of 30-month outcome after perinatal depression: role of proton MRS and socioeconomic factors. Pediatr Res 2002;52(1):71–7.
53. Hanrahan JD, Cox IJ, Edwards AD, et al. Persistent increases in cerebral lactate concentration after birth asphyxia. Pediatr Res 1998;44(3):304–11.
54. Hanrahan JD, Cox IJ, Azzopardi D, et al. Relation between proton magnetic resonance spectroscopy within 18 hours of birth asphyxia and neurodevelopment at 1 year of age. Dev Med Child Neurol 1999;41(2):76–82.
55. Malik GK, Pandey M, Kumar R, et al. MR imaging and in vivo proton spectroscopy of the brain in neonates with hypoxic ischemic encephalopathy. Eur J Radiol 2002;43(1):6–13.

56. Amess PN, Penrice J, Wylezinska M, et al. Early brain proton magnetic resonance spectroscopy and neonatal neurology related to neurodevelopmental outcome at 1 year in term infants after presumed hypoxic-ischaemic brain injury. Dev Med Child Neurol 1999;41(7):436–45.
57. Kadri M, Shu S, Holshouser B, et al. Proton magnetic resonance spectroscopy improves outcome prediction in perinatal CNS insults. J Perinatol 2003;23(3): 181–5.
58. Zarifi MK, Astrakas LG, Poussaint TY, et al. Prediction of adverse outcome with cerebral lactate level and apparent diffusion coefficient in infants with perinatal asphyxia. Radiology 2002;225(3):859–70.
59. Gluckman PD, Wyatt JS, Azzopardi D, et al. Selective head cooling with mild systemic hypothermia after neonatal encephalopahty: multicentre randomised trial. Lancet 2005;365:663–70.
60. Shankaran S, Laptook AR, Ehrenkranz RA, et al. Whole-body hypothermia for neonates with hypoxic-ischemic encephalopathy. N Engl J Med 2005;353(15): 1574–84.
61. Inder TE, Hunt RW, Morley CJ, et al. Randomized trial of systemic hypothermia selectively protects the cortex on MRI in term hypoxic-ischemic encephalopathy. J Pediatr 2004;145(6):835–7.
62. Rutherford MA, Azzopardi D, Whitelaw A, et al. Mild hypothermia and the distribution of cerebral lesions in neonates with hypoxic-ischemic encephalopathy. Pediatrics 2005;116(4):1001–6.
63. Compagnoni G, Pogliani L, Lista G, et al. Hypothermia reduces neurological damage in asphyxiated newborn infants. Biol Neonate 2002;82(4):222–7.
64. L'Abee C, de Vries LS, van der Grond J, et al. Early diffusion-weighted MRI and H-Magnetic resonance spectroscopy in asphyxiated full-term neonates. Biol Neonate 2005;88:306–12.
65. Mercuri E, Rutherford M, Cowan F, et al. Early prognostic indicators of outcome in infants with neonatal cerebral infarction: a clinical, electroencephalogram, and magnetic resonance imaging study. Pediatrics 1999;103:39–46.

Proteomics- and Metabolomics-Based Neonatal Diagnostics in Assessing and Managing the Critically Ill Neonate

Alan R. Spitzer, MD*, Donald Chace, PhD, MSFS

KEYWORDS

• Proteomics • Metabolomics • Neonate • Diagnosis

Mass spectrometry (MS) has occupied an increasingly prominent place in clinical chemistry and laboratory diagnostics during the past few decades.[1] The value of MS has traditionally resided in its ability to measure the mass of bioactive metabolites (e.g., amino acids, fatty acids, organic acids, steroids, lipids, neurotransmitters) in a selective, accurate, and comprehensive manner. Although it continues to be used for the diagnosis of metabolic abnormalities, especially organic acids or acylcarnitines in blood and plasma, we have now entered a new era in which the diagnostic capability of MS is being extended to metabolic processes during active disease states. The examination of rapidly changing proteins, amino acids, and other metabolites during acute disease marks a significant shift in the utility of MS analysis of the blood or other fluids. Furthermore, as this type of analysis continues to emerge, the traditional experts in this field, namely, the metabolic disease specialists, are now being supplemented by individuals from a variety of specialties who have an interest in the various metabolic biomarkers that may be expressed during active clinical conditions. Many of these unique metabolites, often initially analyzed by systems that use some type of physical separation technique, such as gas chromatography (GC) or liquid chromatography (LC) with nonspecific detection (ultraviolet [UV] spectrometry), are now being studied by a more specific and "universal detector," MS. MS increases the number and scope of metabolites detected while concurrently improving the characterization and quantification of metabolites. With more metabolites measured accurately and specifically, often with smaller sample sizes, it is possible to understand the

---

The Center for Research and Education, Pediatrix Medical Group and Pediatrix Analytical Laboratory, 1301 Concord Terrace, Sunrise, FL 33323, USA
* Corresponding author.
E-mail address: alan_spitzer@pediatrix.com (A.R. Spitzer).

Clin Perinatol 35 (2008) 695–716
doi:10.1016/j.clp.2008.07.019 perinatology.theclinics.com

evolution of a disease better. Ideally, as the sciences of proteomics and metabolomics continue to grow, detection of disease markers before the onset of a disease state may become increasingly feasible and an essential component of the practice of medicine. The detection of markers before their secretion reaches a concentration sufficient to disrupt metabolism and result in disease may theoretically, at least, lend itself to new and exciting approaches in preventive medicine.

During the past 2 decades, the pharmaceutical industry, in an attempt to screen more rapidly for therapeutic efficacy, changed its approach to the discovery of new therapeutic agents from a targeted molecular modeling approach to a broader survey of thousands of candidate compounds. The goal of this change was to find a single drug that might exert the desired pharmaceutic effect with a higher margin of safety. The mass spectrometer became a critical tool in this screening process, and the increasing demand of the pharmaceutical companies led to the development of new mass measuring devices that could analyze polar compounds and higher molecular-weight compounds more quickly, more accurately, and in larger numbers. The result of these efforts was the interface of liquid chromatography with MS for polar or large molecules, such as peptides and proteins. The two techniques most often recognized in this field are actually ionization techniques, electrospray ionization (ESI) and matrix-assisted laser desorption ionization (MALDI), which enabled metabolite and protein analysis for the largest variety of compounds possible. The inherent value of this technology can be seen from the Nobel Prizes in chemistry that were awarded recently to two mass spectrometrists for their work in this area (Nobel Prize for Medicine 2003: P.C. Lauterbur and P. Mansfield).

The importance of describing the history of MS in medicine is that it clearly points toward potential future applications. For example, one of the major goals of the pharmaceutical industry is to screen potential aberrations in drug metabolism during a clinical trial. The identification of patients who might have an adverse reaction to a particular drug because of a genetic variation in metabolism could improve the efficacy and safety of a medication. Alternatively, alteration of drug-dosing strategies because of metabolic abnormality seems likely in the near future and may soon herald the age of an approach to medical treatment that is uniquely patient specific (therapeutic tailoring of care). These approaches would represent a major shift in current concepts of medical management, which are now based on the overall general response of the totality of treated patients to a pharmacologic agent.

In the areas of genetics and metabolism, one could also argue that the basic substances of metabolism (e.g., carbohydrates, amino acids, fatty acids) are subject to similar considerations, in that their metabolism can be affected if there is an abnormality of enzyme function. In fact, this approach has been used for decades with organic acid analysis. Basic organic acid analysis was not designed as a population screening tool (testing designed for large numbers of routine tests), however, and it was not indicated for the relatively simple analysis of blood or plasma for metabolites (biomarkers) in unusually high concentrations. Further, questions began to be asked whether certain of these biomarkers might be present before a disease became manifest or could predict whether a patient actually had a specific metabolic alteration of consequence (or, in the pharmaceutic model, would have an adverse event if given a particular drug).

EXPANDED NEWBORN SCREENING

In the late 1980s and early 1990s, it was recognized that carnitine and its fatty acid esters were important in mitochondrial metabolism, specifically β-oxidation.[2]

Furthermore, the presence or absence of these biomarkers seemed to be useful in detecting diseases of fatty acid or organic acid metabolism. Carnitine is a highly polar ionic molecule that can form esters with fatty acids called acylcarnitines. Carnitine and fatty acylcarnitine were not easily analyzed by the GC/MS techniques, even with extensive and complex sample preparation techniques. Newer techniques of MS with their interfaces for unstable and water-soluble compounds, however, led to the development of methods that could readily detect these compounds. Information gathered from the analytic capability of detecting carnitine and acylcarnitine led to further research into the importance of such biomarkers and their utility in detecting inherited disease in the newborn.[3] A specific type of mass spectrometer, a tandem mass spectrometer (tandem MS or MS/MS), was found to be especially useful in that it could selectively detect and quantify many metabolites within a family of compounds, such as acylcarnitines and α-amino acids without the use of time-consuming chromatography. Furthermore, the analysis could be done from the extracts of small quantities of blood and plasma, including dried spots on cards of filter paper. This method, pioneered in the early 1990s, has undergone such substantial improvements in the area of sample preparation, data processing, and result interpretation that it is now considered a standard clinical tool in neonatal metabolic screening and metabolic disease assessment.

In addition to the analysis of amino acids and acylcarnitines, tandem MS can be used to detect and evaluate the presence of many classes of metabolites, including steroids, bile acids, nucleic acids, fatty acids, and lipids.[4–8] Some of these techniques require a chromatographic step, extensive sample purification, or both, and are therefore better suited for diagnostic testing and confirmation than for screening. There are rapid developments on the horizon, however, for new sample preparation systems, and mass spectrometers may be better suited for general population screening in these areas in the near future. It is also worth noting that of the thousands of potential metabolites that can be analyzed from blood, only a few are compounds that correlate with inherited metabolic disease. The addition of one or two biomarkers to the screening process for a single disease that also requires a separate MS assay may be cost-prohibitive if the disease is rare. The model of screening for rare disorders used the concepts of metabolic panels to pick up dozens of diseases. This model is likely to remain in place for screening noninherited disease biomarkers in the future as well if cost considerations and efficiency remain important.

MASS SPECTROMETRY PRIMER

MS is a tool, and like any tool, it is important to understand how it is used and what results can be expected. Most simply stated, MS measures the mass of an "electrically" charged molecule known as an ion. It can detect ionized molecules ranging in size from mass values less than water (mass = 18) to greater than the mass of hemoglobin (mass = 66,980 g/mol). Charged molecules that have not been fragmented (and reflect the native compound) are known as molecular ions or precursor ions. Portions of molecules that have been fragmented are known as fragment ions or product ions. In a mass spectrometric analysis, results may include the mass-to-charge (m/z) values of molecular ions, fragment ions, or both. It is important to note that the mass spectrometer displays the m/z value rather than mass. For metabolites and small molecules, z is usually 1 such that m/z is equal to m. For proteins, however, multiple charging occurs. The m/z values displayed represent this ratio (and this is one reason why the analysis of a protein of 100,000 d can be detected on a mass spectrometer with a mass range of 3000 d; 100 charges produce an m/z value of 1000). Results produced by a mass spectrometer include the mass of the ion and charge (m/z) and the number of these ions. Often, these data are displayed in a chart or graph called a mass spectrum (**Figs. 1** and **2**). The mass spectrum shows the mass value (along the x-axis) and its quantity (along the y-axis), often as bars or vertical lines. Typically, these data are simply represented in a database or spreadsheet format without the spectrum, or they are processed in such a way as to produce a quantitative number (concentration). Most simply stated, from the most common clinical chemistry perspective, what is important is the identification of a compound and its fragments (their presence at particular masses) and its concentration (how much of that compound is present). In certain cases, it is necessary to perform chromatography, which can improve the selectivity and accuracy of an MS analysis.

PROTEOMIC/METABOLOMIC MEDICINE IN CLINICAL CARE

The recent expansion of newborn screening provides clues to the utility of MS in the newer applications of metabolomics and represents a model for future applications of screening in a variety of diseases that affect neonates and adults. These diseases or metabolic abnormalities may result from one or a combination of factors in the areas of genetics, the environment, and nutrition. MS has changed the clinical chemistry/screening model from a single metabolite (single disease detection approach on a relatively large volume of blood) to a multiple metabolite (multiple disease evaluation or panel on a much smaller sample of blood, often just a filter paper spot). In this case, a newborn screening panel might include measurement of several amino acids and

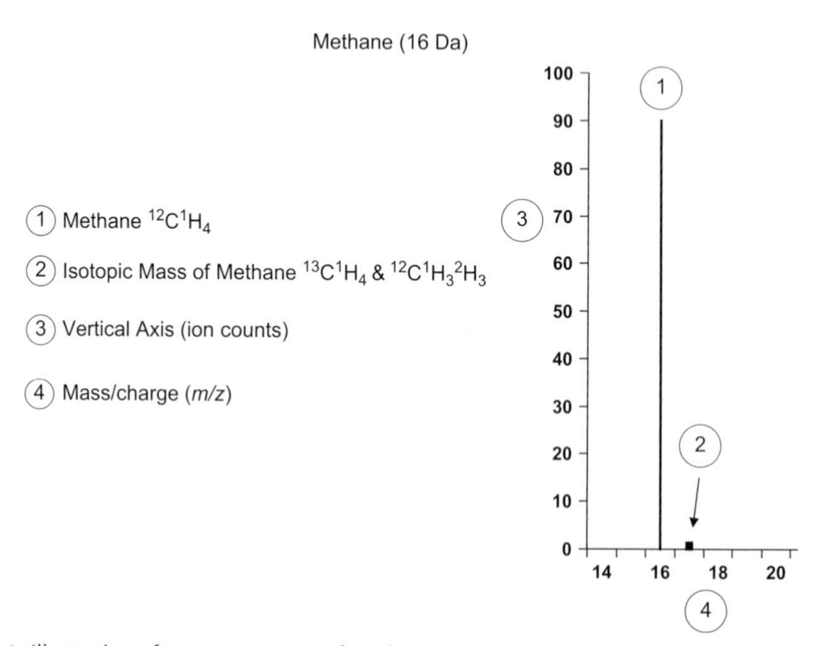

Fig. 1. Illustration of a mass spectrum of methane that would be obtained from electron ionization. The x-axis is mass-to-charge ratio (m/z for mass identification), and the y-axis is ion counts (for mass quantification). The monoisotopic mass of methane is 16 d and is the major peak in the spectrum. It is positioned at m/z 16, because the charge is 1. The natural isotopic contributions of a single carbon-13 or deuterium would be approximately 1.2%; therefore, a peak occurs at m/z 17.

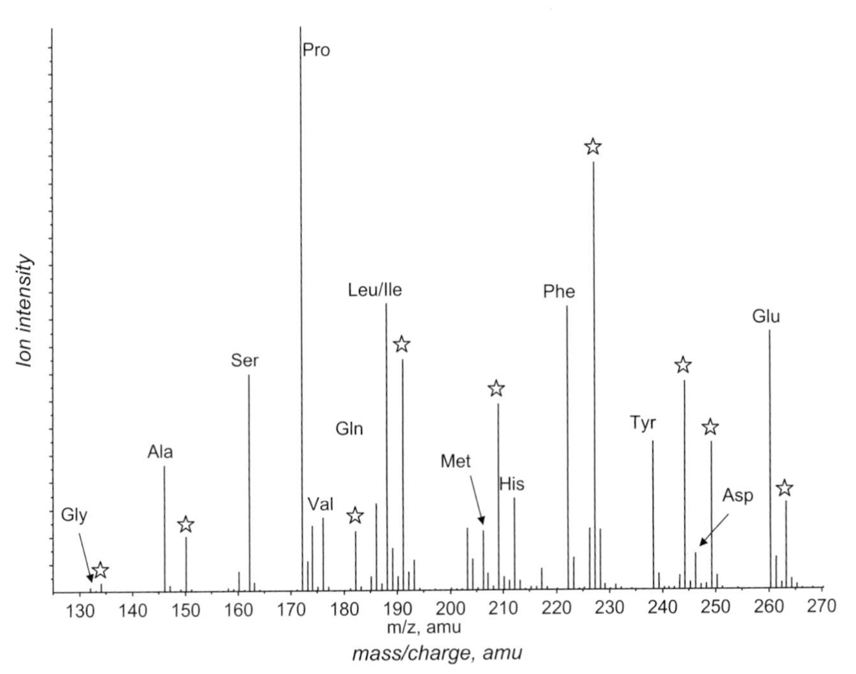

Fig. 2. Tandem mass spectra of dried blood extracts from a normal newborn obtained using neutral loss (NL) of a 102-d scan that detects α-amino acids. The stars represent isotopically labeled amino acids used as reference standards. Ala, alanine; amu, atomic mass unit; Asp, aspartic acid; Gln, glutamine; Glu, glutamic acid; Gly, glycine; His, histidine; Leu/Ile, leucine/Ile; Met, methionine; Phe, phenylalanine; Ser, serine; Tyr, tyrosine; Val, valine.

numerous acylcarnitines. Specific amino acids, such as phenylalanine (Phe) or octanoylcarnitine (an 8-carbon saturated fatty acylcarnitine that is considered a medium-sized fatty acid), are strongly correlated with the genetic diseases, phenylketonuria (PKU), and medium-chain acyl-coA dehydrogenase (MCAD deficiency), respectively. Elevations of these metabolites could also represent transient abnormalities induced by intravenous alimentation with protein or the administration of drugs, such as valproic acid, however. As is often the case, the clinical circumstances of the patient cannot be ignored when attempting to make an appropriate diagnosis with tandem MS.

At first glance in the specific cases of PKU or MCAD deficiency, it seems that there is but a single diagnostic metabolite that the clinician needs to be concerned about.[9] In fact, however, there are often several other metabolites that are characteristic of a specific disease state or environmental factor. In PKU, for example, tyrosine (Tyr) is the other amino acid that is critical for the correct screening of PKU (**Fig. 3**). Its simultaneous measurement by MS/MS permits the calculation of the Phe/Tyr ratio—a well-known index for accurate identification of PKU.[10] Knowledge of metabolic pathways would show that the conversion of Phe to Tyr is deficient in PKU, and one would therefore expect that Phe would be elevated and Tyr would decline. As a consequence of this change, the ratio would increase more rapidly than the elevation of Phe levels alone. With parenteral nutrition, however, the profile that emerges in some infants should be somewhat different. Because the conversion of Phe to Tyr is normal, we would not expect an abnormal ratio, even though we might see elevations

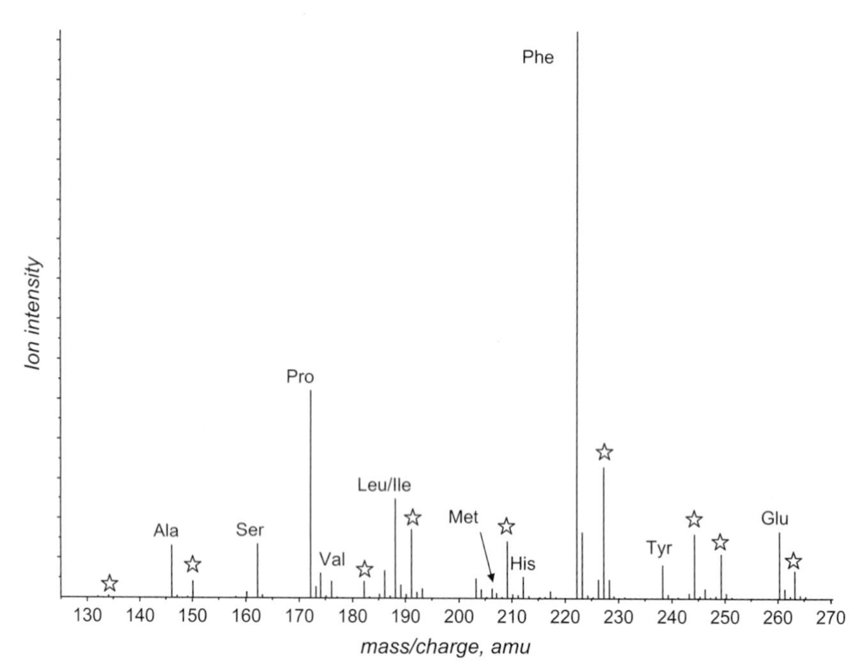

Fig. 3. Tandem mass spectrum of a dried blood extract from a newborn with phenylketonuria (PKU). Note the elevation of Phe (phenylalanine) relative to the internal standard and the slight decrease in the concentration of Tyr. Ala, alanine; amu, atomic mass units; Glu, glutamic acid; His, histidine; Leu/Ile, leucine/Ile; Met, methionine; Pro, proline; Ser, serine; Val, valine.

of Phe attributable to increases in blood Tyr caused by the total parenteral nutrition (TPN) administration. Occasionally, the Tyr content of TPN may be insufficient, resulting in an abnormal Phe/Tyr ratio. Other amino acids, such as Leu, Ala, and Met, may also be elevated with Phe. These multiple elevations of amino acids strongly suggest TPN as the source of the abnormalities on the mass spectrum (**Fig. 4**).

With MCAD deficiency, octanoylcarnitine represents the key diagnostic indicator, but there are important biomarkers that are altered by the enzyme deficiency.[11] These markers include 6- and 10-carbon (saturated and unsaturated) acylcarnitine species. As a result, detection of MCAD deficiency is based, in part, on a generalized pattern or profile of these elevated acylcarnitines. Furthermore, in this genetic disease, fatty acids, which are present in abundance, bind with available free carnitine and are eliminated in urine and bile. This process can result in a secondary carnitine deficiency but also permits the calculation of a ratio of C8 to free carnitine. Ratios may also be helpful in detecting the administration of valproate or medium-chain triglyceride (MCT) oil. The unsaturated fatty acylcarnitine is not seen in valproate or MCT oil metabolism but is seen in MCAD deficiency. Hence, the ratio of C10/C10:1 may be helpful in differentiating MCAD from other causes of these metabolite elevations.[12,13]

With this diagnostic capability, tandem MS has been useful in the measurement of as many as 65 diagnostic metabolites and ratios at the present time.[3] What is most important, however, is that this analysis can be done from a filter paper blood spot, potentially assessing many diseases in a single analysis from one blood spot. Two things are important to note. By measuring multiple metabolites, the cost of screening screen per disease is reduced and greater amounts of information are provided, which

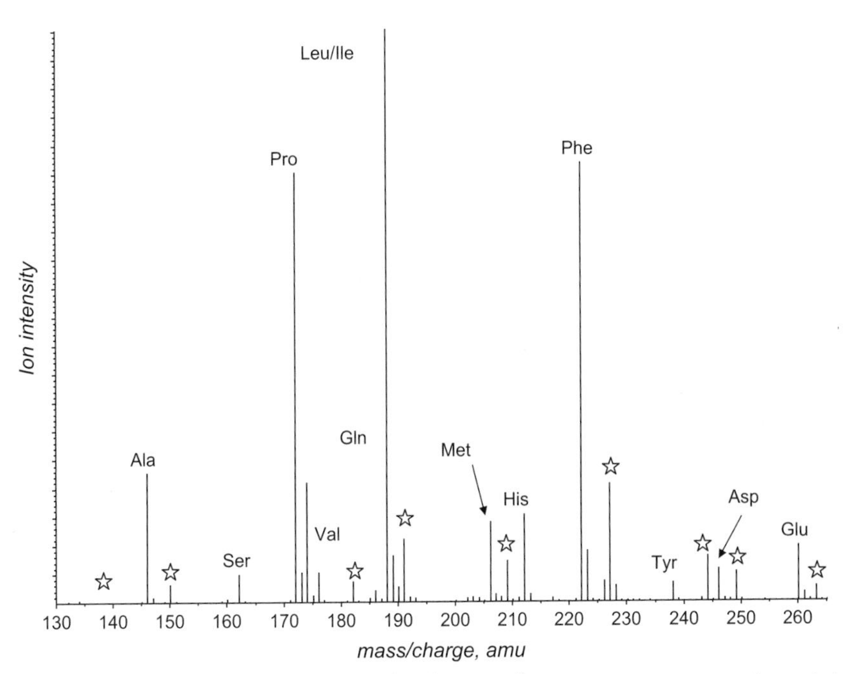

Fig. 4. Tandem mass spectrum of a dried blood extract from a premature neonate on total parenteral nutrition (TPN). Note the elevations of Phe, leucine (Leu), and methionine (Met) relative to their internal standards. It is also interesting to note the decrease in the concentration of Tyr. TPN profiles may or may not have elevated Tyr depending on the formulation. Ala, alanine; amu, atomic mass units; Asp, aspartic acid; Gln, glutamine; Glu, glutamic acid; His, histidine; Pro, proline; Ser, serine; Val, valine.

may be valuable in differentiating genetic or environmental causes of metabolite elevations. In addition, this approach reduces the likelihood of false results through improved pattern recognition, and the patterns can be readily expanded as new validations of metabolites in screening are achieved. Because it is based on a filter paper blood spot, it also reduces the hazards of working with liquid biologic fluids. Finally, shipping costs are reduced, because blood spots can be mailed in an envelope and do not need to be sent in a large box packed with dry ice.

PATHWAYS FOR NEONATAL METABOLIC DIAGNOSIS

Medicine is not always characterized by clear-cut diagnostics based on clinical laboratory tests. In part, this fact is attributable to a traditional focus of relying on the result of individual tests and other diagnostic indicators in an unhealthy state. What about these indicators in a healthy state, however? It is well known, for example, that MCAD deficiency is not diagnosable without a standard clinical chemistry test until a child has become severely hypoglycemic, often comatose, and, occasionally, severely debilitated in a preterminal condition. What is important, however, is that the critical metabolites in MCAD are present in the well state in addition to being present in the disease state. In metabolism and metabolic screening, it is most important that the identifiable metabolic patterns that indicate a disease are detectable before the disease becomes manifest. Although these metabolites may not always be easy to interpret or obvious, they are apparent to the trained eye and are highly predictive of future problems if left untreated.

The analogy of metabolism to a highway on a road map is quite appropriate. For example, if there is an accident on a major freeway, traffic intensity and alternative routes would play a role in determining whether an automobile reaches its destination, in addition to whether these automobiles affect other roads. In the case of a severe accident at rush hour, traffic backs up quickly. Cars are not able to enter the highway ahead of the obstructed road, whereas many cars look for alternative routes. The alternative routes typically are used more heavily than normal, creating other backups along these routes. If the traffic jam is not freed, these routes expand to such a degree that businesses around these routes may be affected and might even have to close if employees cannot get to work. It is easy to imagine how similar circumstances can arise with metabolites. With a metabolic disease, the major pathway of metabolism is blocked and the alternative routes become activated. Many of these routes have adverse effects as certain biochemicals build up, because they were not meant to be so "heavily traveled," (ie, toxic metabolites can be handled efficiently at the normal lower concentrations but not at these suddenly emerging new levels).

In the case of metabolism or MCAD deficiency, for example, as long as there is enough capacity on the alternative pathways, no disease may be detected. Conversely, if there is a major event in which the normal elimination of metabolites is suddenly obstructed on the metabolic highway, backups and traffic jams occur. This circumstance is analogous to what is observed during drug treatments or TPN. What we do not currently understand, however, and is often unknown, is what level of traffic can the highway tolerate? That situation is one in which individual variation occurs and why it may be important to monitor the metabolic traffic under a variety of clinical circumstances.

Finally, the carriers and the environment may ultimately be the most interesting to contemplate. When there is heavy construction on the highway, one lane is closed and backups occur primarily during rush hour. In these instances, the traffic is not persistent and the untoward effects are temporary. The alternative routes are well planned, and there may be no undesired effects. What if there is a problem (another genetic abnormality or partial abnormality) in a minor pathway, however? A multiple carrier or related disease could present a problem in certain uncommon circumstances and would still be detectable based on metabolism but not on the specific gene alone. This concept is the primary advantage, and one of the great challenges, of metabolic screening.

PROTEOMICS IN THE DIAGNOSIS OF NEONATAL-PERINATAL DISEASE

As previously noted, MS technology was first applied in the broad area of metabolic screening for neonatal diseases. The value of this approach has been seen from the fact that it is still used extensively for this purpose around the world. In the United States, tandem MS is currently used in many states, although there is great variability among states with respect to the number of disorders that are examined.[14] Because some states only screen for a small number of disorders, several private laboratories now offer supplemental newborn screening directly to hospitals or parents. The list of possible disorders that are currently tested for in expanded screening with MS/MS technology are delineated in **Box 1**. **Box 2** indicates additional disorders that are examined on the basis of the blood spot but by technologies other than tandem MS at the present time. It should be noted that recent work from the authors' laboratory has evaluated thyroid hormone screening by tandem MS, and the article outlining the merits of this approach and the changes that occur during neonatal intensive care unit (NICU) hospitalization have recently been demonstrated.[15]

The merits of standard neonatal screening are substantial, yet there are some areas of controversy. Some of the disorders tested for at the present time have less than satisfactory treatments (eg, hyperornithinemia with gyral atrophy) and are extremely uncommon. Many physicians may never encounter a child with one of these disorders during their entire clinical career. More significant, perhaps, is the belief that neonatal screening creates a situation in which false-positive test results, a situation inherent in any screening process, only serve to terrify and worry parents and physicians.[16] In general, however, this fear has not emerged as a significant consideration and the American Academy of Pediatrics (AAP), together with the Health Resources and Services Administration (HRSA), has recommended a thoughtfully considered core panel of 29 tests for newborn screening that it believes should be mandated at the state level.[17] In addition, these organizations have designated a specific series of steps that are designed to limit the impact of false-positive results on the family and to provide for enhanced communication between providers and parents. They have also recommended a methodology for continuing to examine the impact of screening, in addition to the further development of screening programs throughout the states.

Beyond neonatal screening, however, proteomic assessment of the neonate, to date, has not been used to any significant degree. Recently, however, this situation has begun to change as the merits of evaluation in acute illnesses have become increasingly apparent. As a physiologically challenged patient, the extremely-low-birth-weight (ELBW) infant is constantly changing; yet, he or she possesses limited volumes of available blood to measure the disease processes that affect these babies before and after birth. Given these circumstances, proteomic assessment by tandem MS would seem to be an ideal methodology for evaluation of the fetal and neonatal patient, and new uses of MS/MS are beginning to appear.

Although genomics has been a primary focus of discussion during the past decade in medicine, and the elegant elaboration of the human genome has been one of the great advances in medical science, the genome has limitations with respect to its ability to diagnose active disease. The identification of the presence of a certain gene, for example, only tells us that the individual has that gene and the potential for a disease to manifest at some future date. It does not indicate, however, whether a specific gene may ever express itself clinically (especially true of the heterozygous state), to what extent it may express itself, and whether the expression is going to result in clinical pathophysiology that produces a medical abnormality. It also does not indicate how an individual patient might respond to therapeutic interventions or metabolize certain drugs.

In contrast, MS detection of abnormal metabolites or protein biomarkers in the blood is far more likely to emerge as a standard for the evaluation of an active disease or pathophysiologic process. In addition, because protein synthesis and metabolism are the primary means through which pathophysiologic processes express themselves in the body, the assessment of protein biomarkers could conceivably anticipate the appearance of an abnormal clinical condition. In other words, the detection of trace amounts of abnormal biomarkers may occur before a disease is clinically apparent. Consequently, medicine may soon evolve to a new paradigm through proteomics. In this situation, one no longer waits for a disease to appear before making a diagnosis; instead, one pursues detection of low-level abnormalities of proteins or other biomarkers and intervenes before the pathophysiology emerges clinically or the patient deteriorates. The future is likely to require an understanding of the genetic potential for disease and a methodology for detecting appropriate biomarkers in the blood during early stages of a disease, such that early intervention can limit morbidity.

Box 1
Disorders currently detected by tandem mass spectrometry

Acylcarnitine profile

Fatty acid oxidation disorders

1. Carnitine/acylcarnitine translocase deficiency
2. Carnitine palmityl transferase deficiency type I
3. 3-Hydroxy long chain acyl-CoA dehydrogenase deficiency
4. 2,4-Dienoyl-CoA reductase deficiency
5. Medium-chain acyl-CoA dehydrogenase deficiency
6. Multiple acyl-CoA dehydrogenase deficiency
7. Neonatal carnitine palmityl transferase deficiency type II
8. Short-chain acyl-CoA dehydrogenase deficiency
9. Short-chain hydroxy Acyl-CoA dehydrogenase deficiency
10. Trifunctional protein deficiency
11. Very-long-chain Acyl-CoA dehydrogenase deficiency

Organic acid disorders

1. 3-Hydroxy-3-methylglutaryl-CoA lyase deficiency
2. Glutaric acidemia type I
3. Isobutyryl-CoA dehydrogenase deficiency
4. Isovaleric acidemia
5. 2-Methylbutryl-CoA dehydrogenase deficiency
6. 3-Methylcrotonyl-CoA carboxylase deficiency
7. 3-Methylglutaconyl-CoA hydratase deficiency
8. Methylmalonic acidemias

Methylmalonyl-CoA mutase deficiency

Some adenosylcobalamin synthesis defects

Maternal vitamin B_{12} deficiency

9. Mitochondrial acetoacetyl-CoA
10. Thiolase deficiency
11. Propionic acidemia
12. Multiple-CoA carboxylase deficiency
13. Malonic aciduria

Amino acid profile

Amino acid disorders

1. Argininemia
2. Argininosuccinic aciduria
3. 5-Oxoprolinuria
4. Carbamoylphosphate synthetase deficiency
5. Citrullinemia

6. Homocystinuria
7. Hypermethioninemia
8. Hyperammonemia, hyperornithinemia,
9. Homocitrullinemia syndrome
10. Hyperornithinemia with gyral atrophy
11. Maple syrup urine disease
12. Phenylketonuria
    Classic/hyperphenylalaninemia
    Biopterin cofactor deficiencies
13. Tyrosinemia

Transient neonatal tyrosinemia

Tyrosinemia type I

Tyrosinemia type II

Tyrosinemia type III

Other uses

1. Hyperalimentation
2. Liver disease
3. Medium-chain triglyceride oil administration
4. Presence of ethylenediaminetetraacetic acid (EDTA) anticoagulants in blood specimen
5. Treatment with benzoate, pyvalic acid, or valproic acid
6. Carnitine uptake deficiency

EMERGING AVENUES FOR FETAL AND NEONATAL ASSESSMENT WITH PROTEOMICS

Fetal Evaluation

Until the modern era of medicine, the fetus has remained a relative black box, in whom any form of intervention meant an immediate demise. With the introduction, however, by Liley[18] of amniotic fluid evaluation of elevated δ optical density (DOD) levels as a marker for hyperbilirubinemia secondary to rhesus (Rh) disease and the initiation of intrauterine transfusion for severe hemolytic disease, the era of fetal evaluation and intervention began. In succeeding years, the fetus has not only been the subject of increasing evaluation for the potential of disease but for interventions as dramatic as fetal surgery for a variety of clinical conditions.[19] As a result, the fetus has emerged as a significant patient, whose well-being should be regarded as vital not only to survival but with respect to active disease states and morbidity. Consequently, the obstetrician and the neonatologist have become increasingly interested in technologies that can assess the status of the fetus.

Fetal assessment, however, is not without risk. In Lee and Harrison's fetal surgical interventions,[20] premature delivery has been an ongoing worry, and it is well documented that even as commonplace an intervention as amniocentesis is associated with a procedural risk of approximately 0.5% for fetal demise or miscarriage.[21] Furthermore, although amniotic fluid is relatively abundant in most pregnancies, fetal blood and tissue are notably sparse, such that access to direct fetal information remains challenging. The difficulty of this situation is helped, however, by the fact that

Box 2
Disorders detected by other technologies (nontandem mass spectrometry)

1. Biotinidase deficiency
   Complete deficiency
   Partial deficiency
2. Congenital adrenal hyperplasia
   Salt wasting 21-hydroxylase deficiency
   Simple virilizing 21-hydroxylase deficiency
3. Congenital hypothyroidism[a] (not valid after 2 months of age)
4. Cystic fibrosis (not valid after 3 months of age)
5. Galactosemia
   Galactokinase deficiency
   Galactose-1-phosphate uridyltransferase deficiency
   Galactose-4-empimerase deficiency
6. Glucose-6-phosphate dehydrogenase deficiency
7. Sickle cell and other hemoglobinopathies
   Hemoglobin S, S/C, S/β-thalassemia, C, and diseases

[a] Tandem mass technology currently being evaluated.

fetal cells, free fetal DNA, and protein do get into the amniotic fluid and the maternal circulation, such that maternal blood or amniotic fluid assessment of the fetus can theoretically occur.[22] In this environment, therefore, the potential for proteomic assessment has held great promise, which is now beginning to emerge.[23,24]

Initial studies have suggested the importance of MS/MS technology in monitoring pregnancy and neonatal care. Gravett and colleagues[25] described the identification of intra-amniotic infection (IAI) through proteomic profiling of novel biomarkers in rhesus monkeys and women with preterm labor (PTL) (**Fig. 5**). Using surface-enhanced laser desorption (SELDI)/time-of-flight (TOF) spectroscopy, they were able to determine unique protein expression profiles in women and rhesus monkeys with IAI. In particular, calgranulin B seemed to be overexpressed in amniotic fluid and blood, in addition to some other novel immunoregulators. These investigators speculated that the ability to identify these biomarkers may ultimately lead to early detection of IAI and interventions that could result in improved pregnancy outcomes. Given the central role of IAI in preterm delivery, the ability to assess and treat such patients early in the course of infection might be one of the primary methods by which preterm deliveries could be reduced. This work was recently confirmed by Ruetschi and colleagues,[26] who found overexpression of 17 proteins in amniotic fluid, more commonly in women with PTL than in those with rupture of membranes. Furthermore, the promise of early detection of congenital abnormalities through similar techniques seems to be on the immediate horizon. The potential changes in the approach to pregnancy that these studies portend cannot be overemphasized.

Most recently, Nagalla and colleagues[28] have expanded the potential for proteomic analysis in a series of publications, using multidimensional liquid chromatography–tandem MS (LC/LC-MS/MS; MudPIT). In a study of novel protein biomarkers for

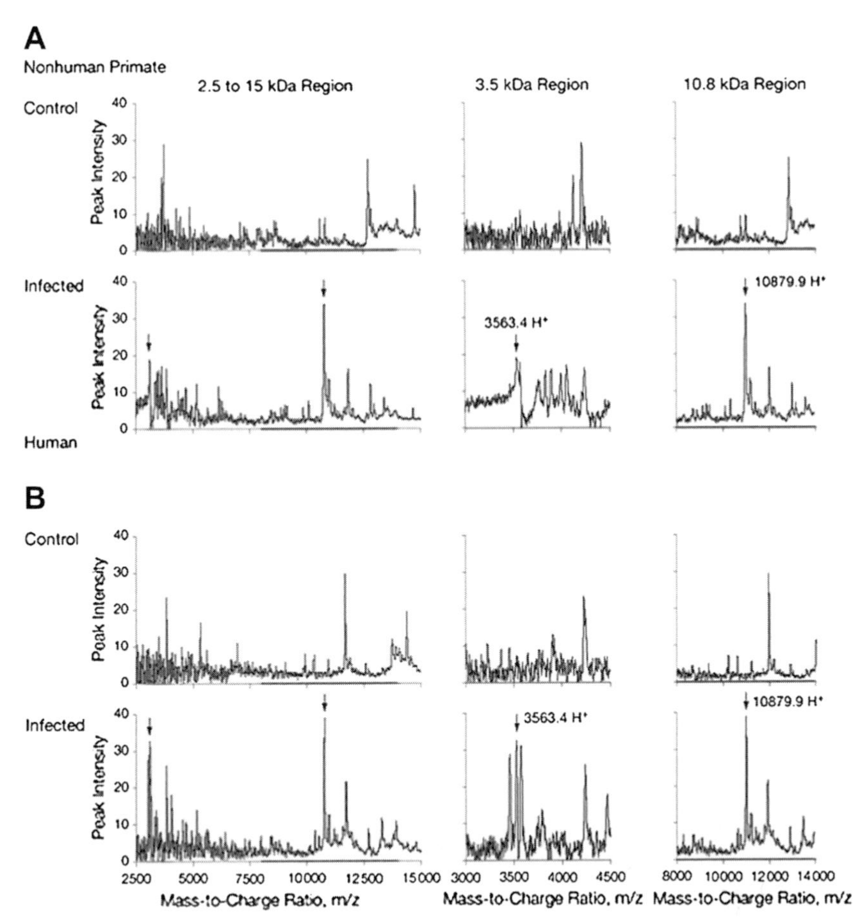

Fig. 5. Surface-enhanced laser desorption (SELDI)/time of flight (TOF) indicates enhanced laser desorption/ionization TOF. Group B *Streptococcus* infection-induced differential protein expression in primate (*A*) and human (*B*) amniotic fluid samples. Detailed spectra show increased expression of the 3.5-kd and 10.8-kd peaks between control and infection. Arrows indicate unique peaks represented by polypeptides overexpressed in infection. (*From* Gravett MG, Novy MJ, Rosenfeld RG, et al. Diagnosis of intraamniotic infection by protein profiling and identification of novel biomarkers. JAMA 2004;292:466; with permission.)

PTL in maternal cervical and vaginal fluid, 28 proteins in cervical-vaginal fluid were determined to be present in differential concentrations in mothers with PTL compared with those with normal pregnancies. Calgranulins, annexins, S-100 calcium-binding protein A7, and epidermal fatty acid–binding protein were abundant in women with PTL, as were serum proteins α_1-antitrypisn, α_1-acid glycoprotein, haptoglobin, serotransferrin, and vitamin D–binding protein.[27] This new insight into prematurity is exciting and portends an era in which mothers might be routinely screened for potential markers of preterm delivery on a regular basis. Should these biomarkers be detected, an aggressive approach to imminent PTL could be initiated and the pregnancy might be sustained for a longer duration.

A second study from this same group examined maternal serum in Down syndrome.[28] In this investigation, first- and second-trimester maternal Trisomy 21 serum specimens were paired with gestational-matched controls. MudPIT LC/LC MS/MS profiling was used, along with MALDI-TOF-MS peptide profiling. Discrimination between Trisomy 21 and nonaffected mothers was achieved with a 96% recognition capability and revealed that most unique biomarkers were serum glycoproteins. Given that the current optimal prenatal assessment for Trisomy 21 achieves only an 80% to 85% recognition rate, proteomic evaluation would represent an important enhancement to early diagnosis of Down syndrome. These findings need to be confirmed in prospective trials, which are currently underway, but clearly indicate what is on the immediate horizon for fetal identification of abnormal processes and genetic diseases. The ability to detect such abnormalities without direct fetal intervention represents a major advance in medical care.

In the immediate future, many other common problems of pregnancy and the fetus are likely to be examined by proteomics as well. Pregnancy-induced hypertension (PIH), growth restriction in utero, the diabetic pregnancy, and placental insufficiency are but a few of the situations in which early proteomic assessment is likely to play a prominent role in the next several years.

Neonatal Evaluation

Few aspects of life define more importantly what it is to be "human" than brain function. It is the ability to reason that distinguishes human beings from all other species; consequently, one of the greatest concerns that any parent has after NICU care is whether there has been any evidence of brain injury. Once a family has asked the question, "Will my baby survive?", the next question is always "How will he or she do?" This question almost inevitably refers to neurodevelopmental outcome. Again, until recently, the physician could only make an educated guess and try to optimize care to achieve the best outcome.

Studies, such as head ultrasounds or MRIs, performed in an attempt to grasp the potential quality of life (and brain function) in an infant, provided only "snapshots" of a baby's status and were far removed from the kind of dynamic evaluation that could truly gauge the neonate's NICU progress or needs. Although these approaches created dramatic enhancements in our understanding of the neonate's condition, they still revealed only a single moment in time and not much about the changing state of the infant. Infant nutrition and its effect on development, in particular, have also been difficult issues to assess, and it is probably a tribute to the neonate that our lack of understanding of nutrition has not obstructed the improvements in outcome observed during the past several decades. Nevertheless, it is apparent that many neonates are malnourished in the NICU, and there is postnatal growth restriction for many infants that is as problematic as in utero growth restriction.[29]

Optimal neonatal nutrition, however, remains an ongoing puzzle and a major concern. Although there is little question that breast milk provides optimal neonatal nutrition for the term infant, the nutritional needs of the premature infant, especially the critically ill patient, are not as obvious. Although there are significant advantages of breast milk with respect to immune protection for the premature neonate, it is well established that breast milk provides insufficient quantities of protein, sodium, calcium, iron, vitamin D, and other nutrients to sustain growth.[30] Neonatologists therefore routinely use human milk fortifier, which supplements breast milk, in an effort to enhance growth in the premature infant.

Not all premature infants, however, can be fed enterally. The ELBW neonate (<1000 g at birth), for a variety of reasons, may go days to weeks before enteral feedings can be initiated. In addition, the risk for necrotizing enterocolitis and common interruptions of enteral feeding in the NICU for a variety of reasons require that intravenous nutrition be provided. Here, the situation becomes even murkier with respect to the provision of protein and fats (glucose is easier to assess, because one can simply follow blood glucose levels to ensure that glucose is being maintained at an appropriate level). Because of the known growth problems in premature infants, there has been a trend during the past decade to push protein to 4 g/kg/d in an effort to maintain known intrauterine protein accretion rates. It is unclear, however, that this approach is safe or appropriate, because amino acid levels have not been commonly measured in preterm infants on TPN and the available solutions for protein administration in a 500-g neonate are essentially the same ones that are used for adults. Needless to say, metabolic differences are quite substantial between these two patient populations.

Recently, in an effort to delineate the effects of parenteral protein administration, Clark and colleagues[31] used MS/MS analysis in a multicenter randomized trial to determine the amino acid levels that were achieved in premature infants receiving TPN. In addition, they tried to verify if increased rates of protein administration during the first month of life could achieve higher growth rates, as has been suggested previously.[32] The results of this study were surprising in that infants who received 33% more protein during the first 28 days of life did not grow at an accelerated rate during that period. In addition, certain amino acids and amino acid acylcarnitines (e.g., isovalerylcarnitine) were elevated to levels that were of concern, whereas other amino acid levels (e.g., alanine) seemed to be inadequate. Essentially, some of the amino acid metabolic pathways in the premature infant seemed to be saturated, whereas others seemed to be undersupplied (**Fig. 6**).

Aggressive protein therapy may therefore result in levels of certain amino acids, such as Phe, isovalerylcarnitine, or other metabolic byproducts, that could produce temporary but important toxicities. Such toxicities, especially if unrecognized and prolonged, may be one of the reasons why some infants, even in the absence of typical types of neurologic injury, such as intraventricular hemorrhage (IVH) or periventricular leukomalacia (PVL), may nevertheless have poorer than expected long-term outcomes. Similarly, low amino acid levels may indicate an unfilled need that current amino acid mixtures are not adequately addressing. These data suggest that the currently available TPN solutions might not be appropriate for the very-low-birth-weight (VLBW) neonate but that with the alteration of amino acid composition, it might actually be possible to increase protein administration in a way to mimic intrauterine growth. The study also indicated the value of the filter paper blood spot to measure a large variety of compounds in the VLBW neonate with little blood loss to the infant, which represents a significant potential technology that could enhance neonatal care in the near future.

A corollary study from that same investigation also looked at a second common nutritional problem of the premature infant receiving parenteral nutrition, cholestatic jaundice.[33] In that trial, 13 (10.7%) of 122 neonates subsequently developed cholestatic jaundice. Amino acid markers of an enhanced likelihood of cholestasis were evidenced by 7 days of life. Citrulline, histidine, methionine, and succinyl carnitine were higher, and serine and glutamate levels were lower in the neonates who developed cholestasis than in those who did not. Thyroxine levels were also lower in neonates who subsequently developed cholestasis. Again, proteomic/metabolomic assessment of acute disease states seems likely to prove to be an increasingly important adjunct to neonatal care in the immediate future.

Other Avenues for Neonatal Critical Care Monitoring with Tandem Mass Spectroscopy

The potential for the use of neonatal MS/MS evaluation is exceptional, and this technology is likely to emerge as a valuable adjunct to care in the next decade. Several

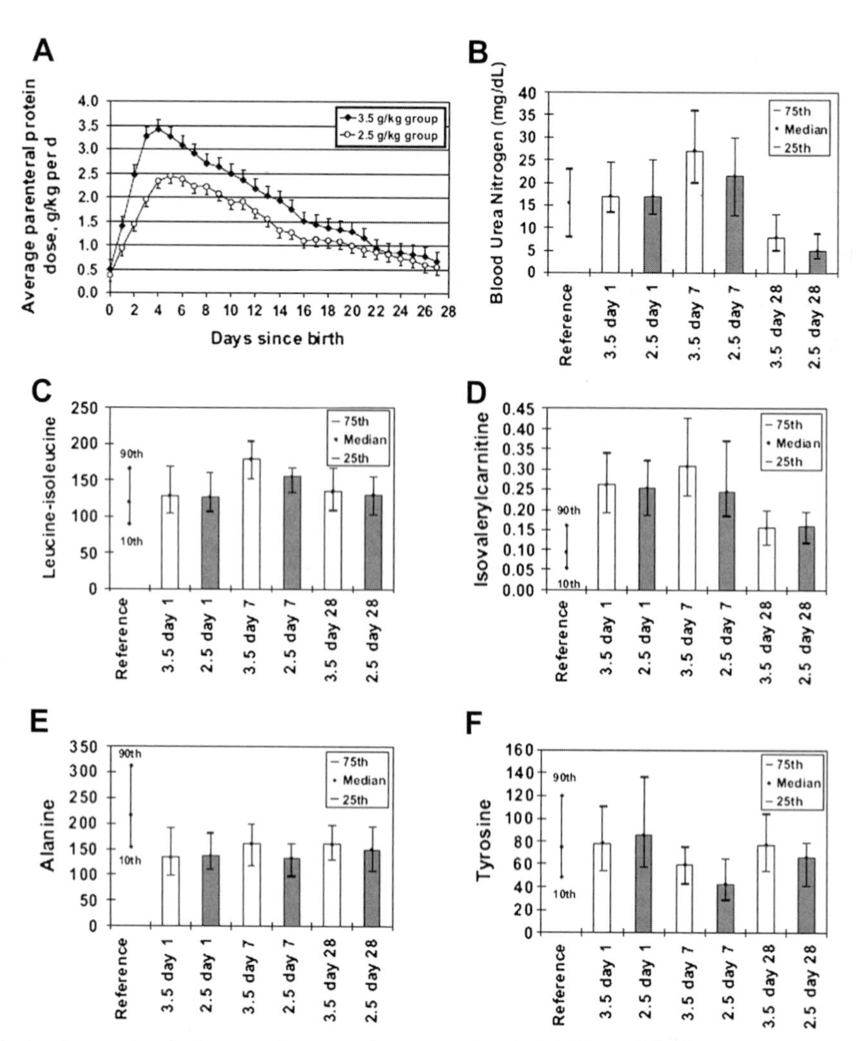

Fig. 6. Comparison between infants receiving protein administration at rates of 2.5 and 3.5 g/kg/d. (*A*) Average ± the standard error of the dose of amino acid over time for both treatment groups. The upper line (*diamonds*) represents the values for the neonates receiving a maximum dose of 3.5 g/kg/d, and the lower line (*open circles*) represents the values for patients receiving a maximum dose of 2.5 g/kg/d. (*B*) Median and quartiles for changes in blood urea nitrogen (mg/dL) over time. (*C–F*) Representative changes in key amino acids and acylcarnitines over time: leucine-isoleucine (*C*), isovalerylcarnitine (*D*), alanine (*E*), and tyrosine (*F*). All values are reported in μmol/L. Graphs represent median, 25th through 75th percentiles for measure values, and median, 10th through 90th percentiles for reference values (*From* Clark RE, Chace DH, Spitzer AR. The effects of two different doses of amino acid administration on growth and blood amino acids in premature neonates admitted to the NICU: a randomized controlled trial. Pediatrics 2007;120:1289; with permission.)

areas of neonatal intensive care would seem to benefit the most from proteomic assessment of the newborn. These include (but are not limited to) the following:

1. Diagnosis and treatment of neonatal septicemia
2. Assessment of the neonate with hypoxic-ischemic or other brain injury

3. Nutritional management of the enterally feeding patient
4. Inflammatory markers in the pathogenesis of chronic lung and liver disease
5. Tailored drug therapy

Neonatal Septicemia

The diagnosis of neonatal infection is one of the most elusive aspects of neonatal intensive care. Although much of the focus in the NICU is on the premature newborn, the most common admitting diagnosis to the NICU is the term newborn with suspected septicemia. Typically, the baby has been born after a somewhat difficult delivery in which the mother has had a fever, raising the suspicion of infection in the newborn. In most instances, maternal fever is simply attributable to dehydration, prolonged labor, or spinal anesthesia, but the cause is often unclear and the concern about the newborn is substantial. In addition to blood culture, which may take 2 days to confirm the diagnosis, other commonly used neonatal diagnostic tests are not always helpful. The complete blood cell count (CBC) in a healthy baby often shows an elevated white blood cell (WBC) count (up to 30,000 cells/mm^3), and in cases of true septicemia in the neonatal period, the WBC count actually decreases as the marrow becomes depressed. C-reactive protein results may also be unclear. Algorithms that attempt to use combinations of these tests to enhance diagnosis have not proved to be as reliable clinically as one would have hoped.[34] Furthermore, neonates rarely run fevers themselves, often becoming hypothermic during infection. As a result, the clinician often makes an educated guess about the likelihood of infection while awaiting a culture result. Antibiotics are used during this period, often unnecessarily, because of the fear that the child may have a life-threatening infection, which is a grave issue in an already immunocompromised patient (which all neonates are). The frequent and prolonged use of antibiotics, however, tends to breed increasingly resistant microorganisms, which may be devastating to future generations of neonates. Therefore, in the same manner as the proteome of maternal infection has been examined, the neonatal proteome during infection also needs assessment. In addition, it is likely that there may be unique protein (and genomic) markers of bacteria, which would indicate the presence of invading microorganisms. To date, no studies have been done to confirm the merits of proteomic assessment, but it seems likely that if maternal infection can be readily detected, neonatal infection should also yield to proteomic evaluation. Such a result would likely enhance the sensitivity and specificity for infection diagnosis.

Hypoxic-Ischemic Brain Injury, Perinatal Asphyxia, and Chronic Lung Disease: the Potential for Proteomic Evaluation

At the present time, the primary methods for the evaluation of brain injury in the neonatal period involve some aspect of brain imaging. Cranial ultrasound,[35] CT, and MRI of a variety of types (e.g., magnetic resonance angiography [MRA],[36] magnetic resonance spectroscopy [MRS],[37] and diffusion-weighted imaging [DWI][38]) are the tools used to define the extent of injury during the neonatal period and the likelihood of residual damage after NICU discharge. More recently, other interesting techniques, such as cerebral function monitoring, have been used to examine brain development in the neonate and the likelihood of neurologic injury.[39,40] For many years, IVH was thought to have the greatest long-term consequence to the VLBW baby.[41] More recently, however, white matter disease (WMD) and PVL, thought to be alternative and related expressions of chronic hypoxic-ischemic injury in the neonate, have attracted attention as the leading events that are likely to produce more permanent neurologic disability in the form of cerebral palsy (CP) and developmental delay.[42] In the term infant, acute hypoxic-ischemic injury and birth trauma seem to be more significant events in the evolution of brain injury.[43] It has been widely recognized, however, that although many neonates who ultimately develop CP sustain their injury during birth or in the NICU, most do not have any evidence of acute neonatal events capable of producing permanent injury.[44–46] In term neonates, most babies with CP have no clearly discernible asphyxial event to which the injury can be attributed.

In the cases in which CP does not seem to be the result of some aspect of neonatal or perinatal care, the obvious question is when and how does it occur? It has become increasingly apparent that some brain injury is initiated before the neonatologist ever sees the patient. In examining those factors that resulted in PTL, Romero and colleagues[47,48] began to notice that certain prostaglandins seemed to be increased in mothers delivering prematurely. They speculated that PTL may be the result of an inflammatory process, with the most likely cause of inflammation being intrauterine infection. This infection, most notably, may not necessarily be clinically apparent, and many women may have subclinical chorioamnionitis, which goes entirely unrecognized until premature labor ensues and the placenta is retrospectively examined. More importantly, they also recognized that if one examined the amniotic fluid of mothers of babies who develop CP, there were significant elevations of cytokines, which were not increased in neonates who did not develop CP.[49,50]

Although these observations may have been comforting to neonatologists who often agonized about what might have occurred to their patient that resulted in white matter injury, even though no clear-cut events in the NICU may have been noted, it made the diagnosis of maternal infection and inflammation that much more important. These initial observations have been confirmed in other studies since that time.[51] Furthermore, it was also recognized that bronchopulmonary dysplasia, an inflammatory pulmonary process of the ventilated premature neonate, most probably had a similar onset before birth, which was subsequently aggravated by a variety of commonplace NICU events.[52] Consequently, the diagnosis of maternal inflammatory disease now occupies a central role in neonatal-perinatal research, and the specific timing of the onset of infection has become increasingly important. Finally, the possibility of early diagnosis of intrauterine infection as a more treatable entity, as noted previously, has emerged as a critical focus of perinatal investigation.

During the same period in which the etiologic factors of white matter injury in the VLBW infant were being examined in depth, new attention began to be focused on the term neonate with hypoxic-ischemic encephalopathy. Few problems have been as troubling to the perinatologist and the neonatologist as birth asphyxia. Because so many of these infants ultimately die or have permanent neurologic injury and so many of these cases result in malpractice litigation, physicians have been desperate to understand the origins of this entity. Even the diagnosis has been an ongoing concern, and the American College of Obstetrics and Gynecology and the AAP have labored repeatedly in an attempt to categorize this entity and the factors that result in an asphyxiated infant better. The primary motivation that drove the increased interest in making a rapid diagnosis of perinatal hypoxic-ischemic injury was the recognition that brain and body cooling seemed to limit the manifestations of the disease process.[53,54] It seemed, however, that brain and body hypothermia needed to be initiated before 6 hours of life to discern any beneficial effect. Later application seemed to have little, if any, value to the asphyxiated newborn.

Several trials have confirmed the benefit of hypothermia after perinatal hypoxic-ischemic injury.[55,56] It has been noted, however, that brain or body cooling has not produced improved outcomes that are as dramatic as those seen in animal studies, when the brain injury can be precisely timed. It is evident then that the most significant variable over which little control could be exerted was the time between the onset of intrauterine hypoxemia and the time of birth. As with the VLBW baby and the development of WMD, one of the principal problems encountered in these trials was the inability to determine accurately the period during which the baby was initially becoming asphyxiated in utero. It seems likely that if a technique could evolve that would provide such information, the use of cooling could be more specifically introduced in selected patients, with a far more favorable outcome. Proteomics or metabolomics would seem to offer a valuable methodology in this respect, and trials to examine the potential role of MS/MS in neurologic injury should be initiated in the near future.

Enteral Nutrition and Proteomics

As noted with intravenous nutrition previously in this article, the science behind neonatal feeding is based on a simple premise, namely, that breast milk is best. For the term newborn, there is no question that this statement is correct, but in the premature neonate, the validity of this statement is not clear. It is well established that the VLBW baby does not grow well on breast milk alone and milk fortifiers are commonly used to supplement breast milk in these babies. Studies must be performed using proteomic and metabolomic assessment during enteral feeding to understand the needs and metabolism of the low-birth-weight newborn better. These are likely to be initiated in the near future.

Neonatal Metabolic Checkup

If many of the concepts in this article are correct, the critically ill neonate seems likely to be an ideal candidate for proteomic/metabolomic screening. Because of the small amount of blood needed for proteomic evaluation, the filter paper spot would seem to be an ideal methodology for examining many simultaneous metabolic processes in the neonate. Nutritional status, risk for sepsis, inflammatory mediators, thyroid hormone levels, central nervous system (CNS) status, and overall hormonal status could all conceivably provide the neonatologist and the perinatologist with a wealth of new information that would have an extraordinarily positive effect on clinical management and ultimate outcome. This possibility may exist in the not too distant future and should herald an exciting new era in newborn medicine.

SUMMARY

The introduction of proteomics and metabolomics into the NICU seems to be a coming event with significant implications for medical practice. This approach is highly likely to have substantial benefits with many positive effects on neonatal outcomes.

REFERENCES

1. Chace DH. Mass spectrometry in the clinical laboratory. Chem Rev 2001;101: 445–77.
2. Millington DS, Terada N, Chace DH, et al. The role of tandem mass spectrometry in the diagnosis of fatty acid oxidation disorders. Prog Clin Biol Res 1992;375: 339–54.
3. Chace DH, Kalas TA, Naylor EW. Use of tandem mass spectrometry for multianalyte screening of dried blood specimens from newborns. Clin Chem 2003;49: 1797–817.
4. Magera MJ, Gunawardena ND, Hahn SH, et al. Quantitative determination of succinylacetone in dried blood spots for newborn screening of tyrosinemia type I. Mol Genet Metab 2006;88:16–21.

5. Lacey JM, Minutti CZ, Magera MJ, et al. Improved specificity of newborn screening for congenital adrenal hyperplasia by second-tier steroid profiling using tandem mass spectrometry. Clin Chem 2004;50:621–5.
6. Griffiths WJ, Jonsson AP, Liu S, et al. Electrospray and tandem mass spectrometry in biochemistry. Biochem J 2001;355:545–61.
7. Bootsma AH, Overmars H, van Rooij A, et al. Rapid analysis of conjugated bile acids in plasma using electrospray tandem mass spectrometry: application for selective screening of peroxisomal disorders. J Inherit Metab Dis 1999;22:307–10.
8. Crain PF, McCloskey JA. Applications of mass spectrometry to the characterization of oligonucleotides and nucleic acids. Curr Opin Biotechnol 1998;9:25–34.
9. Chace DH, Kalas TA. A biochemical perspective on the use of tandem mass spectrometry for newborn screening and clinical testing. Clin Biochem 2005;38:296–309.
10. Chace DH, Sherwin JE, Hillman SL, et al. Use of phenylalanine-to-tyrosine ratio determined by tandem mass spectrometry to improve newborn screening for phenylketonuria of early discharge specimens collected in the first 24 hours. Clin Chem 1998;44:2405–9.
11. Chace DH, Hillman SL, Van Hove JL, et al. Rapid diagnosis of MCAD deficiency: quantitative analysis of octanoylcarnitine and other acylcarnitines in newborn blood spots by tandem mass spectrometry. Clin Chem 1997;43:2106–13.
12. Van Hove JL, Zhang W, Kahler SG, et al. Medium-chain acyl-CoA dehydrogenase (MCAD) deficiency: diagnosis by acylcarnitine analysis in blood. Am J Hum Genet 1993;52:958–66.
13. Iafolla AK, Thompson RJ Jr, Roe CR. Medium-chain acyl-coenzyme A dehydrogenase deficiency: clinical course in 120 children. J Pediatr 1994;124:409–15.
14. Therrell BL, Johnson A, Williams D. Status of newborn screening programs in the United States. Pediatrics 2006;117:S212–52.
15. Kelleher AS, Clark RH, Steinbach M, et al. The influence of amino acid supplementation, gestational age, and time on thyroxine levels in premature neonates. J Perinatology 2008;28:270–4.
16. Tarini BA, Christakis DA, Welch HG. State newborn screening in the tandem mass spectrometry era: more tests, more false positive results. Pediatrics 2006;118:448–56.
17. Watson MS, Mann MY, Lloyd-Puryear MA, et al. Newborn screening: toward a uniform screening panel and system—executive summary. Pediatrics 2006;117:S296–307.
18. Liley AW. Liquor amnil analysis in the management of the pregnancy complicated by rhesus sensitization. Am J Obstet Gynecol 1961;82:1359–70.
19. Harrison MR, Bressack MA, Churg AM, et al. Correction of congenital diaphragmatic hernia in utero. I. The model: intrathoracic balloon produces fatal pulmonary hypoplasia. Surgery 1980;88(1):174–82.
20. Lee H, Harrison MR. Surgery for fetal malformations. In: Spitzer A, editor. Intensive care of the fetus and neonate. 2nd edition. Philadelphia: Elsevier, Inc.; 2005. p. 203–12.
21. Trauffer PM, Wapner RJ, Johnson A. Amniocentesis. In: Spitzer A, editor. Intensive care of the fetus and neonate. 2nd edition. Philadelphia: Elsevier, Inc.; 2005. p. 64.
22. Hyodo M, Samura O, Fujito N, et al. No correlation between the number of fetal nucleated cells and the amount of cell-free fetal DNA in maternal circulation either before or after delivery. Prenat Diagn 2007;27(8):717–21.

23. Van Hove JL, Chace DH, Kahler SG, et al. Acylcarnitines in amniotic fluid: application to the prenatal diagnosis of propionic acidemia. J Inherit Metab Dis 1993; 16:361–7.
24. Shigematsu Y, Hata I, Nakai A, et al. Prenatal diagnosis of organic acidemias based on amniotic fluid levels of acylcarnitines. Pediatr Res 1996;39:680–4.
25. Gravett MG, Novy MJ, Rosenfeld RG, et al. Diagnosis of intra-amniotic infection by proteomic profiling and identification of novel biomarkers. JAMA 2004; 292(4):462–9.
26. Ruetschi U, Rosen A, Karlsson G, et al. Proteomic analysis using protein chips to detect biomarkers in cervical and amniotic fluid in women with intra-amniotic inflammation. J Proteome Res 2005;4(6):2236–42.
27. Pereira L, Reddy AP, Jacob T, et al. Identification of novel protein biomarkers of preterm birth in human cervical-vaginal fluid. J Proteome Res 2007;6:1269–76.
28. Nagalla SR, Canick JA, Jacob T, et al. Proteomic analysis of maternal serum in Down syndrome: identification of novel protein biomarkers. J Proteome Res 2007;6:1245–57.
29. Clark RH, Wagner CL, Merritt RJ, et al. Nutrition in the neonatal intensive care unit: how do we reduce the incidence of extrauterine growth restriction. J Perinatol 2003;23:337–44.
30. Pereira GR, Chan SW. Feeding the critically ill neonate. In: Spitzer A, editor. Intensive care of the fetus and neonate. 2nd edition. Philadelphia: Elsevier, Inc.; 2005. p. 991.
31. Clark RH, Chace DH, Spitzer AR. The effects of two different doses of amino acid administrations on growth and blood amino acids in premature neonates admitted to the NICU: a randomized controlled trial. Pediatrics 2007;120:1286–96.
32. Premji SS, Fenton TR, Sauve RS. Higher versus lower protein intake in formula-fed low birth weight infants. Cochrane Database Syst Rev 2006;(1):CD003959.
33. Steinbach M, Clark RH, Kelleher AS, et al. Demographic and nutritional factors associated with prolonged cholestatic jaundice in the preterm infant. J Perinatol 2008;28:129–35.
34. Gerdes JS. Diagnosis and management of bacterial infections in the neonate. Pediatr Clin North Am 2004;51(4):939–59.
35. Burdjalov V, Srinivasan P, Baumgart S, et al. Handheld, portable ultrasound in the neonatal intensive care nursery: a new, inexpensive tool for the rapid diagnosis of common neonatal problems. J Perinatol 2002;22(6):478–83.
36. Husain AM, Smergel E, Legido A, et al. Comparison of MRI and MRA findings in children with a variety of neurologic conditions. Pediatr Neurol 2000;23(4): 307–11.
37. Vigneron DB. Magnetic resonance spectroscopic imaging of human brain development. Neuroimaging Clin N Am 2006;16(1):75–85.
38. Counsell SJ, Shen Y, Boardman JP, et al. Axial and radial diffusivity in preterm infants who have diffuse white matter changes on magnetic resonance imaging at term-equivalent age. Pediatrics 2006;117(2):376–86.
39. Burdjalov VF, Baumgart S, Spitzer AR. Cerebral function monitoring—a new scoring system for the evaluation of brain maturation in neonates. Pediatrics 2003; 112:855–61.
40. West CR, Groves AM, Williams CE, et al. Early low cardiac output is associated with compromised electroencephalographic activity in very preterm infants. Pediatr Res 2006;59(4):610–5.
41. Papile LA, Burstein J, Burstein R, et al. Incidence and evolution of subependymal and intraventricular hemorrhage: a study of infants with birth weights less than 1,500 gm. J Pediatr 1978;92:529–34.

42. Volpe JJ. Cerebral white matter injury of the premature infant—more common than you think. Pediatrics 2003;112(Pt 1):176–80.
43. Berger R, Garnier Y. Perinatal brain injury. J Perinat Med 2000;28(4):261–85.
44. Tran U, Gray PH, O'Callaghan MJ. Neonatal antecedents for cerebral palsy in extremely preterm babies and interaction with maternal factors. Early Hum Dev 2005;81(6):555–61.
45. Laptook AR, O'Shea TM, Shankaran S, et al. NICHD Neonatal Network. Adverse neurodevelopmental outcomes among extremely low birth weight infants with a normal head ultrasound: prevalence and antecedents. Pediatrics 2005; 115(3):673–80.
46. Wood NS, Costeloe K, Gibson AT, et al. EPICure Study Group. The EPICure study: associations and antecedents of neurological and developmental disability at 30 months of age following extremely preterm birth. Arch Dis Child Fetal Neonatal Ed 2005;90(2):F134–40.
47. Romero R, Parvizi ST, Oyarzun E, et al. Amniotic fluid interleukin-1 in spontaneous labor at term. J Reprod Med 1990;35(3):235–8.
48. Romero R, Avila C, Santhanam U, et al. Amniotic fluid interleukin 6 in preterm labor. Association with infection. J Clin Invest 1990;85(5):1392–400.
49. Yoon BH, Romero R, Yang SH, et al. Interleukin-6 concentrations in umbilical cord plasma are elevated in neonates with white matter lesions associated with periventricular leukomalacia. Am J Obstet Gynecol 1996;174(5):1433–40.
50. Yoon BH, Jun JK, Romero R, et al. Amniotic fluid inflammatory cytokines (interleukin-6, interleukin-1beta, and tumor necrosis factor-alpha), neonatal brain white matter lesions, and cerebral palsy. Am J Obstet Gynecol 1997;177(1):19–26.
51. Ellison VJ, Mocatta TJ, Winterbourn CC, et al. The relationship of CSF and plasma cytokine levels to cerebral white matter injury in the premature newborn. Pediatr Res 2005;57(2):282–6.
52. Dammann O, Leviton A, Bartels DB, et al. Lung and brain damage in preterm newborns. Are they related? How? Why? Biol Neonate 2004;85(4):305–13.
53. Bona E, Hagberg H, Loberg EM, et al. Protective effects of moderate hypothermia after neonatal hypoxia-ischemia: short- and long-term outcome. Pediatr Res 1998;43(6):738–45.
54. Gunn AJ, Gluckman PD, Gunn TR. Selective head cooling in newborn infants after perinatal asphyxia: a safety study. Pediatrics 1998;102(4 Pt 1):885–92.
55. Gluckman PD, Wyatt JS, Azzopardi D, et al. Selective head cooling with mild systemic hypothermia after neonatal encephalopathy: multicentre randomised trial. Lancet 2005;365(9460):663–70.
56. Shankaran S, Laptook AR, Ehrenkranz RA, et al. For the National Institute of Child Health and Human Development Neonatal Research Network. Whole-body hypothermia for neonates with hypoxic-ischemic encephalopathy. N Engl J Med 2005; 353(15):1574–84.

Hypothermia for Hypoxic-Ischemic Encephalopathy

Rakesh Sahni, MD*, Ulana M. Sanocka, MD

KEYWORDS

- Cooling • Neuroprotection • Asphyxia
- Newborn infant • Brain injury

Hypoxic-ischemic encephalopathy (HIE) is an important cause of acute neurologic injury at birth, affecting approximately two to three cases per 1000 full-term live births in developed countries, with a higher incidence in less developed countries.[1] Despite advancements in many aspects of neonatal intensive care, the outcome for infants with hypoxic–ischemic brain injury remains poor. Fifteen percent to twenty-five percent of infants with severe HIE die, and 25% to 30% of survivors have major long-term disabilities.[2,3] Historically, interventions to improve outcomes in this population have been disappointing. The treatment of infants who have HIE is generally supportive and includes resuscitation techniques that follow the latest Neonatal Resuscitation Program guidelines,[4] attention to glucose, fluid and electrolyte homeostasis, maintenance of $PaCO_2$ within a normal range, correction of hypotension, and treatment of seizures. A wide variety of neuroprotective strategies have been studied in experimental animals and infants with HIE. These include fluid restriction, prophylactic phenobarbital, oxygen free radical scavengers or antagonists, excitatory amino acid antagonists, nitric oxide synthase antagonists, calcium channel blockers, magnesium, N-methyl-D-aspartate (NMDA) receptor blockers, strategies to reduce cerebral edema (dexamethasone, furosemide, hyperventilation, and mannitol), and hypothermia. Despite some initially promising results with some of these strategies (mostly in experimental animals), only hypothermia appears to be a safe and effective intervention.[5,6]

Interest in cooling the whole body or a body part dates back millennia; however, it was not until the late 1940s that Miller and colleagues,[7] made the observation that newborn animals tolerated anoxia longer if their body temperature was reduced. Between 1959 and 1972, 288 term or near-term infants were cooled as an adjunct to standard resuscitation.[8] Infants who were not breathing spontaneously 5 minutes after birth were immersed in cold water until respiration resumed and then allowed to slowly spontaneously rewarm. Although mortality was reduced, there was no systematic

Department of Pediatrics, College of Physicians and Surgeons, Columbia University, 630 W. 168th Street, New York, NY 10032, USA
* Corresponding author.
E-mail address: rs62@columbia.edu (R. Sahni).

Clin Perinatol 35 (2008) 717–734
doi:10.1016/j.clp.2008.07.016
perinatology.theclinics.com

neurologic follow-up of cooled infants compared with a control group. Clinical interest in cooling infants diminished as reports associated mild hypothermia with increased oxygen requirement and greater mortality in preterm infants <1500 g,[9] and the disappointing outcome of delayed cooling after near drowning.[10] More recently, experiments have found that reduction in brain temperature of 2 °C to 5 °C applied after perinatal hypoxia–ischemia can improve neuropathologic,[11–15] cerebral energetic,[16,17] electrophysiologic,[13,18] and functional outcomes.[14] In 1998, Gunn and colleagues,[19] showed the safety of prolonged hypothermia in a study of 22 newborns. To date, only three randomized clinical trials (RCTs) of therapeutic hypothermia in the neonate have been published;[20–22] however, several more trials are underway. This article reviews the rationale for therapeutic hypothermia and the current status of hypothermic neuroprotection in the treatment of infants with HIE.

PATHOGENESIS AND PHASES OF HYPOXIC ISCHEMIC ENCEPHALOPATHY

Impaired cerebral blood flow (CBF) is the principal pathogenetic mechanism underlying most of the neuropathology attributed to intrapartum hypoxia–ischemia.[23] The alteration in CBF most likely occurs as a consequence of interruption in placental blood flow and gas exchange that may be acute or intermittent.[24] The fetal circulatory and noncirculatory adaptive responses preserve cerebral perfusion and thus oxygen delivery. However, when the disruption is severe or the adaptive mechanisms fail, neuronal cell death follows. The degree of CBF impairment caused by this insult dictates the timing and mode of cell death as well as the ensuing degree and type of brain injury. This brain injury may occur in two phases: during the acute insult and during a recovery period after restoration in circulation termed *reperfusion injury*. The pathophysiology of HIE begins with the initial hypoxic–ischemic insult and unfolds throughout the infant's recovery period. Disrupted CBF leads in sequence to the phase of primary energy failure, the immediate reperfusion period, the latent phase, and, finally, the secondary phase of energy failure (**Fig. 1**).

The initial response of the fetus to a hypoxic–ischemic event is preservation of CBF by increased cerebral vasodilation (secondary to hypercapnia and hypoxemia), loss of cerebral autoregulation, and redistribution of organ blood flow. Increased CBF, however, is quickly superseded by impairment in CBF, with concomitant bradycardia and decreased blood pressure.[25]

At the cellular level, the disruption of CBF leads to a primary energy failure, and the activation of cell death processes.[26] Energy failure induced by severe, acute asphyxia rapidly results in neuronal death via necrosis, characterized by plasma membrane swelling and rupture, which releases intracellular toxins into the local milieu. In contrast, energy loss after less severe or prolonged hypoxic–ischemic insult leads to apoptosis, a slower form of neuronal death often described as cell suicide.[27]

During primary phase energy failure, decreased levels of high-energy phosphate compounds, such as phosphocreatine (PCr), the principal storage form of high-energy phosphate, and adenosine triphosphate (ATP), promote mitochondrial dysfunction (**Fig. 2**). Under healthy conditions, the cell's ATP is mitochondrially generated via oxidative phosphorylation, which is tightly coupled to glucose metabolism. However, after energy failure, ATP production relies primarily on anaerobic glycolysis.[28] A critical function of ATP is to maintain sodium (Na^+), potassium (K^+), and calcium (Ca^{2+}) ionic gradients across membranes.[29] After ATP loss, K^+ leaks out of the affected cell, inducing depolarization and a massive release of glutamate, an excitatory amino acid.[30] Glutamate accumulates in the proximal synapses partly because of decreased glutamate removal from the synapses by ATP-dependent glial glutamate

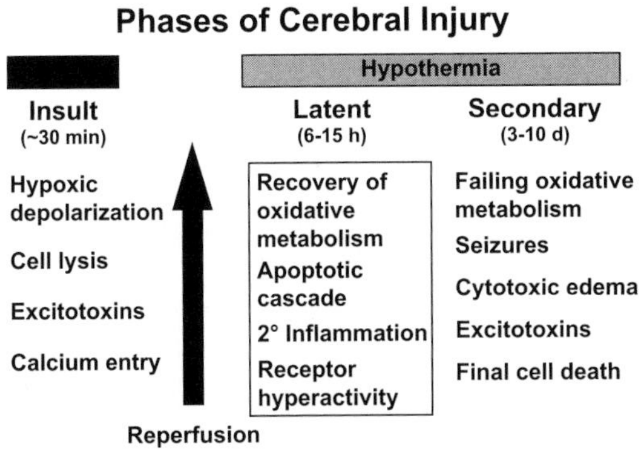

Phases of Cerebral Injury

Hypothermia

Insult (~30 min)
Hypoxic depolarization
Cell lysis
Excitotoxins
Calcium entry

Reperfusion

Latent (6-15 h)
Recovery of oxidative metabolism
Apoptotic cascade
2° Inflammation
Receptor hyperactivity

Secondary (3-10 d)
Failing oxidative metabolism
Seizures
Cytotoxic edema
Excitotoxins
Final cell death

Fig. 1. Flow diagram shows the relationship between the phases of cerebral injury after a severe but reversible period of hypoxia–ischemia. During reperfusion after the insult, there is a period of approximately 30 to 60 minutes during which cellular energy metabolism is restored, with progressive resolution of the acute cell swelling secondary to hypoxic depolarization. This is followed by a latent phase, during which oxidative metabolism has normalized, but there is hyperactivity of glutaminergic receptors, the intracytoplasmic components of the apoptotic cascade are activated, and the secondary inflammatory reaction is initiated. This may be followed by secondary deterioration leading to ultimate delayed neuronal death after 3 days. As indicated by the bar, treatment with cerebral hypothermia needs to be initiated as early as possible in the latent phase before the onset of secondary deterioration, and then continued for more than 48 hours for long lasting neuroprotection. (*From* Gunn AJ, Gluckman PD. Head cooling for neonatal encephalopathy: the state of the art. Clin Obstet Gynecol 2007;50(3):636–51; with permission.)

transporters.[31] The accumulated glutamate overstimulates the NMDA receptors resulting in a rapid influx of Ca^{2+} into the intracellular space. The type of cell death that follows excessive Ca^{2+} influx is concentration dependent; necrosis requires higher levels of intracellular Ca^{2+} than apoptosis.[32] Thus, through this glutamate-mediated

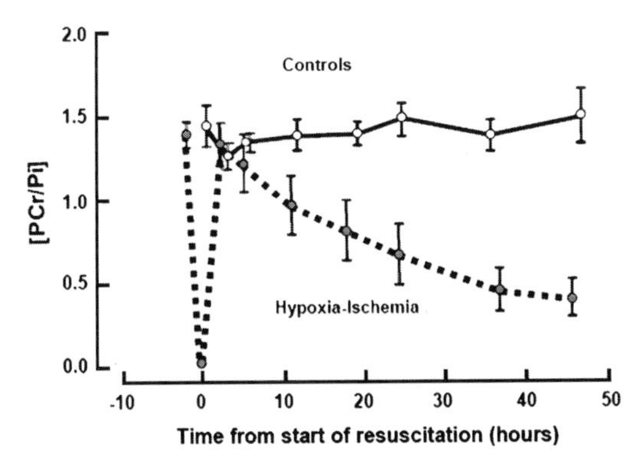

Fig. 2. The ratio of phosphocreatine (PCr), the principle storage form of high-energy phosphate to monophosphate after hypoxic-ischemic injury. Phosphocreatine levels precipitously decrease immediately after the hypoxic–ischemic event. After resuscitation, levels are comparable to those of the controls. However, throughout the neonate's recovery period, levels decrease gradually, indicative of the secondary energy failure. (*From* Lorek A, Takei Y, Cady EB, et al. Delayed ("secondary") cerebral energy failure after acute hypoxia-ischemia in the newborn piglet: continuous 48-hour studies by phosphorus magnetic resonance spectroscopy. Pediatr Res 1994;36:699–706; with permission.)

neurodegenerative process, primary energy failure can activate cell death pathways before restoration of CBF.

The return of CBF demarcates the immediate reperfusion period. This period is characterized by normal blood pressure and intracellular pH, a transient improvement in cytotoxic edema, and an absence of seizures.[33,34] Experimental animal models suggest that the immediate reperfusion period rapidly transitions into the latent phase during which electroencephalogram (EEG) intensity is depressed. Within the cell, mitochondrial metabolism is nearly restored.[13,35]

Neuroprotective strategies are most effective if implemented during the first 6 hours after reperfusion.[33,36] After this temporal window, however, the affected infant experiences a second phase of energy failure.[33] Once again, levels of ATP as well as PCr decrease, whereas cytotoxic edema increases.[34,37] Unlike the primary phase energy failure, intracellular pH remains unchanged, and the infant's cardiorespiratory status is usually stable.[37]

The cellular response to secondary phase energy failure is similar to that of the primary phase energy failure in that excitatory amino acids are released from cells, leading to necrotic and apoptotic cell death. Much of the cell death is delayed, occurring slowly (hours to days) during the infant's recovery period.[38] The severity of the secondary phase energy failure is strongly correlated with adverse neurodevelopmental outcomes at 1 and 4 years of age.[39] CBF increases during the phase of secondary energy failure, and the infant begins to experience seizures.[33] In general, early seizures prognosticate poor long-term neurodevelopmental outcome.

NEUROPROTECTION AND HYPOTHERMIA

Pharmacology of Neuroprotection with Hypothermia

Modest systemic or selective hypothermia of the brain by as little as 2 °C to 4 °C has been shown to reduce the extent of tissue injury in experimental as well as human studies after events such as stroke, trauma, or cardiac arrest.[40–50] Before initiating hypothermia as a treatment strategy in newborn infants with HIE, several factors determining effective neuroprotection with hypothermia need to be considered: duration of therapy (brief versus prolonged), timing for initiation of therapy, degree of cooling, and method of achieving hypothermia.

Duration of therapy: brief versus prolonged

Brief periods (0.5–3 hours) of mild to moderate hypothermia immediately after hypoxic–ischemic injury results in only partial or temporary neuroprotection in most experimental animals.[13,40–48] Findings suggest that such brief cooling may be most effective only after relatively mild insults.[51–53] Prolonging hypothermia from 24 to 72 hours after hypoxia–ischemia attenuates brain damage and improves behavioral performance.[13,44,48] More critically, this protection appears to be lost if hypothermia is delayed by as little as 15 to 45 minutes after the primary insult.[54–56] Such an extreme sensitivity to delay is consistent with the hypothesis that hypothermia might act to suppress reperfusion injury.[57] Alternatively, this strategy may effectively represent intervention at the end of the primary phase of energy failure, when cerebrovascular perfusion is being re-established, and cell function is starting to recover.[13] A more recent approach has been to try to suppress the secondary encephalopathic processes by maintaining hypothermia throughout the course of the secondary phase of energy failure. Supporting this concept, extended periods of cooling, of between 5 and 72 hours, appear to be more consistently effective.[12,16,53,58,59]

Timing for initiation of therapy

The sooner hypothermia can be initiated, the more likely it is to be successful. Hypothermia is most effective when administered during the latent phase of the injury, before the onset of the secondary phase of energy failure.[60] Short durations of cooling are associated with extreme sensitivity to delay. In contrast, extended periods of hypothermia may be effective after significant delays between the primary insult and the start of cooling. Moderate selective cerebral hypothermia initiated within 90 minutes and continued until 72 hours after ischemia has been shown to prevent secondary cytotoxic edema and improve electroencephalographic recovery in the fetal sheep.[13] There was also concomitant substantial reduction in parasagittal cortical infarction and improvement in neuronal loss scores in all regions assessed. Though markedly reduced, significant neuroprotection was still observed when the delay was extended to 5.5 hours.[44] Data from various adult models also support this hypothermia-induced neuroprotective concept.[40,42,43] These studies performed at various stages of maturation in a range of species strongly support several conclusions. First, that a sufficient duration of cooling is required in relation to the type and severity of the primary insult, suggesting that such delayed cooling is acting via sustained suppression of cytotoxic events in the secondary phase of energy failure. Second, that although the window of opportunity for prolonged cooling after global insults (or reversible focal injury) may be up to 6 hours or even longer in some circumstances, the degree of neuroprotection progressively declines if cooling is initiated more than a few hours after insult.

Degree of cooling

Moderate hypothermia at brain temperatures of 32 °C to 34 °C initiated immediately or within a few hours after reperfusion and continued for 24 to 72 hours has been shown to favorably affect outcome in newborn and adult animals.[13,44] It is highly likely that there is a critical depth of hypothermia required for effective neuronal rescue. In turn, the required threshold may be modified by the severity of the initial insult, how soon hypothermia is started after the insult, and how long cooling is continued.[52,53,59] There is an obvious trade-off between the adverse systemic effects of cooling, which increase markedly below a core temperature of 32 °C to 34 °C, and the potential cerebral benefit. The potential systemic adverse effects of hypothermia in newborn infants include increased mortality; particularly in preterm infants, hypoglycemia; reduction of cardiac contractility and cardiac output; sinus bradycardia; hypotension; ventilation-perfusion mismatch; increased blood viscosity; coagulopathy; acid, base, and electrolyte imbalance; and an increased risk of infections.[48,61]

Method of achieving hypothermia

Selective brain cooling is attractive, because it can provide adequate neuroprotection with minimal risk of systemic adverse effects, but it is associated with differential gradients within the brain.[62] In contrast, total body cooling is more likely to be associated with adverse effects but causes fewer gradients within the brain. In a small, observational study, Rutherford and colleagues,[63] have recently reported a decreased incidence of severe cortical lesions on magnetic resonance imaging in infants treated with selective head cooling and modest systemic hypothermia compared with those with whole-body cooling.

Protective Mechanisms

Moderate (35.5 °C) and profound (21 °C and 28 °C) hypothermia maintained during the hypoxic–ischemic insult results in absence of histologic injury and preservation of motor function.[42,47,64–66] Postischemic hypothermia is also neuroprotective through the reduction of secondary cortical cytotoxic edema, cortical infarction, and neuronal loss.[13–15,17,67] The most important target for hypothermia is the reduction in cerebral energy metabolism. Cooling the brain during hypoxia–ischemia ameliorates the change in energy metabolites resulting in less brain damage.[64] A potential mechanism for preservation of energy metabolites is a decrease in brain energy use rate and consequent preservation of brain ATP levels.[68] The neuroprotection afforded by hypothermia may be through the inhibition of apoptosis;[11,69] studies have found a reduction in caspase-3 like activity and a reduction in the phosphorylation of Akt.[70,71] Hypothermia has also been shown to inhibit glutamate release,[72,73] preserve endogenous antioxidants and reduce nitric oxide production,[73] decrease free radical production,[57,74] improve protein synthesis,[75] preserve N-acetylaspartate, and reduce glutathione levels.[76]

Clinical Trials

Pilot trials

Although Westin and colleagues,[77] first reported the beneficial effects of hypothermia in perinatal asphyxia in 1955, only in the last decade have systematic studies been performed to address the efficacy and safety of hypothermia in HIE.[19,78–81] These studies described the methodology for cooling the head or the whole body for up to 72 hours without serious short-term complications. The results from these studies showed that although bradycardia occurred commonly, other acute complications did not occur with mild hypothermia for 72 hours. In a multicenter, randomized, controlled, pilot trial of whole-body cooling to a rectal temperature of 33 °C $\pm$ 0.5 °C for 48 hours in neonates (n = 65) after a hypoxic–ischemic event, Eicher and colleagues,[20] reported a lower combined outcome of death or severe neuromotor disability in the hypothermia group (52%) than in the normothermia group (84%). The mortality rate was 31% in those treated with hypothermia compared with 42% in the controls. There was higher incidence of bradycardia and greater use of inotropic agents in the hypothermia group compared with the control subjects. The cumulative evidence from the numerous animal studies and reassuring results of short-term safety and feasibility studies in human infants with HIE fostered the development of larger RCTs.

Large-scale clinical trials

Two large randomized, multicenter trials in term infants with HIE, using either selective or systemic modest hypothermia have recently been completed. The first study (Cool-Cap Trial)[21] used selective head cooling and mild systemic hypothermia and included 234 infants with moderate to severe neonatal encephalopathy and abnormal amplitude-integrated electroencephalogram (aEEG). The stepwise biochemical/clinical, neurologic, and electroencephalography (EEG) criteria for entry were as follows: >36 weeks' gestation; an Apgar score <5 at 10 minutes after birth or a continued need for resuscitation at 10 minutes after birth; or a pH < 7.0 or base deficit >16 mmol/L in the umbilical blood or venous blood sample within 60 minutes of birth; and a modified Sarnat score and aEEG criteria consistent with a diagnosis of moderate to severe HIE. Infants were randomly selected to head cooling and mild systemic hypothermia (rectal temperature 34–35 °C) or normothermia for 72 hours and were then rewarmed at a rate of <0.5 °C per hour over a period of 4 hours. The primary outcome was death or severe disability at 18 months. Of the 218 infants (93%), 66% of the controls and 55% of the cooled infants had an unfavorable primary outcome (odds ratio, 0.61; 95% CI, 0.32–1.09; *P* = .1). A logistic regression analysis controlling for baseline aEEG severity, presence of seizures, and age at randomization indicated a possible treatment effect from hypothermia (odds ratio, 0.57; 95% CI, 0.32–1.01; *P* = .05). There were no differences in frequency of clinically important complications.

In a predefined subgroup analysis, head cooling was beneficial to those with less severe prerandomization aEEG changes (n = 172; odds ratio, 0.42; 95% CI, 0.22–0.80; *P* = .009) compared with those with severe changes (n = 46). On further post hoc analysis, when baseline clinical severity was added to the regression model, a significant protective effect from hypothermia was observed for the entire cohort (odds ratio 0.52, 95% CI, 0.28–0.70; *P* = .04).[21]

In the second large randomized controlled clinical trial, performed in the National Institute of Child Health and Human Development (NICHD) Neonatal Research Network Centers, Shankaran and colleagues,[22] tested the effect of whole-body hypothermia in moderate to severe HIE. The study enrolled 208 infants ≥36 weeks' gestation, admitted to a neonatal intensive care unit at <6 hours of age, with either a diagnosis of encephalopathy or poor respiratory effort at birth requiring resuscitation. Eligibility criteria were similar to those in the CoolCap Trial and included a pH of 7.0 or less or a base deficit of 16 mmol/L or more in a sample of umbilical cord blood or any blood during the first hour after birth. If, during this interval, the pH was between 7.01 and 7.15, a base deficit was between 10 and 15.9 mmol/L, or a blood gas level was not available, the presence of additional criteria could qualify the patient for consideration. These additional criteria included the existence of an acute perinatal event (like late or variable decelerations, cord rupture, cord prolapse, uterine rupture, maternal trauma, hemorrhage, or cardiorespiratory arrest) and either a 10-minute Apgar score of <5 or assisted ventilation initiated at birth and continued for at least 10 minutes. Once these criteria were met, all infants underwent a standardized neurologic evaluation performed by a certified examiner. Infants were eligible candidates when seizures or moderate or severe encephalopathy was present; no aEEG was used. Infants randomly selected to undergo whole-body hypothermia (n = 102) were placed on a precooled blanket (5 °C) connected to a cooling system, and the esophageal temperature was reduced to and maintained at 33.5 °C ± 0.5 °C for 72 hours followed by slow rewarming by on-site research personnel using the Cincinnati Sub-Zero System, while the control infants (n = 106) were given standard intensive care. The primary outcome was a combined end point of death or moderate to severe disability at 18 to 22 months of age. Of the 205 infants (98%), those who underwent hypothermia had significantly lower incidence of death or moderate/severe disability at 18 months (44% vs 66%; relative risk, 0.72; 95% CI, 0.54–0.95; *P* = .01), indicating six infants need to be treated on average to result in one additional infant with a better outcome. There were no differences between the two groups in the incidence of mortality alone, disabling cerebral palsy, blindness, severe hearing impairment, and Bayley Mental Development Index or Psychomotor Development Index scores.

Taken together, the remarkably similar effect sizes in the above RCTs strongly suggest that induced hypothermia is associated with a significant reduction in death or disability. Edwards and Azzopardi,[82] in a recent speculative meta-analysis of these three studies, [20–22] have reported an overall rate of death or disability in 118 of 237 infants treated with hypothermia compared with 158 of 241 normothermic infants, giving a relative risk (RR) of 0.76 (0.65–0.89), *P* = .001, that is, a 24% reduction in risk, with a number needed to treat of six (**Fig. 3**). There is a potential of achieving relatively greater improvements if the therapy with hypothermia can be targeted more effectively.

Other ongoing trials

In the Total Body Cooling Trial (TOBY) from England, infants with moderate-to-severe HIE were randomly assigned to receive whole-body cooling or standard intensive care. This multicenter trial has enrolled 325 infants between December 2002 and

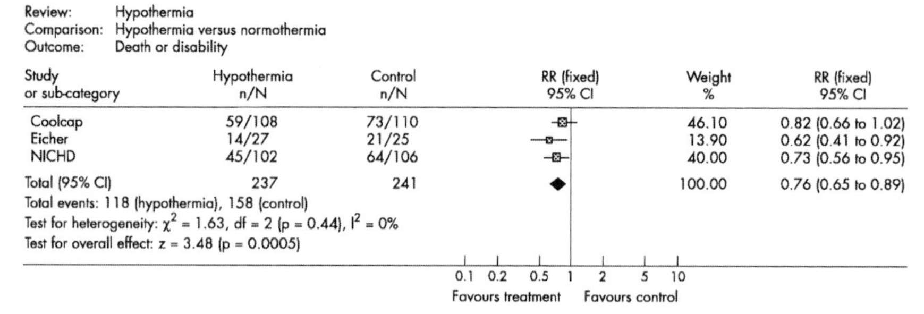

Fig. 3. Speculative meta-analysis of the effect of mild hypothermia on death or disability after perinatal asphyxia. The CoolCap study used selective head cooling with systemic cooling to 34.5 °C for 72 hours, and outcome assessed as death or severe disability at 18 months;[21] the Eicher trial was a pilot study of whole-body cooling to 33 °C for 48 hours with outcome assessed at 12 months;[20] and the NICHD trial used whole-body cooling to 33.5 °C for 72 hours with assessment of death or moderate or severe disability at 18 months.[22] (*From* Edwards AD, Azzopardi DV. Therapeutic hypothermia following perinatal asphyxia. Arch Dis Child Fetal Neonatal Ed 2006;91:F127–31; with permission.).

November 2006, and currently the outcomes at 18 months are being assessed.[83] Because the entry criteria for this trial were similar to those of the CoolCap trial, the findings from the TOBY trial can be effectively compared with those of CoolCap to assess the relative benefits from whole-body versus selective head cooling in HIE. The ICE (Infant Cooling Evaluation) aimed to enroll 276 infants from a wide geographic region (19 centers in Australia, Canada, the United States, and New Zealand) using simplified protocols.[84,85] Hypothermia in this trial was achieved by turning off the ambient heating systems and by applying "Hot-Cold" gel packs (at 10 °C) under the infant's head, back, or across the chest, so that the rectal temperature was maintained between 33 °C and 34 °C The results from the ICE trial are likely to be more generalizable than those in currently published trials.[84] In addition, they will provide information on the feasibility and safety of a pragmatic approach to whole-body cooling during transport.

Current Controversies and Unanswered Questions

Is hypothermia safe in infants with hypoxic-ischemic encephalopathy?

Cold-injury syndrome, a potential complication of therapeutic hypothermia, can result in sclerema, hypovolemia, glucose instability, pulmonary hypertension, and multisystem organ damage (especially pulmonary hemorrhage, renal failure, and disseminated intravascular coagulopathy).[86,87] The safety of mild hypothermia in HIE is well established, as no serious adverse safety issues have been reported to date in both the initial pilot trials and the RCTs.[19–22,78–81,84,88,89] However, all trials noted reversible cardiovascular effects, specifically sinus bradycardia and hypotension. Thoresen and Whitelaw reported that some concurrent medications exacerbated adverse cardiovascular effects during both cooling and rewarming in an early pilot study.[61] Gluckman and colleagues,[21] reported elevated liver enzymes, and Eicher and colleagues,[81] noted an increase in late coagulopathy (several days after rewarming) and more persistent pulmonary hypertension that required inhaled nitric oxide treatment in the hypothermia-treated infants.

Effective therapeutic window—how late is too late?

The effective therapeutic window of opportunity for initiation of hypothermia, or any other potential therapy, is not clearly defined. The experimental treatment studies used very carefully standardized insults, occurring at a precisely known time. In contrast, the precipitating insult in neonatal encephalopathy is a well-defined sentinel event, such as placental abruption that is terminated at birth, in only approximately 25% of cases.[90] In other cases, the preceding insults seem to evolve over hours during labor, and, in at least some cases, perhaps 10% of the total, the infants seem to have been compromised even before the onset of labor.[90] Thus, it is very likely that the effective window of opportunity to initiate hypothermia treatment for HIE, in some cases, may be somewhat less than suggested experimentally. The two large RCTs were unable to determine the effect of time of initiation on outcome, perhaps because cooling of most infants was started relatively late in the time window in both trials, between 4 and 5 hours after birth.[21,22] However, there are no human data to support efficacy of hypothermia initiated more than 6 hours after birth. Because mild hypothermia does not significantly suppress aEEG activity, it may be that future treatment could be initiated more rapidly for outborn infants by delaying aEEG evaluation after cooling has been started and then either continuing or withdrawing therapy once that information is available. Moreover, because mild hypothermia is relatively safe, one could argue that a liberal interpretation of this window is reasonable until more information becomes available.

How to select infants most likely to benefit?

Data from RCTs suggest that neuroprotection with hypothermia as currently used is only partial, and many patients die of neural injury or survive with disability despite hypothermia.[21,50] Given the underlying pathophysiology of HIE, it may be impossible to rescue the brains of all affected infants. Hence, one would like to identify the potentially treatable case in advance, to target treatment to those who are most likely to benefit and avoid offering false hope. Post hoc analysis from the CoolCap trial[21] and the NICHD body cooling trial[22] indicate that although clinical evaluation of the severity of encephalopathy using modified Sarnat criteria was highly predictive of the risk of death or disability, the relative improvement after hypothermia treatment was remarkably similar for infants with moderate and severe encephalopathy. Data from the NICHD body cooling trial has been examined further to determine whether there were clinical and laboratory variables available within 6 hours of birth that could be incorporated into either a scoring scheme or a decision tree scheme to determine which infants were likely to benefit from cooling and which would not.[91] Although both approaches identify score ranges of infants who are unlikely to benefit from hypothermia, very few infants (2%–3%) had such scores. Thus, the authors do not recommend using these scoring systems as a tool for excluding infants from hypothermic intervention until these approaches are validated prospectively. Similarly, the investigators from the CoolCap trial do not advocate use of aEEG criteria to exclude infants from cooling.[1] Currently, the best that can be said, based on common sense and consistency with clinical trial protocols, is that the hypothermia treatment should not be offered to infants judged to be in extremis. Future clinical and experimental studies will likely identify components of clinical examination, biochemical tests, or electrophysiological patterns that might be more predictive of timing of HIE, rather than severity, and response to hypothermia treatment.

What is the most appropriate target temperature?

It is highly likely that there is a critical depth of hypothermia required for effective neuronal rescue. Despite the experimental evidence that moderate hypothermia at brain temperatures of 32 °C to 34 °C initiated immediately or within a few hours after reperfusion and continued for 24 to 72 hours favorably affect outcome in newborn and adult animals,[13,44] there is uncertainty about the precise temperature reduction that provides most optimal neuroprotection. Furthermore, it is also unclear whether different regions or cell types in the brain are protected uniformly by similar reduction in temperature. Experimental data suggest that 5 °C of cooling is superior than a reduction of 3 °C (comparable to a rectal temperature of 32 °C vs 34 °C in humans).[92] Clinical trials of hypothermia down to a target esophageal temperature of around 33.5 °C have been relatively safe, but some clinical side effects have been suggested by studies using lower temperatures.[81] These data suggest that currently the upper extreme of the ideal temperature range is being targeted and that a slightly increased degree of hypothermia may provide greater neuroprotection. Further, selective head cooling using slightly lower temperature than the current target ranges may result in deeper cooling of the cortex compared with other areas of the brain. Only clinical trials of deeper systemic cooling can help to resolve these issues.

Should an electroencephalogram be used in identifying infants suitable for hypothermic neuroprotection?

The CoolCap study protocol recommends aEEG as an additional selection criterion for identification of infants eligible for hypothermic neuroprotection.[21] However, it is not known whether this improves the specificity of selecting infants at risk for significant hypoxic–ischemic brain injury and those that may benefit from hypothermia. Sarkar and colleagues[93] recently reported poor correlation between aEEG obtained shortly after perinatal HIE and short-term adverse outcomes, with a sensitivity of 54.8% and negative predictive value of only 44%. Moreover, artifacts on a raw EEG may also influence the correct interpretation of aEEG. With the advent of new digital monitors that simultaneously display raw EEG and aEEG, artifacts caused by movement or electrical interference have been noted to occur in as many as 12% of the aEEG recordings.[94] Both types of artifacts influence the voltage and width of the aEEG band. Thus, if an abnormal aEEG is used as a prerequisite for qualifying for hypothermia, some infants who could potentially benefit from this therapy would be excluded. Therefore, not only should aEEG be used with caution as a screening tool in selecting candidates for neuroprotective interventions, but it is essential to examine the underlying raw EEG for artifacts at the beginning of a recording or when there is a sudden change in the appearance of the aEEG trace.

Is head cooling better than whole-body cooling?

Ideally, for adequate neuroprotection with minimal risk of systemic adverse effects in unstable and sick infants, only the brain should be cooled. This approach has been well accomplished in animals with relatively smaller heads,[95] but is difficult to achieve in human infants. However, selective head cooling can be achieved using a cooling cap over the scalp while the body is warmed by an overhead warmer to limit the degree of systemic hypothermia, as demonstrated by the CoolCap trial.[21] Moreover, the mild systemic hypothermia is desirable during selective head cooling, as it helps in preventing scalp edema or injury from excessively cold cap temperatures[88] and provides some degree of cooling for deeper cerebral structures such as brain stem.[62] Recent data from studies in piglets have shown that head cooling is associated with considerable and sustained decrease in deep intracerebral temperature at the level of the basal ganglia compared with the rectal temperature.[96] It is difficult to make a distinction whether head cooling is superior to whole-body cooling in humans based on the results of hypothermia RCTs because the overall effect sizes were similar.[21,22] Interestingly, recent short-term recovery studies in the piglets suggest that the optimal degree of cooling needed for neuroprotection may be greater in the cortex than in the basal ganglia.[97] Given that during head cooling of the piglet there was an approximately 6 °C gradient between the superficial and deep brain, whereas whole-body cooling resulted in less than 0.6 °C difference between the warmest (basal ganglia) and the coldest parts of the brain (the cortex), it is possible that head cooling may provide a more effective balance of cooling to these structures than whole-body cooling. As a result, a relatively better protective effect in the cortex would be provided, with better preservation of cognitive function. As mentioned earlier, in a small, observational study, Rutherford and colleagues[63] have recently reported a decreased incidence of severe cortical lesions on magnetic resonance imaging in infants treated with selective head cooling and modest systemic hypothermia compared with those with whole-body cooling. Also, both modes of hypothermia were associated with a decrease in basal ganglia and thalamic lesions that were significant in infants with a moderate aEEG finding but not in those with a severe aEEG finding.[63] These data suggest that infants treated with selective head cooling may benefit more in long-term cognitive rather than motor function compared with those with whole-body cooling.

Does hypothermia affect long-term neurodevelopmental outcomes?

The long-term effects of hypothermia as a neuroprotective therapy for HIE at school age and later are not yet known. Furthermore, whether cortical cooling with head cooling results in better cognitive outcomes or whether more consistent brainstem cooling with the whole body approach is associated with reduced neuromotor dysfunction also remains unknown. Participants at a recent NICHD workshop suggested that if therapeutic hypothermia is to be implemented outside of an RCT, clinicians should follow published protocols, ensure systematic follow-up of survivors using validated neurodevelopmental tests, and preferably submit information on patient data to national or international registries.[98] This approach will help answer some of the above questions and allow for continued refinement in the therapy. The age of follow-up for infants enrolled in hypothermia trials is a critical issue in evaluating the efficacy of these therapies. In all the recent hypothermia trials, the primary outcome of death or disability was examined at 18 months of age, the earliest age at which major disability can be ruled out with a high level of confidence. For assessments of effects beyond 18 months, it is necessary to evaluate the relationship of intervention to early childhood outcome, because hypothermia may influence not only major neurologic sequelae detected at 18 months, but also potential sequelae of brain injury in childhood.[3,99] Further, the relationship between the degree of cooling in hypothermia trials and outcome may be discernable only on detailed evaluations of cognitive, executive, and fine motor ability beyond 18 months of age. These evaluations should include behavior, learning, fine motor development, executive function and attention, and psychosocial outcomes. Moreover, the differences in efficacy between selective head cooling and whole body cooling may only be discernable after careful evaluation of deep brain function, as deep brain temperatures have less fluctuation and are more easily achievable with whole body cooling compared with selective head cooling.[62] The CoolCap and the NICHD Neonatal Research Network is currently evaluating subjects between 6 and 7 years of age. One may still have concerns as to whether the benefits of cooling will be evident when the current study subjects reach school age, as these trials were not powered to address those issues.

Should hypothermia be the standard of care for infants with hypoxic-ischemic encephalopathy?

Various national bodies have declared that hypothermia should still be considered experimental until the results of current ongoing trials and information on long-term follow-up of survivors are available.[98,100–102] Others may argue that although many additional questions about how hypothermia should be used need to be addressed, its basic efficacy is now well established. They suggest that even if at one extreme there was no apparent effect of cooling among the next 400 children to be randomly selected, then the cumulative meta-analysis would continue to show a significant overall effect (RR 0.85, 95% CI 0.76–0.96, $P = .01$).[103] Given the high probability of adverse outcome with HIE and no other therapy currently available (along with the evidence for benefit from current meta-analyses, the remarkable safety profile, the strong foundation in basic science, and supporting evidence from related disease states such as encephalopathy after cardiac arrest) it may be unethical not to offer hypothermia treatment to infants with HIE.[104]

FUTURE DIRECTIONS

HIE remains a challenging problem for clinicians. Currently, hypothermia is the only intervention that shows promise in improving neurologic outcome in full-term newborn infants after HIE. One in six babies will garner some benefit from this treatment, especially those with milder degrees of encephalopathy. However, for infants with severe HIE, outcome remains bleak despite cooling.

As our understanding of the mechanism of hypoxic–ischemic brain injury has evolved, a variety of neuroprotective strategies have emerged targeting the different pathways leading to cell death. Extensive experimental data from both adult and neonatal animals strongly support the use of pharmacologic agents with postischemic hypothermia in ameliorating brain injury. Some of the candidate agents for improving neuroprotection in combination with hypothermia include N-acetylcysteine, a glutathione precursor and a potent free radical scavenger;[105,106] allopurinol, an antioxidant that inhibits xanthine oxidase and scavenges hydroxyl free radicals;[107–109] erythropoietin, an endogenous cytokine with neuroprotective role in high doses;[110–112] deferoxamine, an iron-chelating agent that reduces the formation of free radicals;[109,113,114] topiramate, a broad-spectrum anticonvulsant;[115,116] xenon, a noble gas with anesthetic properties; N-methyl-D-aspartate receptor antagonist;[117,118] and a variety of caspase inhibitors believed to play a role in apoptotic cell death.[70,119,120]

The outcome data from the above studies is heartening and it is hoped that the beneficial effects observed in animal models will be translated successfully into human studies. To date, human therapeutic experience with any of these agents is limited except for allopurinol. The focus of ongoing research should be directed at establishing safety profiles and optimal treatment regimens; studies should be conducted on appropriate animal models whose brain development and pattern of neuronal injury is similar to that of a newborn human infant. We are entering an era in which hypothermia will be used in combination with other novel neuroprotective interventions. The targeting of multiple sites in the cascade leading to brain injury may prove to be a more effective treatment strategy after HIE in newborn infants than hypothermia alone.

REFERENCES

1. Wyatt JS, Gluckman PD, Liu PY, et al. Determinants of outcomes after head cooling for neonatal encephalopathy. Pediatrics 2007;119:912–21.
2. Dixon G, Badawi N, Kurinczuk JJ, et al. Early developmental outcomes after newborn encephalopathy. Pediatrics 2002;109:26–33.
3. Robertson CM, Finer NN, Grace MG. School performance of survivors of neonatal encephalopathy associated with birth asphyxia at term. J Pediatr 1989;114:753–60.

4. Kattwinkel J, editor. Textbook of neonatal resuscitation. 5th edition. American Academy of Pediatrics/American Heart Association; 2006.
5. Vannucci RC, Perlman JM. Interventions for perinatal hypoxic-ischemic encephalopathy. Pediatrics 1997;100:1004–14.
6. Volpe J. Neurology of the newborn. 4th edition. Philadelphia: W.B. Saunders Company; 2001.
7. Miller JA. Factors in neonatal resistance to anoxia. I. Temperature and survival of newborn guinea pigs under anoxia. Science 1949;110:113–4.
8. Miller JA Jr, Miller FS, Westin B. Hypothermia in the treatment of asphyxia neonatorum. Biol Neonat 1964;20:148–63.
9. Silverman WA, Sinclair JC. Temperature regulation in the newborn infant. N Engl J Med 1966;274:146–8.
10. Bohn DJ, Biggar WD, Smith CR, et al. Influence of hypothermia, barbiturate therapy, and intracranial pressure monitoring on morbidity and mortality after near-drowning. Crit Care Med 1986;14:529–34.
11. Edwards AD, Yue X, Squier MV, et al. Specific inhibition of apoptosis after cerebral hypoxia-ischaemia by moderate post-insult hypothermia. Biochem Biophys Res Commun 1995;217:1193–9.
12. Sirimanne ES, Blumberg RM, Bossano D, et al. The effect of prolonged modification of cerebral temperature on outcome following hypoxic ischemic injury in the infant rat. Pediatr Res 1996;39:591–7.
13. Gunn AJ, Gunn TR, de Haan HH, et al. Dramatic neuronal rescue with prolonged selective head cooling after ischemia in fetal lambs. J Clin Invest 1997;99:248–56.
14. Bona E, Hagberg H, Loberg EM, et al. Protective effects of moderate hypothermia after neonatal hypoxia-ischemia: short- and long-term outcome. Pediatr Res 1998;43:738–45.
15. Tooley JR, Satas S, Porter H, et al. Head cooling with mild systemic hypothermia in anesthetized piglets is neuroprotective. Ann Neurol 2003;53:65–72.
16. Thoresen M, Penrice J, Lorek A, et al. Mild hypothermia after severe transient hypoxia-ischemia ameliorates delayed cerebral energy failure in the newborn piglet. Pediatr Res 1995;37:667–70.
17. Wagner BP, Nedelcu J, Martin E. Delayed postischemic hypothermia improves long-term behavioral outcome after cerebral hypoxia-ischemia in neonatal rats. Pediatr Res 2002;51:354–60.
18. Gunn AJ. Cerebral hypothermia for prevention of brain injury following perinatal asphyxia. Curr Opin Pediatr 2000;12:111–5.
19. Gunn AJ, Gluckman PD, Gunn TR. Selective head cooling in newborn infants after perinatal asphyxia: a safety study. Pediatrics 1998;102:885–92.
20. Eicher DJ, Wagner CL, Katikaneni LP, et al. Moderate hypothermia in neonatal encephalopathy: efficacy outcomes. Pediatr Neurol 2005;32:11–7.
21. Gluckman PD, Wyatt JS, Azzopardi D, et al. Selective head cooling with mild systemic hypothermia after neonatal encephalopathy multicenter randomized trial. Lancet 2005;365:663–70.
22. Shankaran S, Laptook AR, Ehrenkranz RA, et al. Whole-body hypothermia for neonates with hypoxic-ischemic encephalopathy. N Engl J Med 2005;353:1574–84.
23. Shalak L, Perlman JM. Hypoxic-ischemic brain injury in the term infant-current concepts. Early Hum Dev 2004;80:125–41.
24. Cowan F, Rutherford M, Groenendaal F, et al. Origin and timing of brain lesions in term infants with neonatal encephalopathy. Lancet 2003;361:736–42.

25. Hankins GD, Speer M. Defining the pathogenesis and pathophysiology of neonatal encephalopathy and cerebral palsy. Obstet Gynecol 2003;102:628–36.
26. Vannucci RC. Cerebral carbohydrate and energy metabolism in perinatal hypoxic-ischemic brain damage. Brain Pathol 1992;2:229–34.
27. Nakajima W, Ishida A, Lange MS, et al. Apoptosis has a prolonged role in the neurodegeneration after hypoxic ischemia in the newborn rat. J Neurosci 2000;20:7994–8004.
28. Vannucci RC, Brucklacher RM, Vannucci SJ. Glycolysis and perinatal hypoxic-ischemic brain damage. Dev Neurosci 2005;27:185–90.
29. Somjen GG, Aitken PG, Czeh G, et al. Cellular physiology of hypoxia of the mammalian central nervous system. Res Publ Assoc Res Nerv Ment Dis 1993;71: 51–65.
30. Jabaudon D, Scanziani M, Gahwiler BH, et al. Acute decrease in net glutamate uptake during energy deprivation. Proc Natl Acad Sci U S A 2000;97:5610–5.
31. Choi DW. Glutamate neurotoxicity and diseases of the nervous system. Neuron 1988;1:623–34.
32. Halestrap AP. Calcium, mitochondria and reperfusion injury: a pore way to die. Biochem Soc Trans 2006;34:232–7.
33. Gunn AJ, Gunn TR. The ‘pharmacology’ of neuronal rescue with cerebral hypothermia. Early Hum Dev 1998;53:19–35.
34. Nedelcu J, Klein MA, Aguzzi A, et al. Biphasic edema after hypoxic-ischemic brain injury in neonatal rats reflects early neuronal and late glial damage. Pediatr Res 1999;46:297–304.
35. Puka-Sundvall M, Wallin C, Gilland E, et al. Impairment of mitochondrial respiration after cerebral hypoxia-ischemia in immature rats: relationship to activation of caspase-3 and neuronal injury. Brain Res Dev Brain Res 2000;125:43–50.
36. Roth SC, Baudin J, Cady E, et al. Relation of deranged neonatal cerebral oxidative metabolism with neurodevelopmental outcome and head circumference at 4 years. Dev Med Child Neurol 1997;39:718–25.
37. Lorek A, Takei Y, Cady EB, et al. Delayed (“secondary”) cerebral energy failure after acute hypoxia-ischemia in the newborn piglet: continuous 48-hour studies by phosphorus magnetic resonance spectroscopy. Pediatr Res 1994;36: 699–706.
38. Sarnat HB, Sarnat MS. Neonatal encephalopathy following fetal distress. A clinical and electroencephalographic study. Arch Neurol 1976;33:696–705.
39. Martin E, Buchli R, Ritter S, et al. Diagnostic and prognostic value of cerebral 31P magnetic resonance spectroscopy in neonates with perinatal asphyxia. Pediatr Res 1996;40:749–58.
40. Minamisawa H, Smith ML, Siesjo BK. The effect of mild hyperthermia and hypothermia on brain damage following 5, 10, and 15 minutes of forebrain ischemia. Ann Neurol 1990;28:26–33.
41. Yager J, Towfighi J, Vannucci RC. Influence of mild hypothermia on hypoxic-ischemic brain damage in the immature rat. Pediatr Res 1993;34:525–9.
42. Laptook AR, Corbett RJ, Sterett R, et al. Modest hypothermia provides partial neuroprotection for ischemic neonatal brain. Pediatr Res 1994;35:436–42.
43. Thoresen M, Bagenholm R, Loberg EM, et al. Posthypoxic cooling of neonatal rats provides protection against brain injury. Arch Dis Child Fetal Neonatal Ed 1996;74:F3–9.
44. Gunn AJ, Gunn TR, Gunning MI, et al. Neuroprotection with prolonged head cooling started before post ischemic seizures in fetal sheep. Pediatrics 1998; 102:1098–106.

45. Colbourne F, Sutherland G, Corbett D. Postischemic hypothermia: A critical appraisal with implications for clinical treatment. Mol Neurobiol 1997;14:171–201.
46. Edwards AD, Wyatt JS, Thoresen M. Treatment of hypoxic-ischaemic brain damage by moderate hypothermia. Arch Dis Child Fetal Neonatal Ed 1998;78:F85–8.
47. Towfighi J, Housman C, Heitjan DF, et al. The effect of focal cerebral cooling on perinatal hypoxic ischemic brain damage. Acta Neuropathol 1994;87:598–604.
48. Laptook AR, Corbett RJ. The effects of temperature on hypoxic-ischemic brain injury. Clin Perinatol 2002;29:623–49.
49. Marion DW, Penrod LE, Kelsey SF, et al. Treatment of traumatic brain injury with moderate hypothermia. N Engl J Med 1997;336:540–6.
50. Bernard SA, Gray TW, Buist MD, et al. Treatment of comatose survivors of out-of-hospital cardiac arrest with induced hypothermia. N Engl J Med 2002;346:557–63.
51. Haaland K, Loberg EM, Steen PA, et al. Posthypoxic hypothermia in newborn piglets. Pediatr Res 1997;41:505–12.
52. Chopp M, Chen H, Dereski MO, et al. Mild hypothermic intervention after graded ischemic stress in rats. Stroke 1991;22:37–43.
53. Colbourne F, Corbett D. Delayed and prolonged post-ischemic hypothermia is neuroprotective in the gerbil. Brain Res 1994;654:265–72.
54. Busto R, Dietrich WD, Globus MY, et al. Postischemic moderate hypothermia inhibits CA1 hippocampal ischemic neuronal injury. Neurosci Lett 1989;101:299–304.
55. Shuaib A, Trulove D, Ijaz MS, et al. The effect of post-ischemic hypothermia following repetitive cerebral ischemia in gerbils. Neurosci Lett 1995;186:165–8.
56. Kuboyama K, Safar P, Radovsky A, et al. Delay in cooling negates the beneficial effect of mild resuscitative cerebral hypothermia after cardiac arrest in dogs: a prospective, randomized study. Crit Care Med 1993;21:1348–58.
57. Zhao W, Richardson JS, Mombourquette MJ, et al. Neuroprotective effects of hypothermia and U-78517f in cerebral ischemia are due to reducing oxygen-based free radicals—an electron paramagnetic resonance study with gerbils. J Neurosci Res 1996;45:282–8.
58. Carroll M, Beek O. Protection against hippocampal CA1 cell loss by post-ischemic hypothermia is dependent on delay of initiation and duration. Metab Brain Dis 1992;7:45–50.
59. Coimbra C, Wieloch T. Moderate hypothermia mitigates neuronal damage in the rat brain when initiated several hours following transient cerebral ischemia. Acta Neuropathol 1994;87:325–31.
60. Gunn AJ, Bennet L, Gunning MI, et al. Cerebral hypothermia is not neuroprotective when started after postischemic seizures in fetal sheep. Pediatr Res 1999;46:274–80.
61. Thoresen M, Whitelaw A. Cardiovascular changes during mild therapeutic hypothermia and rewarming in infants with hypoxic-ischemic encephalopathy. Pediatrics 2000;106:92–9.
62. Laptook AR, Shalak L, Corbett RJ. Differences in brain temperature and cerebral blood flow during selective head versus whole-body cooling. Pediatrics 2001;108:1103–10.
63. Rutherford MA, Azzopardi D, Whitelaw A, et al. Mild hypothermia and the distribution of cerebral lesions in neonates with hypoxic-ischemic encephalopathy. Pediatrics 2005;116:1001–6.
64. Williams GD, Dardzinski BJ, Buckalew AR, et al. Modest hypothermia preserves cerebral energy metabolism during hypoxia-ischemia and correlates with brain

damage: a 31P nuclear magnetic resonance study in unanesthetized neonatal rats. Pediatr Res 1997;42:700–8.
65. Young RS, Olenginski TP, Yagel SK, et al. The effect of graded hypothermia on hypoxic-ischemic brain damage: a neuropathologic study in the neonatal rat. Stroke 1983;14:929–34.
66. Young RS, Kolonich J, Woods CL, et al. Behavioral performance of rats following neonatal hypoxia-ischemia. Stroke 1986;17:1313–6.
67. Tomimatsu T, Fukuda H, Endoh M, et al. Long-term neuroprotective effects of hypothermia on neonatal hypoxic-ischemic brain injury in rats, assessed by auditory brainstem response. Pediatr Res 2003;53:57–61.
68. Laptook AR, Corbett RJ, Sterett R, et al. Quantitative relationship between brain temperature and energy utilization rate measured in vivo using 31P and 1H magnetic resonance spectroscopy. Pediatr Res 1995;38:919–25.
69. Zhu CL, Wang XY, Cheng XY, et al. Neuroprotective effect and mechanisms of hypothermia in neonatal rat cerebral hypoxic-ischemic damages. Zhonghua Er Ke Za Zhi 2003;41:911–5.
70. Adachi M, Sohma O, Tsuneishi S, et al. Combination effect of systemic hypothermia and caspase inhibitor administration against hypoxic-ischemic brain damage in neonatal rats. Pediatr Res 2001;50:590–5.
71. Tomimatsu T, Fukuda H, Endo M, et al. Effects of hypothermia on neonatal hypoxic-ischemic brain injury in the rat: phosphorylation of Akt, activation of caspase-3-like protease. Neurosci Lett 2001;312:21–4.
72. Eilers H, Bickler PE. Hypothermia and isoflurane similarly inhibit glutamate release evoked by chemical anoxia in rat cortical brain slices. Anesthesiology 1996;85:600–7.
73. Thoresen M, Satas S, Puka-Sundvall M, et al. Post-hypoxic hypothermia reduces cerebrocortical release of NO and excitotoxins. Neuroreport 1997;8:3359–62.
74. Lei B, Adachi N, Arai T. The effect of hypothermia on H2O2 production during ischemia and reperfusion: a microdialysis study in the gerbil hippocampus. Neurosci Lett 1997;222:91–4.
75. Bergstedt K, Hu BR, Wieloch T. Postischaemic changes in protein synthesis in the rat brain: effects of hypothermia. Exp Brain Res 1993;95:91–9.
76. Brooks KJ, Hargreaves I, Bhakoo K, et al. Delayed hypothermia prevents decreases in N-acetylaspartate and reduced glutathione in the cerebral cortex of the neonatal pig following transient hypoxia-ischaemia. Neurochem Res 2002;27:1599–604.
77. Westin B, Einhorning G. An experimental study of the human fetus with special reference to asphyxia neonatorum. Acta Paediatr 1955;44:79–81.
78. Azzopardi D, Robertson NJ, Cowan FM, et al. Pilot study of treatment with whole body hypothermia for neonatal encephalopathy. Pediatrics 2000;106:684–94.
79. Shankaran S, Laptook A, Wright LL, et al. Whole-body hypothermia for neonatal encephalopathy: animal observations as a basis for a randomized, controlled pilot study in term infants. Pediatrics 2002;110:377–85.
80. Simbruner G, Haberl C, Harrison V, et al. Induced brain hypothermia in asphyxiated human newborn in fants: a retrospective chart analysis of physiological and adverse effects. Intensive Care Med 1999;25:1111–7.
81. Eicher DJ, Wagner CL, Katikaneni LP, et al. Moderate hypothermia in neonatal encephalopathy: safety outcomes. Pediatr Neurol 2005;32:18–24.
82. Edwards AD, Azzopardi DV. Therapeutic hypothermia following perinatal asphyxia. Arch Dis Child Fetal Neonatal Ed 2006;91:F127–31.
83. TOBY Trial. Available at: http://www.npeu.ox.ac.uk/toby/. Accessed July 16, 2008.

84. Jacobs SE, Stewart M, Inder TE, et al. Progress of the pragmatic Australian "ICE" (Infant Cooling Evaluation) randomised controlled trial of whole body cooling for term newborns with hypoxic-ischemic encephalopathy. Presented at the Hot Topics in Neonatology; December 3–5, 2006; Washington, DC.
85. Kirpalani H, Barks J, Thorlund K, et al. Cooling for neonatal hypoxic ischemic encephalopathy: do we have the answer? Pediatrics 2007;120:1126–30.
86. Bower BD, Jones LF, Weeks MM. Cold injury in the newborn: a study of 70 cases. Br Med J 1971;5169:303–9.
87. Culic S. Cold injury syndrome and neurodevelopmental changes in survivors. Arch Med Res 2005;36:532–8.
88. Battin MR, Dezoete JA, Gunn TR, et al. Neurodevelopmental outcome of infants treated with head cooling and mild hypothermia after perinatal asphyxia. Pediatrics 2001;107:480–4.
89. Battin MR, Penrice J, Gunn TR, et al. Treatment of term infants with head cooling and mild systemic hypothermia (35.0 °C and 34.5 °C) after perinatal asphyxia. Pediatrics 2003;111:244–51.
90. Westgate JA, Gunn AJ, Gunn TR. Antecedents of neonatal encephalopathy with fetal acidaemia at term. Br J Obstet Gynaecol 1999;106:774–82.
91. Ambalavanan N, Carlo WA, Shankaran S, et al. Predicting outcomes of neonates diagnosed with hypoxemic-ischemic encephalopathy. Pediatrics 2006;118:2084–93.
92. Gunn AJ, Thoresen M. Hypothermic neuroprotection. NeuroRx 2006;3:154–69.
93. Sarkar S, Barks JD, Donn SM. Should amplitude-integrated electroencephalography be used to identify infants suitable for hypothermic neuroprotection? J Perinatol 2008;28:117–22.
94. Hagmann CF, Robertson NJ, Azzopardi D. Artifacts on electroencephalograms may influence the amplitude-integrated EEG classification: a qualitative analysis in neonatal encephalopathy. Pediatrics 2006;118:2552–4.
95. Tooley JR, Eagle RC, Satas S, et al. Significant head cooling can be achieved while maintaining normothermia in the newborn piglet. Arch Dis Child Fetal Neonatal Ed 2005;90:F262–6.
96. Thoresen M, Simmonds M, Satas S, et al. Effective selective head cooling during posthypoxic hypothermia in newborn piglets. Pediatr Res 2001;49:594–9.
97. Iwata O, Thornton JS, Sellwood MW, et al. Depth of delayed cooling alters neuroprotection pattern after hypoxia-ischemia. Ann Neurol 2005;58:75–87.
98. Higgins RD, Raju TN, Perlman J, et al. Hypothermia and perinatal asphyxia: executive summary of the National Institute of Child Health and Human Development workshop. J Pediatr 2006;148:170–5.
99. Shankaran S, Woldt E, Koepke T, et al. Acute neonatal morbidity and long-term central nervous system sequelae of perinatal asphyxia in term infants. Early Hum Dev 1991;25:135–48.
100. Blackmon LR, Stark AR. American Academy of Pediatrics, Committee on Fetus and Newborn. Hypothermia: a neuroprotective therapy for neonatal hypoxic-ischemic encephalopathy. Pediatrics 2006;117:942–8.
101. American Heart Association. 2005 American Heart Association (AHA) guidelines for cardiopulmonary resuscitation (CPR) and emergency cardiovascular care (ECC) of pediatric and neonatal patients: pediatric basic life support. Pediatrics 2006;117(5). Available at: www.pediatrics.org/cgi/content/full/117/5/e989. Accessed July 16, 2008.
102. International Liaison Committee on Resuscitation. The International Liaison Committee on Resuscitation (ILCOR) consensus on science with treatment

recommendations for pediatric and neonatal patients: pediatric basic and advanced life support. Pediatrics 2006;117(5). Available at: www.pediatrics.org/cgi/content/full/117/5/e955. Accessed July 16, 2008.

103. Gunn AJ, Gluckman PD. Head cooling for neonatal encephalopathy: the state of the art. Clin Obstet Gynecol 2007;50:636–51.
104. Gunn AJ, Hoehn T, Hansmann G, et al. Hypothermia: an evolving treatment for neonatal hypoxic ischemic encephalopathy. Pediatrics 2008;121:648–9.
105. Jatana M, Singh I, Singh AK, et al. Combination of systemic hypothermia and N-acetylcysteine attenuates hypoxic-ischemic brain injury in neonatal rats. Pediatr Res 2006;59:684–9.
106. Wang X, Svedin P, Nie C, et al. N-acetylcysteine reduces lipopolysaccharide-sensitized hypoxic-ischemic brain injury. Ann Neurol 2007;61:263–71.
107. Clancy RR, McGaurn SA, Goin JE, et al. Allopurinol neurocardiac protection trial in infants undergoing heart surgery using deep hypothermic circulatory arrest. Pediatrics 2001;108:61–70.
108. Peeters-Scholte C, Braun K, Koster J, et al. Effects of allopurinol and deferoxamine on reperfusion injury of the brain in newborn piglets after neonatal hypoxia-ischemia. Pediatr Res 2003;54:516–22.
109. Pacher P, Nivorozhkin A, Szabó C. Therapeutic effects of xanthine oxidase inhibitors: renaissance half a century after the discovery of allopurinol. Pharmacol Rev 2006;58:87–114.
110. Gonzalez FF, McQuillen P, Mu D, et al. Erythropoietin enhances long-term neuroprotection and neurogenesis in neonatal stroke. Dev Neurosci 2007;29:321–30.
111. Juul SE, McPherson RJ, Bammler TK, et al. Recombinant erythropoietin is neuroprotective in a novel mouse oxidative injury model. Dev Neurosci 2008;30:231–42.
112. McPherson RJ, Juul SE. Recent trends in erythropoietin-mediated neuroprotection. Int J Dev Neurosci 2008;26:103–11.
113. Hamrick SE, McQuillen PS, Jiang X, et al. A role for hypoxia-inducible factor-1 alpha in desferoxamine neuroprotection. Neurosci Lett 2005;379:96–100.
114. Mu D, Chang YS, Vexler ZS, et al. Hypoxia-inducible factor 1alpha and erythropoietin upregulation with deferoxamine salvage after neonatal stroke. Exp Neurol 2005;195:407–15.
115. Liu Y, Barks JD, Xu G, et al. Topiramate extends the therapeutic window for hypothermia-mediated neuroprotection after stroke in neonatal rats. Stroke 2004;35:1460–5.
116. Schubert S, Brandl U, Brodhun M, et al. Neuroprotective effects of topiramate after hypoxia-ischemia in newborn piglets. Brain Res 2005;1058:129–36.
117. Ma D, Hossain M, Chow A, et al. Xenon and hypothermia combine to provide neuroprotection from neonatal asphyxia. Ann Neurol 2005;58:182–93.
118. Hobbs C, Thoresen M, Tucker A, et al. Xenon and hypothermia combine additively, offering long-term functional and histopathologic neuroprotection after neonatal hypoxia/ischemia. Stroke 2008;39:1307–13.
119. Han BH, Xu D, Choi J, et al. Selective, reversible caspase-3 inhibitor is neuroprotective and reveals distinct pathways of cell death after neonatal hypoxic-ischemic brain injury. J Biol Chem 2002;277:30128–36.
120. Feng Y, Fratkin JD, LeBlanc MH. Inhibiting caspase-8 after injury reduces hypoxic-ischemic brain injury in the newborn rat. Eur J Pharmacol 2003;481:169–73.

Brain Cooling for Preterm Infants

Alistair Jan Gunn, MB, ChB, PhD[a,b,c,*], Laura Bennet, PhD[a]

KEYWORDS

- Therapeutic hypothermia • Fetal sheep • Preterm infant
- Periventricular leukomalacia

Advances in neonatal care have led to a progressive improvement in the survival of preterm, low birth weight babies over the past 2 decades. Unfortunately, in the 1990s improved survival was associated with increased risk for neurodevelopmental impairment.[1] The increasing success of newborn intensive care has been associated with a moderate rise in the childhood prevalence of cerebral palsy,[2] although there is some evidence that disability rates among very low birth weight infants have now stabilized and may be improving.[3] In the United States, the direct costs of caring for premature infants were estimated in 2005 to be at least $26 billion per year.[4] The major cause of this huge personal and societal burden is the profoundly increased risk for physical handicap (including cerebral palsy and retinopathy) and long-term learning, cognitive, and behavioral difficulties.[5,6] Thus, the importance of improving understanding of the underlying pathogenesis of brain damage in preterm infants, and finding ways to prevent or treat it, cannot be overstated.[7]

The seminal insight that underpinned development of potential neuroprotective therapies for term newborn infants and at older ages was that after global injuries, such as hypoxia-ischemia, the brain's mitochondrial function, and thus, oxidative capacity, recovered fully in many cases, in a so-called latent phase lasting many hours, only to secondarily deteriorate.[8,9] There is now compelling empiric evidence that this secondary mitochondrial failure corresponds to overt cell death[10] or, at the very least, to an irreversible stage in the processes leading to delayed cell death.[11] It is this delay that offered the tantalizing possibility that intervention could alleviate long-term damage. Experimental[11] and clinical studies[12–16] have demonstrated that

This work was supported by grants from the Health Research Council of New Zealand, the March of Dimes Birth Defects trust, the Auckland Medical Research Foundation, and Lottery Health New Zealand.

[a] Department of Physiology, Faculty of Medical and Health Sciences, University of Auckland, Private Bag 92019, Auckland, New Zealand
[b] Department of Paediatrics, University of Auckland, Private Bag 92019, Auckland, New Zealand
[c] Starship Children's Hospital, Private Bag 92024, Auckland, New Zealand
* Corresponding author. Department of Physiology, Faculty of Medical and Health Sciences, University of Auckland, Private Bag 92019, Auckland, New Zealand.
E-mail address: aj.gunn@auckland.ac.nz (A.J. Gunn).

Clin Perinatol 35 (2008) 735–748
doi:10.1016/j.clp.2008.07.012 **perinatology.theclinics.com**

prolonged, moderate cerebral hypothermia initiated within a few hours after severe hypoxia-ischemia and continued until resolution of the acute phase of delayed cell death can reduce subsequent neuronal loss and improve behavioral recovery.

A key clinical issue is that there is as yet no specific diagnostic marker for when evolving cell death becomes irreversible. Empirically, as recently reviewed, there is strong evidence that the latent phase before the onset of secondary energy failure represents the realistic window of opportunity for intervention.[11] Studies at term and in adult animals suggest that there is rapid loss of effect as treatment delay is increased, and little or no protection when hypothermia was initiated after the onset of delayed seizures.[17,18]

IS COOLING RELEVANT TO PRETERM INFANTS?

The obvious question is whether or not induced therapeutic hypothermia could help reduce neural injury in preterm newborns. Direct translation of hypothermia to preterm infants is unwise without specific preclinical and clinical studies because of differences in the pattern of injury and their greater potential susceptibility to the adverse effects of hypothermia. Historical data suggest that mild hypothermia is associated with increased mortality in preterm newborns weighing less than 1500 g.[19–21] This review summarizes what has been learned about the causes and timing of preterm brain injury, the recent evidence from preterm fetal sheep that this injury evolves over time and can be interrupted by induced hypothermia, and, finally, the potential for harm with hypothermia.

HOW SIMILAR IS PRETERM BRAIN INJURY TO HYPOXIC-ISCHEMIC INJURY AT TERM?

The classic feature of brain injury in preterm infants is white matter injury, predominantly in the periventricular tracts (periventricular leukomalacia [PVL]). Although cystic PVL is now uncommon,[22] diffuse white matter injury, with selective loss of immature (premyelination) oligodendrocytes, remains a nearly universal problem.[23–26] This white matter injury is consistently and strongly associated with the high risk for cerebral palsy and neurodevelopmental impairment in survivors of premature birth.[27,28] In many ways, however, this is a paradoxic finding, because intellectual function and many aspects of motor coordination derive from neuronal activity rather than white matter per se.[29] Strikingly, there has been no apparent improvement in neurodevelopmental outcomes of premature infants, despite the progressive reduction in the incidence of the severe, cystic form of PVL over the past 10 years.[22]

More recently, it has become apparent that PVL is only part of the story. Imaging studies have shown that PVL is associated not only with reduced white matter volumes and ventricular enlargement but also reduced volume and complexity of cerebral cortical gray matter[30,31] and reduced size of subcortical nuclei.[26,32,33] The poor neurodevelopmental outcomes of ex-preterm neonates[34] are strongly associated with reduced brain growth.[35,36] There is increasing evidence that this chronic impairment is at least in part related to acute subcortical gray matter injury occurring in association with white matter damage. MRI of preterm infants known to have had profound perinatal asphyxia show a consistent pattern of acute subcortical damage involving the thalamus and basal ganglia and cerebellar infarction combined with diffuse periventricular white matter injury but sparing of the cortex.[26,37–40] MRI does not reliably detect selective neuronal loss clinically or experimentally;[41,42] thus, milder cases of acute injury may be missed.

Supporting this hypothesis, postmortem studies of infants dying in the early neonatal period also strongly suggest a significant incidence of acute subcortical neuronal injury, including increased apoptosis, gliosis, and neuronal necrosis in the basal ganglia, hippocampus, and brainstem.[41,43] A population-based, postmortem survey found a 32% incidence of neuronal loss in preterm infants, particularly in the pons.[44] Similarly, a subsequent series of 41 premature infants found that more than a third of infants who had PVL had associated acute neuronal cell death, particularly in the basal ganglia and cerebellum,[29] and more than half had gray matter astrogliosis suggestive of milder local injury. Electroencephalogram (EEG) abnormalities in preterm infants in the perinatal period are highly predictive of long-term outcome.[45] Given that in near midgestation fetal sheep EEG changes after severe cerebral ischemia were closely associated with the severity of neuronal damage and not with white matter injury,[46] these findings also point to the presence of acute neuronal injury.

ANTECEDENTS OF PRETERM BRAIN INJURY

The etiology of acute neural injury in preterm infants is complex and still not fully understood. There is increasing evidence, however, that key events include exposure to hypoxia around the time of birth and pre- and postnatal exposure to infection/inflammation.[47,48] Although it is more difficult to clinically assess encephalopathy in very low birth weight infants, older premature infants (31 to 36 weeks' gestation) who have metabolic acidosis on cord blood show evolving clinical encephalopathy after birth, which in turn is associated with adverse neurologic outcome.[49] Metabolic acidosis is more common in premature infants than at term,[50] and adverse neonatal and long-term outcomes are strongly associated with evidence of exposure to perinatal hypoxia as shown by metabolic acidosis, active labor, abnormal heart rate traces in labor, and subsequent low Apgar scores.[44,47,51] The epidemiologic association of adverse outcomes with exposure to chorioaminonitis may be directly mediated by inflammatory injury[52–54] but may well be indirectly mediated through increased susceptibility to damage during perinatal hypoxia.[55]

PRETERM MODEL OF HYPOXIC-ISCHEMIC INJURY

To explore the possible treatment of preterm brain injury more closely, the authors have established a clinically relevant model of hypoxic-ischemic injury induced by complete occlusion of the umbilical cord in preterm fetal sheep, at the neural equivalent of 28- to 32-week-old infants,[56] for defined periods.[57–59] This insult results in severe injury to the subventricular germinal zone and subcortical structures, including the striatum and hippocampus, but sparing of the cortex after 3 days' recovery,[57] with diffuse loss of immature oligodendrocytes in the periventricular region.[58,60]

Timing of Secondary Deterioration After Hypoxic-Ischemic in the Preterm Fetus

As discussed previously, it is critical to identify the onset of this secondary phase when treatment is likely no longer effective. **Fig. 1** shows that the preterm fetus demonstrates a similar pattern of initial recovery of mitochondrial function as shown by levels of cytochrome oxidase measured by near infrared spectroscopy, followed by a progressive secondary deterioration beginning approximately 3 hours after asphyxia, with a significant reduction in cytochrome oxidase levels compared with sham controls by 10 hours (see **Fig. 1**).[59] Intracerebral oxygenation (measured as the difference between oxygenated and deoxygenated hemoglobin concentrations) fell transiently at 3 and 4 hours after asphyxia despite normal blood pressure and blood oxygen levels,[59] followed by a substantial increase to well over sham control levels, consistent with impairment of oxidative metabolism (see **Fig. 1**). In the early hours after reperfusion, the fetal EEG was highly suppressed, and delayed seizures

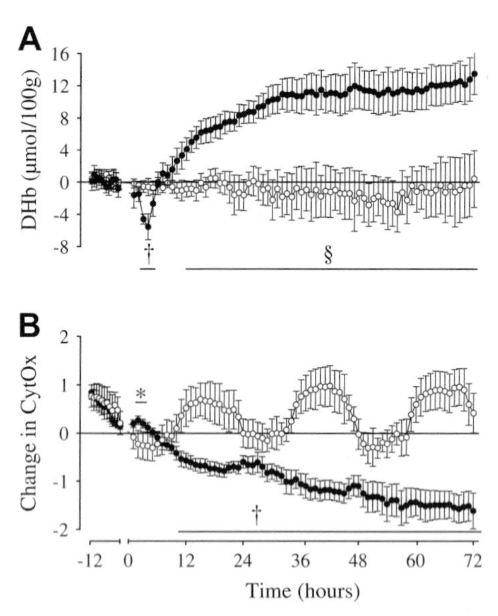

Fig. 1. Evidence of delayed mitochondrial dysfunction after severe hypoxia-ischemia in preterm fetal sheep. This figure shows the time sequence of acute concentration changes in fetal delta hemoglobin (DHb, [*panel A*] the difference between oxygenated and deoxygenated hemoglobin), a measure of relative intracerebral oxygenation, and cytochrome oxidase (CytOx [*panel B*]). Both were measured by near infrared spectroscopy before and after asphyxia induced by 25 minutes of umbilical cord occlusion (filled circles, n = 7) or sham occlusion (open circles, n = 7) in preterm fetal sheep. Occlusion data not shown. Data are mean ± SEM hourly averages. *, $P<.05$; †, $P<.01$; §, $P<.001$; occlusion group versus sham occlusion group, analysis of variance. (*Data derived from* Bennet L, Roelfsema V, Pathipati P, et al. Relationship between evolving epileptiform activity and delayed loss of mitochondrial activity after asphyxia measured by near-infrared spectroscopy in preterm fetal sheep. J Physiol 2006;572:141.)

were seen from a mean of 8 hours. Cytochrome oxidase is the terminal electron acceptor of the mitochondrial electron transport chain; thus, these data strongly indicate that severe asphyxia leads to delayed, evolving loss of mitochondrial oxidative metabolism, accompanied by late seizures and relative luxury cerebral perfusion.

Hypothermia and Post-Asphyxial Brain Injury

In this experimental paradigm, moderate, delayed cerebral hypothermia started 90 minutes after umbilical cord occlusion and continued for 3 days was associated with markedly reduced loss of neurons and immature oligodendrocytes (**Fig. 2**).[60] After 3 days' recovery from umbilical cord occlusion, carotid blood flow was significantly greater in the hypothermia-occlusion group than in the normothermia-occlusion group, and EEG frequency, although not amplitude, was significantly improved to sham control levels.[60] These hemodynamic and electrophysiologic improvements were reflected in greater histologic neuronal survival in many nuclei of the basal ganglia and the cornu ammonis regions of the hippocampus, with suppression of induction of activated caspase-3 and of microglia.[60] Further, mild to moderate cerebral cooling, to a mean ± standard error of the mean (SEM) core body temperature of 37.5°C ± 0.7°C versus 39.3°C ± 0.1°C in sham controls, was associated with selective protection of particular phenotypic striatal projection neurons, including a significant reduction in loss of neurons immunopositive for calbindin-28 kd and neuronal nitric

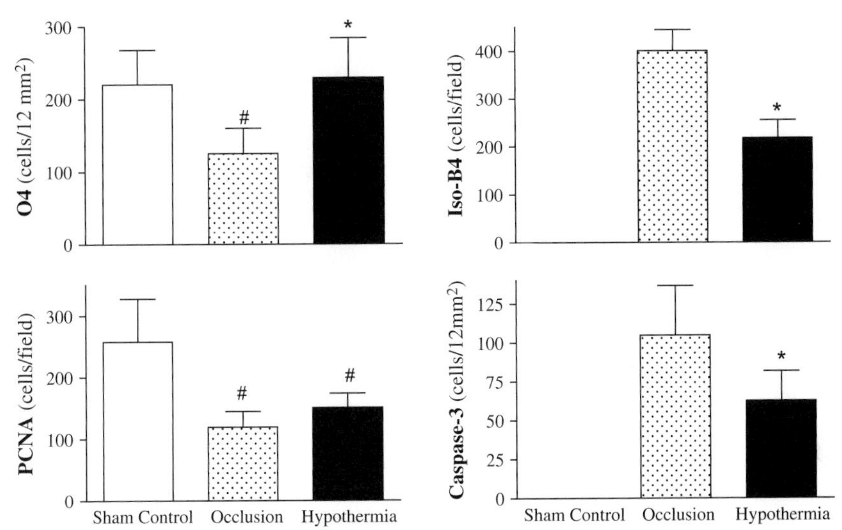

Fig. 2. The effect of hypothermia on numbers of O4-positive, immature oligodendrocytes, activated caspase-3 (Asp175), isolectin-B4–labeled activated microglia, and proliferating cell nuclear antigen (PCNA)–positive cells in the periventricular white matter after 3 days' recovery from 25 minutes of umbilical cord occlusion in preterm fetal sheep. #, $P<.05$ versus sham control group; *, $P<.05$ versus normothermia-occlusion group. (*Data derived from* Bennet L, Roelfsema V, George S, et al. The effect of cerebral hypothermia on white and grey matter injury induced by severe hypoxia in preterm fetal sheep. J Physiol 2007;578:491.)

oxide synthase. This was not true for neurons immunopositive for glutamic acid decarboxylase. These findings suggest that hypothermia might reduce cerebral palsy in some premature infants.[61]

White matter injury, with loss of O4-positive immature oligodendrocytes, was associated with induction of activated caspase-3 and of microglia, as shown in **Fig. 2**.[60] Fluorescent labeling studies confirmed that the great majority of caspase-3–positive cells in the periventricular white matter after severe hypoxia co-localized with the oligodendrocytes.[62] Hypothermia was associated with suppression of activated caspase-3 and microglia in white matter (see **Fig. 2**), consistent with previous reports that hypothermia potently suppresses post-hypoxic/ischemic apoptosis and inflammation.[11]

Despite this improvement, the number of proliferating cells in the periventricular region remained suppressed in both occlusion groups (see **Fig. 2**).[60] The reduction in proliferation in the normothermia-occlusion group presumably reflects the balance between profound loss of proliferating immature oligodendrocytes but an increase in proliferation by microglia.[63,64] The improved survival of O4-positive cells in the hypothermia-occlusion group and marked reduction in numbers of reactive microglia were not accompanied by recovery in the numbers of proliferating cells. This continued reduction likely reflects suppression by hypothermia of overall glial proliferation,[65] not just microglia.[63] Further studies are needed to better define whether or not post-hypoxic cooling alters long-term proliferation of progenitor cells and immature oligodendrocytes and whether or not the acute neuroprotection seen with acute hypothermia is sufficient to restore ultimate brain growth.

Hypothermia and Excitotoxicity?

Classically, cell death resulting from abnormal glutamate receptor activation (excitotoxicity) is related to pathologically elevated levels of extracellular glutamate, as occurs in gray matter during hypoxia-ischemia,[66] although there is evidence that this does not occur in white matter.[67] After reperfusion, extracellular glutamate levels in gray matter rapidly return to control values;[68] thus, it might be predicted that excitotoxicity should not be important after reperfusion. More recent data, however, show that pathologic hyperexcitability of glutamate receptors can continue for many hours after hypoxia-ischemia and that receptor blockade can suppress this activity and improve neuronal outcome.[69]

Although overall EEG activity is profoundly suppressed for many hours after asphyxia in near-midgestation fetal sheep regardless of whether or not injury later developed or not, epileptiform EEG transient activity was only seen in the early recovery phase after a profound insult that was associated with severe injury.[57] Further, the frequency of transients was correlated with the severity of neuronal loss in the striatum and hippocampus (**Fig. 3**).[60,70] These events occur in the early recovery phase before secondary failure of mitochondrial function, raising the possibility that these early events may be an in vivo analog of glutamate receptor hyperactivity and directly contribute to injury.[71] Clearly, these events could be simply a manifestation of injury. A possible causal relationship is supported by the observations that suppression of EEG transients with a glutamate receptor antagonist reduces cell loss[58] and, conversely, that increased EEG transient activity during blockade of inhibitory α_2-adrenergic receptor activity was associated with increased neuronal loss.[70] Supporting this interpretation, neuroprotection with postasphyxial moderate cerebral hypothermia in the preterm fetal sheep was associated with a marked reduction in numbers of epileptiform transients in the first 6 hours after asphyxia (see **Fig. 3**) and reduced amplitude but not numbers of delayed seizures.[72] Thus, this abnormal activity in the early recovery phase may be an important therapeutic target.

ADVERSE EFFECTS OF HYPOTHERMIA

Silverman and colleagues[19] demonstrated in 1958 that the thermal environment has a critical effect on the survival of newly born premature infants less than 1500 g birth weight. Subsequent controlled trials confirmed the importance of maintaining premature infants within a strict normothermic environment.[20,21] The specific complications leading to this greater mortality are unclear, and it is unknown whether or not these problems would be affected by modern intensive care.

Mild to moderate hypothermia (to mean rectal temperatures of 33°C to 34.5°C) has had a strikingly good safety record in term infants who have acute encephalopathy in intensive care.[14,15] In meta-analysis, the only consistent changes were benign, including physiologic bradycardia, mild thrombocytopenia,[73] and a possible increase in inotrope requirements.[74] Similarly, the only consistent minor adverse effect of head cooling was scalp edema under the cap, which resolved rapidly before or after removal of the cap.[14] Nevertheless, the known systemic effects of hypothermia[75] suggest theoretic concerns that hypothermia might promote hypotension, increase oxygen consumption, decrease surfactant production, increase pulmonary vascular resistance, or promote free fatty acid release and so increase the risk for jaundice or reduce resistance to infection.

CardioRespiratory Effects of Hypothermia

Although deep hypothermia (<30°C) can cause ventricular arrhythmias, in a clinically acceptable range (33°C–35°C) hypothermia is associated with slowing of the atrial pacemaker and intracardiac conduction, with sinus bradycardia,[14,15] decreased left ventricular contractility,[76] and cardiac output.[77] The reduction in cardiac output is

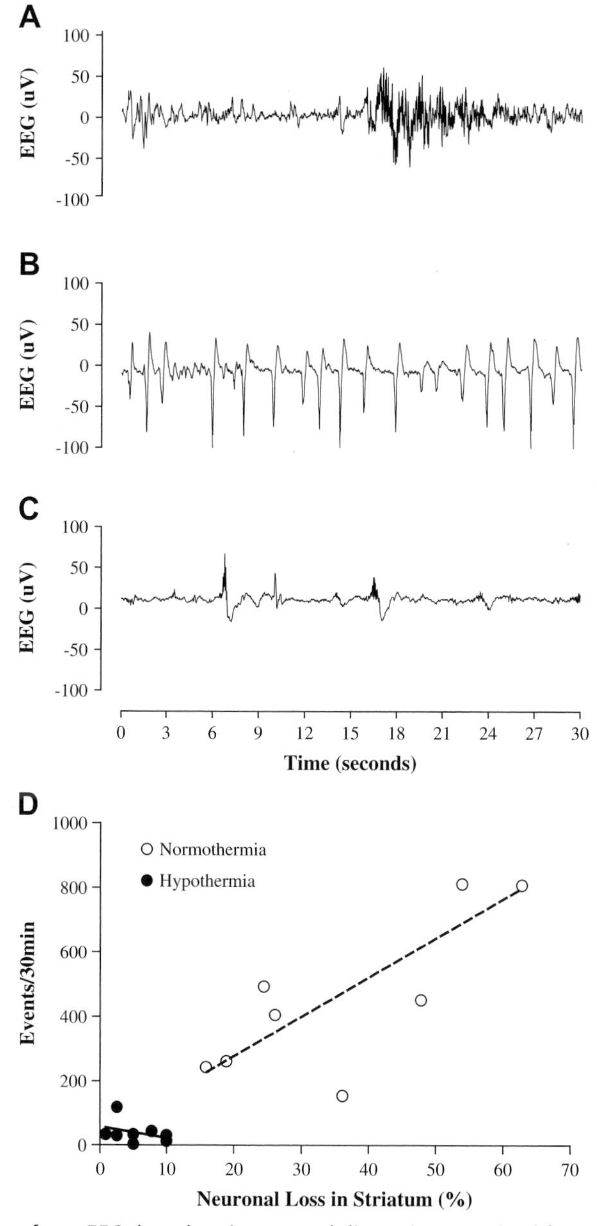

Fig. 3. Examples of raw EEG data showing normal discontinuous mixed frequency EEG activity (*A*), epileptiform transients superimposed on a suppressed EEG background at 3 hours post occlusion (*B*), and marked suppression of EEG transients during hypothermia at 3 hours post occlusion (*C*). The bottom panel (*D*) shows the relationship between maximal frequency of EEG epileptiform transient events in 30-minute intervals in the first 6 hours after umbilical cord occlusion, and neuronal loss in the striatum after 3 days' recovery ($r^2 = 0.65$, $P = .008$). (*Data derived from* Bennet L, Dean JM, Wassink G, et al. Differential effects of hypothermia on early and late epileptiform events after severe hypoxia in preterm fetal sheep. J Neurophysiol 2007;97:572.)

largely linearly proportional to decreased metabolic need;[78] thus, these physiologic effects per se have not required treatment. A few term infants have markedly prolonged QT duration above the 98th percentile corrected for age and heart rate, without arrhythmia. These changes resolve with rewarming.[79]

Respiration could be compromised by reduced surfactant production,[75] increased pulmonary vascular resistance,[80] and increased oxygen consumption.[75] One case series in term infants has suggested that hypothermia was associated with a modest but consistent increase in required fraction of inspired oxygen,[81] although this finding has not been supported by subsequent clinical trials.[74]

Metabolic and Endocrine Effects

Unlike adults, infants respond to cooling with intense nonshivering thermogenesis, which is associated with release of free fatty acids and increased oxygen consumption. Historically, there has been concern that this could lead to displacement of unconjugated bilirubin, increasing the risk for kernicertus.[82] It is likely that routine phototherapy attenuates this theoretic risk.[83] A recent study in newborn piglets suggested that mild systemic hypothermia significantly attenuated changes in cerebral cortical cell membrane Na(+), K(+)-ATPase activity, and lipid peroxidation products during hyperbilirubinemia, raising the possibly that hypothermia actually may be protective.[84]

Hypothermia has been associated with transient mild hyperglycemia in adults, neonates,[13,14] and preterm fetal sheep,[60] likely reflecting catecholamine release. There was no increase in hypoglycemia,[14,15] but one study in piglets suggested that if cooling was continued, increased glucose administration became necessary to maintain normal levels.[85]

Hypokalemia occurs in animal models during deep hypothermia but corrects spontaneously during rewarming, suggesting that this change is the result of intracellular redistribution.[86] This has not been a issue, however, with the mild to moderate hypothermia used in the large randomized controlled trials in term infants.[74] Cold suppresses antidiuretic hormone,[75] and in newborn rabbits, mild hypothermia has been associated with decreased renal blood flow and glomerular filtration rate.[87] No effects on renal function were reported in term infants, however.[14] Some preterm infants may have poor cortisol responses to stress, which may contribute to their risk for hypotension.[88] A recent study in preterm fetal sheep has shown, however, that cerebral hypothermia with mild systemic cooling after severe hypoxia neither suppressed the normal robust pituitary and adrenal response nor triggered an exaggerated rise in cortisol.[89] Similarly, hypothermia had no adverse effects on the responses of the insulin-like growth factor system to asphyxia.[90]

Hematologic and Immunologic Effects

Very low birth weight infants have a high risk for intraventricular hemorrhage, which can have devastating consequences.[91] Because hypothermia is associated with significant coagulation changes, including platelet dysfunction and sequestration and physicochemical delay of the clotting cascade,[92] there must be a substantive concern that mandates cautious testing. Reassuringly, meta-analysis suggests that there was no overall increase in hemorrhagic complications during cooling of term infants,[74] with a small reduction in platelet counts. Although a smaller study from Eicher and colleagues[93] suggested a clinically manageable increase in bleeding problems, they did not find increased intracranial bleeding. Potentially, this result could have been related to the lower rectal temperatures in that trial (33°C) or could be a chance finding. In the piglet, even deeper cooling of the cortex (to <30 °C) was not associated with cerebral hemorrhage.[94]

A further major issue that should concern pediatricians is suppression of immune function, including impaired leukocyte mobility and phagocytosis, which have been reported during mild hypothermia.[75] Although there was no increase in the rate of post-randomization infection in cooled term newborn infants, these large randomized trials included routine treatment for possible perinatal infection.[14,15] In older adults, induced hypothermia is associated with increased risk for infective complications, such as pneumonia,[75] and this possibility must be a significant potential issue given the high rate of acquired infection in preterm infants,[95] along with the potential deleterious effects of infection on the brain.[55]

SUMMARY

In conclusion, the most striking concepts to emerge from recent clinical studies of premature infants are that disability is closely associated with injury to gray and white matter and that a substantial proportion of significant injury seems to occur in the immediate perinatal period. Experimental studies in preterm fetal sheep suggest that, consistent with experience at term, a prolonged period of moderate cerebral hypothermia can significantly reduce white and gray matter injury. Although therapeutic hypothermia has had a remarkably favorable safety profile in clinical studies,[74] and no adverse effects were suggested by the studies in the preterm fetal sheep, the known profile of effects of hypothermia suggests the potential for adverse effects on intracranial hemorrhage, nosocomial infection, and potentially respiratory management. It may well be that hypothermia would have an unacceptable risk profile in the most immature preterm infants. How then to proceed?

As suggested by Salhab and Perlman,[49] hypothermia and other innovative therapies should first be tested in older preterm infants, at 31 to 36 weeks, who have metabolic acidosis and clinical encephalopathy. These infants present the closest clinical parallel to term infants who have acute encephalopathy and thus are the most likely to benefit while being least at risk for intracranial hemorrhage.[91] It is now time to consider careful safety studies and then large randomized trials in this highly vulnerable population.

REFERENCES

1. Wilson-Costello D, Friedman H, Minich N, et al. Improved survival rates with increased neurodevelopmental disability for extremely low birth weight infants in the 1990s. Pediatrics 2005;115:997–1003.
2. Bhushan V, Paneth N, Kiely JL. Impact of improved survival of very low birth weight infants on recent secular trends in the prevalence of cerebral palsy. Pediatrics 1993;91:1094–100.
3. Wilson-Costello D, Friedman H, Minich N, et al. Improved neurodevelopmental outcomes for extremely low birth weight infants in 2000–2002. Pediatrics 2007;119:37–45.
4. Committee on Understanding Premature Birth and Assuring Healthy Outcomes. In: Behrman RE, Butler AS, editors. Preterm birth: causes, consequences, and prevention. Washington, DC: Institute of Medicine of the National Academies; 2007.
5. Marlow N, Wolke D, Bracewell MA, et al. Neurologic and developmental disability at six years of age after extremely preterm birth. N Engl J Med 2005;352:9–19.
6. Saigal S, den Ouden L, Wolke D, et al. School-age outcomes in children who were extremely low birth weight from four international population-based cohorts. Pediatrics 2003;112:943–50.
7. Paneth N. Classifying brain damage in preterm infants. J Pediatr 1999;134:527–9.

8. Hanrahan JD, Sargentoni J, Azzopardi D, et al. Cerebral metabolism within 18 hours of birth asphyxia: a proton magnetic resonance spectroscopy study. Pediatr Res 1996;39:584–90.
9. Roth SC, Baudin J, Cady E, et al. Relation of deranged neonatal cerebral oxidative metabolism with neurodevelopmental outcome and head circumference at 4 years. Dev Med Child Neurol 1997;39:718–25.
10. Vannucci RC, Towfighi J, Vannucci SJ. Secondary energy failure after cerebral hypoxia-ischemia in the immature rat. J Cereb Blood Flow Metab 2004;24: 1090–7.
11. Gunn AJ, Gluckman PD. Head cooling for neonatal encephalopathy: the state of the art. Clin Obstet Gynecol 2007;50:636–51.
12. The Hypothermia after Cardiac Arrest Study Group. Mild therapeutic hypothermia to improve the neurologic outcome after cardiac arrest. N Engl J Med 2002;346: 549–56.
13. Bernard SA, Gray TW, Buist MD, et al. Treatment of comatose survivors of out-of-hospital cardiac arrest with induced hypothermia. N Engl J Med 2002;346: 557–63.
14. Gluckman PD, Wyatt JS, Azzopardi D, et al. Selective head cooling with mild systemic hypothermia to improve neurodevelopmental outcome following neonatal encephalopathy. Lancet 2005;365:663–70.
15. Shankaran S, Laptook AR, Ehrenkranz RA, et al. Whole-body hypothermia for neonates with hypoxic-ischemic encephalopathy. N Engl J Med 2005;353: 1574–84.
16. Eicher DJ, Wagner CL, Katikaneni LP, et al. Moderate hypothermia in neonatal encephalopathy: efficacy outcomes. Pediatr Neurol 2005;32:11–7.
17. Gunn AJ, Bennet L, Gunning MI, et al. Cerebral hypothermia is not neuroprotective when started after postischemic seizures in fetal sheep. Pediatr Res 1999;46: 274–80.
18. Thoresen M, Satas S, Loberg EM, et al. Twenty-four hours of mild hypothermia in unsedated newborn pigs starting after a severe global hypoxic-ischemic insult is not neuroprotective. Pediatr Res 2001;50:405–11.
19. Silverman WA, Fertig JW, Berger AP. The influence of the thermal environment upon the survival of newly born premature infants. Pediatrics 1958;22:876–86.
20. Day RL, Caliguiri L, Kamenski C, et al. Body temperature and survival of premature infants. Pediatrics 1964;34:171–81.
21. Buetow KC, Klein SW. Effect of maintenance of "normal" skin temperature on survival of infants of low birth weight. Pediatrics 1964;34:163–70.
22. Hamrick SE, Miller SP, Leonard C, et al. Trends in severe brain injury and neurodevelopmental outcome in premature newborn infants: the role of cystic periventricular leukomalacia. J Pediatr 2004;145:593–9.
23. Inder TE, Anderson NJ, Spencer C, et al. White matter injury in the premature infant: a comparison between serial cranial sonographic and MR findings at term. AJNR Am J Neuroradiol 2003;24:805–9.
24. Inder T, Huppi PS, Zientara GP, et al. Early detection of periventricular leukomalacia by diffusion-weighted magnetic resonance imaging techniques. J Pediatr 1999;134:631–4.
25. Maalouf EF, Duggan PJ, Rutherford MA, et al. Magnetic resonance imaging of the brain in a cohort of extremely preterm infants. J Pediatr 1999;135:351–7.
26. Yokochi K. Thalamic lesions revealed by MR associated with periventricular leukomalacia and clinical profiles of subjects. Acta Paediatr 1997;86:493–6.

27. Woodward LJ, Anderson PJ, Austin NC, et al. Neonatal MRI to predict neurodevelopmental outcomes in preterm infants. N Engl J Med 2006;355:685–94.
28. Miller SP, Ferriero DM, Leonard C, et al. Early brain injury in premature newborns detected with magnetic resonance imaging is associated with adverse early neurodevelopmental outcome. J Pediatr 2005;147:609–16.
29. Pierson CR, Folkerth RD, Billiards SS, et al. Gray matter injury associated with periventricular leukomalacia in the premature infant. Acta Neuropathol 2007;114:619–31.
30. Ajayi-Obe M, Saeed N, Cowan FM, et al. Reduced development of cerebral cortex in extremely preterm infants. Lancet 2000;356:1162–3.
31. Inder TE, Huppi PS, Warfield S, et al. Periventricular white matter injury in the premature infant is followed by reduced cerebral cortical gray matter volume at term. Ann Neurol 1999;46:755–60.
32. Argyropoulou MI, Xydis V, Drougia A, et al. MRI measurements of the pons and cerebellum in children born preterm; associations with the severity of periventricular leukomalacia and perinatal risk factors. Neuroradiology 2003;45:730–4.
33. Lin Y, Okumura A, Hayakawa F, et al. Quantitative evaluation of thalami and basal ganglia in infants with periventricular leukomalacia. Dev Med Child Neurol 2001;43:481–5.
34. Bhutta AT, Cleves MA, Casey PH, et al. Cognitive and behavioral outcomes of school-aged children who were born preterm: a meta-analysis. JAMA 2002;288:728–37.
35. Bhutta AT, Anand KJ. Abnormal cognition and behavior in preterm neonates linked to smaller brain volumes. Trends Neurosci 2001;24:129–30.
36. Woodward LJ, Edgin JO, Thompson D, et al. Object working memory deficits predicted by early brain injury and development in the preterm infant. Brain 2005;128:2578–87.
37. Johnsen SD, Tarby TJ, Lewis KS, et al. Cerebellar infarction: an unrecognized complication of very low birthweight. J Child Neurol 2002;17:320–4.
38. Barkovich AJ, Sargent SK. Profound asphyxia in the premature infant: imaging findings. AJNR Am J Neuroradiol 1995;16:1837–46.
39. de Vries LS, Smet M, Goemans N, et al. Unilateral thalamic haemorrhage in the pre-term and full-term newborn. Neuropediatrics 1992;23:153–6.
40. Leijser LM, Klein RH, Veen S, et al. Hyperechogenicity of the thalamus and basal ganglia in very preterm infants: radiological findings and short-term neurological outcome. Neuropediatrics 2004;35:283–9.
41. Felderhoff-Mueser U, Rutherford MA, Squier WV, et al. Relationship between MR imaging and histopathologic findings of the brain in extremely sick preterm infants. AJNR Am J Neuroradiol 1999;20:1349–57.
42. Fraser M, Bennet L, Helliwell R, et al. Regional specificity of magnetic resonance imaging for cerebral ischemic changes in preterm fetal sheep. Reprod Sci 2007;14:182–91.
43. Takizawa Y, Takashima S, Itoh M. A histopathological study of premature and mature infants with pontosubicular neuron necrosis: neuronal cell death in perinatal brain damage. Brain Res 2006;1095:200–6.
44. Bell JE, Becher JC, Wyatt B, et al. Brain damage and axonal injury in a Scottish cohort of neonatal deaths. Brain 2005;128:1070–81.
45. Hayakawa M, Okumura A, Hayakawa F, et al. Background electroencephalographic (EEG) activities of very preterm infants born at less than 27 weeks

gestation: a study on the degree of continuity. Arch Dis Child Fetal Neonatal Ed 2001;84:F163–7.
46. Fraser M, Bennet L, Gunning M, et al. Cortical electroencephalogram suppression is associated with post-ischemic cortical injury in 0.65 gestation fetal sheep. Brain Res Dev Brain Res 2005;154:45–55.
47. de Vries LS, Eken P, Groenendaal F, et al. Antenatal onset of haemorrhagic and/or ischaemic lesions in preterm infants: prevalence and associated obstetric variables. Arch Dis Child Fetal Neonatal Ed 1998;78:F51–6.
48. Becher JC, Bell JE, Keeling JW, et al. The Scottish perinatal neuropathology study: clinicopathological correlation in early neonatal deaths. Arch Dis Child Fetal Neonatal Ed 2004;89:F399–407.
49. Salhab WA, Perlman JM. Severe fetal acidemia and subsequent neonatal encephalopathy in the larger premature infant. Pediatr Neurol 2005;32:25–9.
50. Low JA. Determining the contribution of asphyxia to brain damage in the neonate. J Obstet Gynaecol Res 2004;30:276–86.
51. Weinberger B, Anwar M, Hegyi T, et al. Antecedents and neonatal consequences of low Apgar scores in preterm newborns: a population study. Arch Pediatr Adolesc Med 2000;154:294–300.
52. Yoon BH, Park CW, Chaiworapongsa T. Intrauterine infection and the development of cerebral palsy. BJOG 2003;110(Suppl 20):124–7.
53. Duncan JR, Cock ML, Scheerlinck JP, et al. White matter injury after repeated endotoxin exposure in the preterm ovine fetus. Pediatr Res 2002;52:941–9.
54. Mallard C, Welin AK, Peebles D, et al. White matter injury following systemic endotoxemia or asphyxia in the fetal sheep. Neurochem Res 2003;28:215–23.
55. Wang X, Hagberg H, Nie C, et al. Dual role of intrauterine immune challenge on neonatal and adult brain vulnerability to hypoxia-ischemia. J Neuropathol Exp Neurol 2007;66:552–61.
56. Barlow RM. The foetal sheep: morphogenesis of the nervous system and histochemical aspects of myelination. J Comp Neurol 1969;135:249–62.
57. George S, Gunn AJ, Westgate JA, et al. Fetal heart rate variability and brainstem injury after asphyxia in preterm fetal sheep. Am J Physiol Regul Integr Comp Physiol 2004;287:R925–33.
58. Dean JM, George SA, Wassink G, et al. Suppression of post hypoxic-ischemic EEG transients with dizocilpine is associated with partial striatal protection in the preterm fetal sheep. Neuropharmacology 2006;50:491–503.
59. Bennet L, Roelfsema V, Pathipati P, et al. Relationship between evolving epileptiform activity and delayed loss of mitochondrial activity after asphyxia measured by near-infrared spectroscopy in preterm fetal sheep. J Physiol 2006;572:141–54.
60. Bennet L, Roelfsema V, George S, et al. The effect of cerebral hypothermia on white and grey matter injury induced by severe hypoxia in preterm fetal sheep. J Physiol 2007;578:491–506.
61. George S, Scotter J, Dean JM, et al. Induced cerebral hypothermia reduces post-hypoxic loss of phenotypic striatal neurons in preterm fetal sheep. Exp Neurol 2007;203:137–47.
62. Barrett RD, Bennet L, Davidson J, et al. Destruction and reconstruction: hypoxia and the developing brain. Birth defects res C Embryo Today 2007;81:163–76.
63. Si QS, Nakamura Y, Kataoka K. Hypothermic suppression of microglial activation in culture: inhibition of cell proliferation and production of nitric oxide and superoxide. Neuroscience 1997;81:223–9.

64. Guan J, Bennet L, George S, et al. Insulin-like growth factor-1 reduces postischemic white matter injury in fetal sheep. J Cereb Blood Flow Metab 2001;21:493–502.
65. Lee KS, Lim BV, Jang MH, et al. Hypothermia inhibits cell proliferation and nitric oxide synthase expression in rats. Neurosci Lett 2002;329:53–6.
66. Johnston MV. Excitotoxicity in perinatal brain injury. Brain Pathol 2005;15:234–40.
67. Fraser M, Bennet L, van Zijl PL, et al. Extracellular amino acids and peroxidation products in the periventricular white matter during and after cerebral ischemia in preterm fetal sheep. J Neurochem 2008;105:2214–23.
68. Tan WK, Williams CE, During MJ, et al. Accumulation of cytotoxins during the development of seizures and edema after hypoxic-ischemic injury in late gestation fetal sheep. Pediatr Res 1996;39:791–7.
69. Jensen FE, Wang C, Stafstrom CE, et al. Acute and chronic increases in excitability in rat hippocampal slices after perinatal hypoxia In vivo. J Neurophysiol 1998; 79:73–81.
70. Dean JM, Gunn AJ, Wassink G, et al. Endogenous alpha(2)-adrenergic receptor-mediated neuroprotection after severe hypoxia in preterm fetal sheep. Neuroscience 2006;142:615–28.
71. Bennet L, Roelfsema V, Dean J, et al. Regulation of cytochrome oxidase redox state during umbilical cord occlusion in preterm fetal sheep. Am J Physiol Regul Integr Comp Physiol 2007;292:R1569–76.
72. Bennet L, Dean JM, Wassink G, et al. Differential effects of hypothermia on early and late epileptiform events after severe hypoxia in preterm fetal sheep. J Neurophysiol 2007;97:572–8.
73. Shah PS, Ohlsson A, Perlman M. Hypothermia to treat neonatal hypoxic ischemic encephalopathy: systematic review. Arch Pediatr Adolesc Med 2007;161:951–8.
74. Jacobs S, Hunt R, Tarnow-Mordi W, et al. Cooling for newborns with hypoxic ischaemic encephalopathy. Cochrane Database Syst Rev 2007; CD003311.
75. Schubert A. Side effects of mild hypothermia. J Neurosurg Anesthesiol 1995;7: 139–47.
76. Greene PS, Cameron DE, Mohlala ML, et al. Systolic and diastolic left ventricular dysfunction due to mild hypothermia. Circulation 1989;80:III44–8.
77. Gebauer CM, Knuepfer M, Robel-Tillig E, et al. Hemodynamics among neonates with hypoxic-ischemic encephalopathy during whole-body hypothermia and passive rewarming. Pediatrics 2006;117:843–50.
78. Walter B, Bauer R, Kuhnen G, et al. Coupling of cerebral blood flow and oxygen metabolism in infant pigs during selective brain hypothermia. J Cereb Blood Flow Metab 2000;20:1215–24.
79. Gunn TR, Wilson NJ, Aftimos S, et al. Brain hypothermia and QT interval. Pediatrics 1999;103:1079.
80. Benumof JL, Wahrenbrock EA. Dependency of hypoxic pulmonary vasoconstriction on temperature. J Appl Phys 1977;42:56–8.
81. Thoresen M, Whitelaw A. Cardiovascular changes during mild therapeutic hypothermia and rewarming in infants with hypoxic-ischaemic encephalopathy. Pediatrics 2000;106:92–9.
82. Ahdab-Barmada M, Moossy J. The neuropathology of kernicterus in the premature neonate: diagnostic problems. J Neuropathol Exp Neurol 1984;43:45–56.
83. Newman TB, Liljestrand P, Jeremy RJ, et al. Outcomes among newborns with total serum bilirubin levels of 25 mg per deciliter or more. N Engl J Med 2006; 354:1889–900.

84. Park WS, Chang YS, Chung SH, et al. Effect of hypothermia on bilirubin-induced alterations in brain cell membrane function and energy metabolism in newborn piglets. Brain Res 2001;922:276–81.
85. Satas S, Loberg EM, Porter H, et al. Effect of global hypoxia-ischaemia followed by 24 h of mild hypothermia on organ pathology and biochemistry in a newborn pig survival model. Biol Neonate 2003;83:146–56.
86. Sprung J, Cheng EY, Gamulin S, et al. The effect of acute hypothermia and serum potassium concentration on potassium cardiotoxicity in anesthetized rats. Acta Anaesthesiol. Scandia 1992;36:825–30.
87. Guignard JP, Gillieron P. Effect of modest hypothermia on the immature kidney. Acta Paediatr 1997;86:1040–1.
88. Ng PC, Lee CH, Lam CW, et al. Transient adrenocortical insufficiency of prematurity and systemic hypotension in very low birthweight infants. Arch Dis Child Fetal Neonatal Ed 2004;89:F119–26.
89. Davidson JO, Fraser M, Naylor AS, et al. The effect of cerebral hypothermia on cortisol and ACTH responses after umbilical cord occlusion in preterm fetal sheep. Pediatr Res 2008;63:51–5.
90. Roelfsema V, Gunn AJ, Breier BH, et al. The effect of mild hypothermia on Insulin-like Growth Factors after severe asphyxia in the preterm fetal sheep. J Soc Gynecol Investig 2005;12:232–7.
91. Perlman JM. White matter injury in the preterm infant: an important determination of abnormal neurodevelopment outcome. Early Hum Dev 1998;53:99–120.
92. Rohrer MJ, Natale AM. Effect of hypothermia on the coagulation cascade. Crit Care Med 1992;20:1402–5.
93. Eicher DJ, Wagner CL, Katikaneni LP, et al. Moderate hypothermia in neonatal encephalopathy: Safety outcomes. Pediatr Neurol 2005;32:18–24.
94. Tooley JR, Eagle RC, Satas S, et al. Significant head cooling can be achieved while maintaining normothermia in the newborn piglet. Arch Dis Child Fetal Neonatal Ed 2005;90:F262–6.
95. Sharek PJ, Horbar JD, Mason W, et al. Adverse events in the neonatal intensive care unit: development, testing, and findings of an NICU-focused trigger tool to identify harm in North American NICUs. Pediatrics 2006;118:1332–40.

Supportive Care During Neuroprotective Hypothermia in the Term Newborn: Adverse Effects and Their Prevention

Marianne Thoresen, MD, PhD

KEYWORDS

• Asphyxia • Encephalopathy • Newborn
• Hypodermic • Neuroprotection • Adverse effects

WHICH INFANTS SHOULD BE COOLED?

The entry criteria in the two large published trials,[1–5] the CoolCap trial[2] and National Institute of Child Health and Human Development (NICHD) trial,[3] recruited infants of similar severity (moderate and severe encephalopathy). As such, the percentages of poor outcome in the untreated arm in the two trials were 66% and 62%, respectively. A series of feasibility studies undertaken in New Zealand[5] and the United Kingdom[6] led to the CoolCap trial, which recruited 235 infants. These studies combined selective head cooling (SHC; circulating cold water in a cap fitted around the head) with mild body hypothermia to 34.5°C rectal temperature, using a protocol that was then applied in the CoolCap trial (and, later, the Whole Body Hypothermia for Perinatal Asphyxial Encephalopathy [TOBY] trial).[7] In the United States, the NICHD used total body hypothermia by means of two cooling blankets, reducing infant temperatures to a rectal temperature of 33.5°C in its 2005 trial (n = 204).[3]

Currently, we are awaiting the outcome of 650 randomized infants from three international studies, with the largest being the United Kingdom–led TOBY trial (Primary Investigator: Dennis Azzopardi)[6,7] with 325 infants recruited. Two other trials were stopped prematurely because of lack of equipoise among the participants: the Australian Infant Cooling Evaluation (ICE) trial (n = 204, Primary Investigator: Sue Jacobs) and the European, induced hypothermia in asphyxiated newborns trial (Neo nEuro Network) (n = 121, Primary Investigator: George Simbrunner). Many centers have decided to delay introducing hypothermia treatment into their protocols until these

Child Health, St. Michael 's Hospital, Level D, University of Bristol, Southwell Street, BS2 8 EG Bristol, UK
E-mail address: marianne.thoresen@bris.ac.uk

Clin Perinatol 35 (2008) 749–763
doi:10.1016/j.clp.2008.07.018 perinatology.theclinics.com

outcome data are available. It is important, however, to note that the current published data support cooling with a relative risk (RR) of 0.76 (95% confidence interval [CI]: 0.54–0.86) and a number needed to treat number to treat (NTT) to prevent 1 case of death or severe disability of 6. In a recent commentary, the point was made that even if the three trials named previously with 650 infants did not show any positive effect, the RR would still have a CI less than 1.0 and the NNT would increase to 15.[4,6]

In the United Kingdom, infants who currently undergo therapeutic hypothermia are registered to an anonymized data set, the "TOBY register".[8] The TOBY register protocol and data sheets are freely available linked to the Web site.

DELAY AND DURATION OF COOLING: DIFFERENT METHODS IN USE

It is strongly recommended to follow the trial protocols[2,3] with regard to the selection of infants, the therapeutic window for initiation of treatment, and the duration of hypothermia. There are limited safety data available for infants that do not fit these entry criteria; that is, infants who were younger than 36 weeks of age, were more than 6 hours old when cooling was initiated, or had a core temperature less than 33.5°C during cooling. Eicher and colleagues[1] cooled infants to 33.0°C and included infants as premature as 35 weeks of gestation. These investigators reported more adverse effects than the CoolCap or NICHD trial. An Italian feasibility study cooled infants to 32°C or 34°C and reported no increase in adverse effects[9] in the 32°C group.

MANAGEMENT OF THE ASPHYXIATED INFANT IN THE DELIVERY ROOM

If severe, clinical asphyxia is apparent and the child fulfils the entry criteria, cooling therapy should be considered. The overhead heater should be turned off during resuscitation as soon as adequate ventilation and heart rate are obtained. The decision to turn off external heating is made by the medical staff as a treatment decision. Active heating is also turned off in the transport incubator. A rectal probe should be inserted to 6 cm to monitor core temperature within 20 minutes after birth, whether this occurs during transport or in the NICU. **Fig. 1** shows the relationship between the deep brain (basal ganglia), superficial brain, scalp skin temperature, and rectal temperature

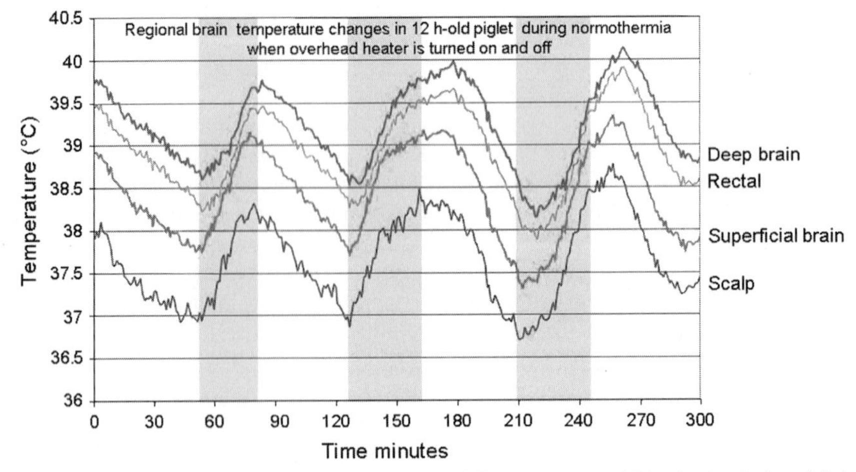

Fig. 1. Continuous temperature recordings from different areas within the brain in addition to skin and rectal temperature at normothermia (which is 39°C for piglets). The shaded boxes indicate when the overhead heater is turned on.

in a 12-hour-old piglet when the overhead heater is turned on and off at regular intervals. There is a parallel increase in all temperatures within minutes after the heater is turned on.

COOLING AND MONITORING DURING TRANSPORT

It is not a simple matter to predict how fast a baby 's temperature is going to drop once the external heating is turned off. The classic study by Dahm and James[10] shows that a healthy baby who is dried and wrapped drops from a rectal temperature of 37.5°C (at birth, newborns are approximately 0.5°C warmer than their mother) to 36.0°C by 30 minutes after birth. If the baby is mildly asphyxiated and self-ventilating, the temperature drops to 34.5°C by 30 minutes.[11] Therefore, "active cooling" is rarely indicated after birth, because the reduced metabolism and heat production in an asphyxiated infant reduce core temperature. Adding active cooling may inadvertently lead to "overcooling." This illustrates the importance of rectal temperature monitoring.

Fig. 2 illustrates serious overcooling. A term newborn was resuscitated for 30 minutes after placental abruption. The active heating was turned off, and cooling was initiated without continuous rectal temperature monitoring; only intermittent axillary temperature measurements were done. The arriving transport team recorded a core temperature of 30°C, and, although rewarming was started during transport to the cooling center, the temperature continued to drop to 27.7°C. The heart rate dropped to approximately 70 beats per minute (however, there was no cardiac arrhythmia), and moderate hypotension to a mean arterial blood pressure (MABP) of 30 mm Hg and significant hypocapnia to 2.4 kPa occurred. These changes are as expected and reflect the low metabolism and low temperature. The ventilator settings used were typical for

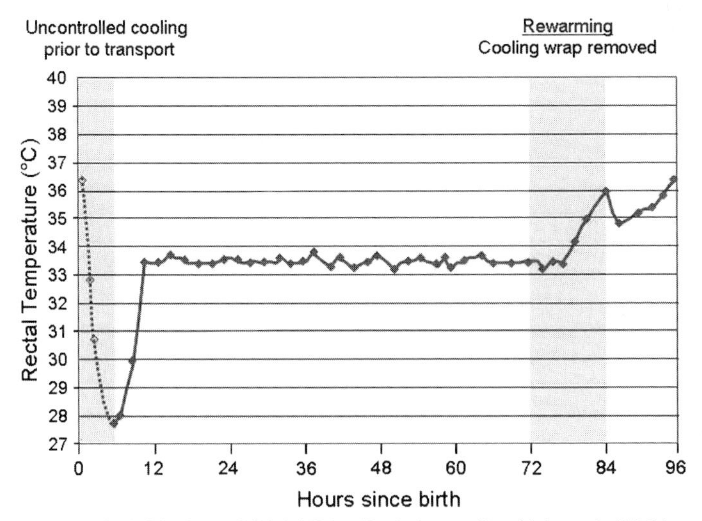

Fig. 2. Overcooling of a term newborn when a rectal probe was not used until arrival in the cooling center, at which time the temperature was found to be 27.7°C. The open symbols represent axillary temperature. After rewarming to 36°C at 84 hours, the cooling wrap was removed. The temperature dropped 1°C because the infant could not maintain the core temperature in a bed preheated to 29°C. GA, gestational age; HR, heart rate; Hb, hemoglobin.

a term normothermic newborn; however, hypothermia reduced metabolism and carbon dioxide (CO_2) production and severe hypocapnia occurred.

Fig. 2 also shows a common problem at the end of rewarming: when the cooling equipment is removed, the newborn often becomes hypothermic, because it is difficult to anticipate a baby's individual, external heating needs.

METHODS OF COOLING AND STABILITY OF TEMPERATURES

In 1998, the Thoresen and Whitelaw[12] placed gloves filled with cold water around the infant as a method of cooling. This approach was followed by the CoolCap procedure, which was developed in New Zealand.[5] A cap circulating with cold water is fitted onto the head to make cooling "selective" (ie, cooling the head more than the rest of the body). The body is simultaneously heated using an overhead heater to "balance" the cooling so that the rectal temperature is only moderately hypothermic (34.5°C). The CoolCap equipment is now approved by the US Food and Drug Administration (FDA) for neuroprotective therapy.[13]

For many years while recruiting to the TOBY trial, the author and her colleagues used a cooling blanket circulated with a coolant fluid for manual temperature regulation. For the past year, however, a servo-controlled system for cooling with a "body wrap" around the trunk and legs circulating with cold water has been used. This device records rectal and skin (forehead)[14] temperature to run an algorithm that automatically adjusts the water temperature to maintain a steady rectal temperature. Since

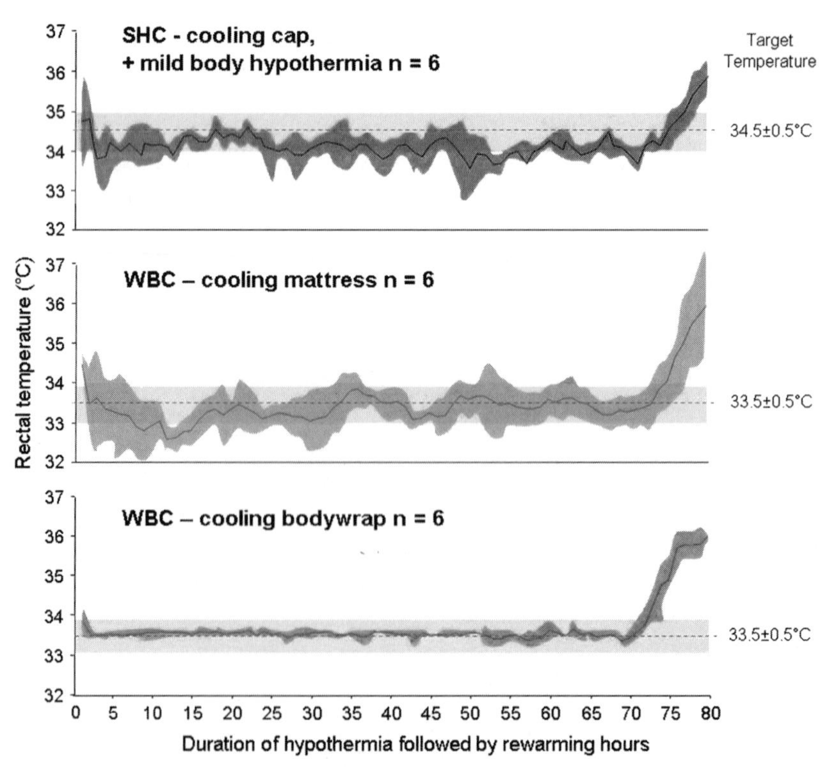

Fig. 3. Mean temperature with SD (shaded) during hypothermia treatment in three groups of term newborns cooled with different methods. SHC, selective head cooling; WBC, whole-body cooling.

using this equipment, no manual temperature adjustment has been necessary. **Fig. 3** shows mean temperatures from six randomly chosen infants cooled with these three methods. It is not known whether large swings in temperature are damaging in themselves or whether a gradient of temperatures throughout the brain, as is likely to occur with SHC, is beneficial. What we do know is that SHC and total body cooling gave significant and similar neuroprotection in the two large trials.

In a piglet cooling study, the animals were randomized between 24 hours of SHC, blanket cooling, or normothermia starting 3 hours after the insult. There was no difference in neuroprotection obtained between the cooling methods, and, in fact, no protective effect of cooling was observed when the cooling was started with a 3-hour delay.[15]

In experimental models, one is able to cool the brain, particularly the cortex, more than the core (rectal) temperature.[16] For obvious reasons, invasive brain temperature data are not available in infants, and it has been suggested that it is not possible to cool the deep brain in a large infant head more than the body core temperature. There is some observational evidence that the cortex may be better protected by SHC.[17]

TOO HOT OR TOO COLD: CLINICAL EXAMPLES OF DIFFICULTIES IN CONTROLLING CORE TEMPERATURE

Fig. 4 shows a case in which the rectal temperature was grossly hyperthermic to 39.5°C before transport to a cooling center could take place. Active, manually controlled cooling resulted in "overcooling" to 30.5°C during treatment. **Fig. 5** shows stable temperature during cooling (body wrap with servo-control) until the wrap was removed before transport to the MRI scanner. Without rectal temperature monitoring during transport and in the scanner, the temperature had dropped to 29.6°C on return to the neonatal intensive care unit (NICU). The corresponding physiological data on return were a heart rate of 76 beats per minute and blood pressure of 62 mm Hg.

Another example where temperature instability may arise is when seizures are stopped with anticonvulsants. **Fig. 6** shows that when phenobarbital is given, the rectal temperature drops. When seizures stop, heat production is reduced. Phenobarbital also reduces metabolism per se.

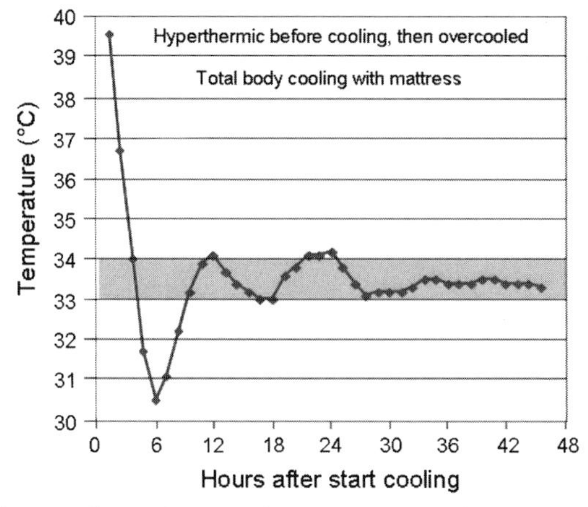

Fig. 4. Newborn who was hyperthermic after resuscitation followed by overcooling. With large temperature swings, it is difficult to obtain steady temperatures with manual control of the cooling device.

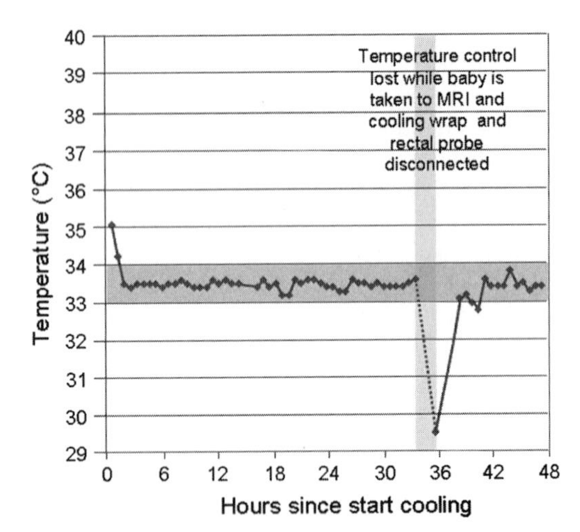

Fig. 5. Stable rectal temperature with servo-controlled total body cooling. During the trip to the MRI scanner, the rectal cooling probe was removed and active temperature control was halted. On return, the temperature was 29.6°C.

REWARMING AFTER RESUSCITATION AND REWARMING AFTER 72 HOURS OF HYPOTHERMIA

Fig. 7 shows rewarming of an infant brought in cold and in poor condition after a home delivery. Rapid rewarming in a preheated incubator after resuscitation brought the temperature from 32°C to 37°C within 1.5 hours, followed by a rapid overshoot to 39°C. The temperature was difficult to maintain within the normal range by changing incubator temperature, and long hyperthermic periods occurred coinciding with seizure activity. There is ample evidence, experimentally[18–21] and clinically,[22,23] that hyperthermia increases injury after hypoxia-ischemia. The children randomized to normothermia within the trials have had a rectal temperature tightly controlled to 37.0°C ± 0.2°C. The asphyxiated children who the author and her colleagues treated during a 12-month period between the CoolCap and TOBY trials had significantly worse temperature control, with an average temperature of 37.4°C ± 0.8°C. Analysis of temperatures in the noncooled infants in their CoolCap trial showed that even one measurement of rectal temperature greater than 38.0°C increased the risk of a poor outcome.[23]

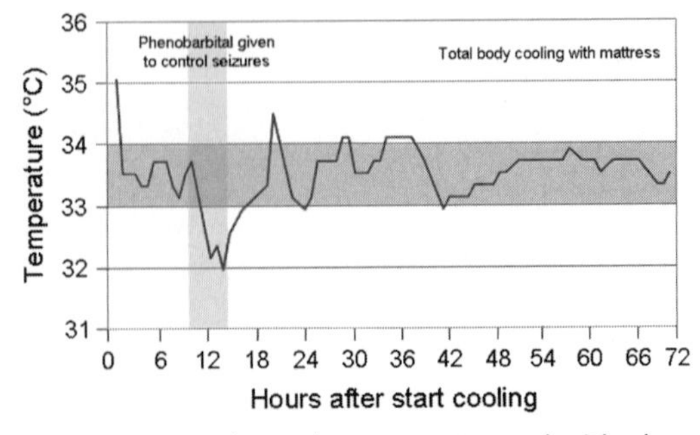

Fig. 6. Effect on core temperature when seizures are stopped with phenobarbital. Heat production is reduced and the temperature drops.

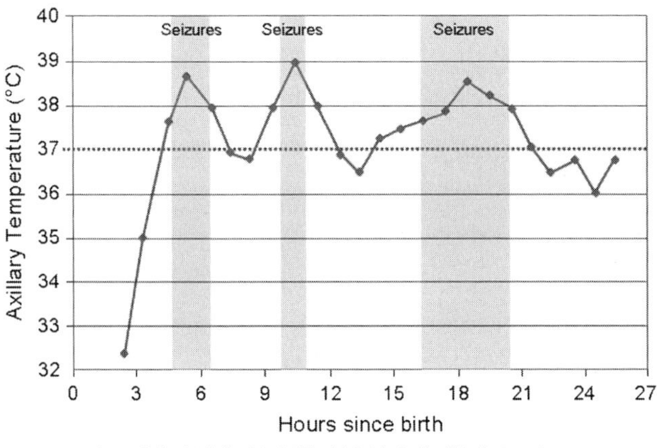

Fig. 7. Newborn had seizures during the periods of background shading on the trace, which coincided with high temperature. Rectal temperature would be expected to be 0.5°C higher than axillary temperature.

PARTICULAR PROBLEMS DURING REWARMING

Seizures are more likely to occur during rewarming.[24] Recently, in 17 infants rewarmed after 72 hours of hypothermia in the author's center, seizures occurred in 4; in 3 infants, the seizures were nonconvulsive only (diagnosed on amplitude-integrated electroencephalograpy [aEEG]), an example of which is shown in shown in **Fig. 8**. This child had a grade 3 encephalopathy with early seizures that responded to phenobarbital at a dose of 20 mg/kg administered twice and was seizure free until 3 hours into rewarming at 0.5°C per hour. The nonconvulsive seizures were first recognized after 3 hours and stopped by clonazepam at a dose of 100 μg/kg; rewarming was stopped and resumed slowly after a delay with no further seizures. Continuous aEEG monitoring allows detection of nonconvulsive seizures and the effect of anticonvulsive treatment. Evidence is lacking as to whether these seizures are damaging in themselves, although experimental data suggest that postinsult seizures increase brain injury.[25]

During rewarming, the vasoconstricted skin dilates and intravascular blood volume increases. If the vascular bed is underfilled, hypotension may occur. Echocardiography

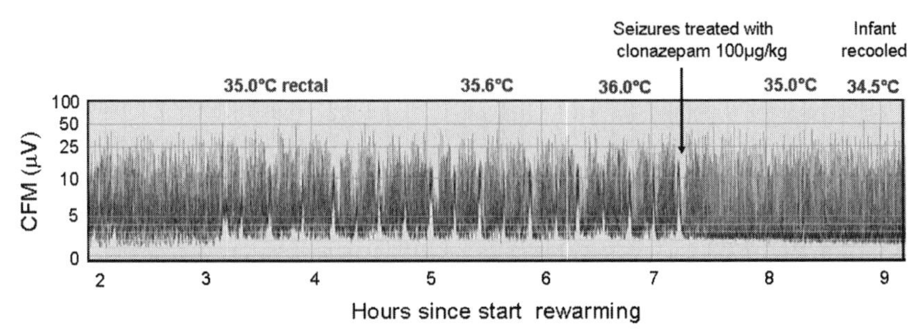

Fig. 8. aEEG trace during rewarming and the occurrence of nonconvulsive seizures that stopped after treatment (clonazepam). The core temperature was reduced again, and rewarming was halted for 3 hours. There were no further seizures, and the total rewarming time was 11 hours in this baby. CFM, cerebral function monitor.

is the definitive way of answering this question. The author and her colleagues give volume of 0.9% NaCl, or albumin at a dose of 10 mL/kg if the albumin value is low (<28 g per 100 mL) at the discretion of the attending physician as soon as there is a drop of 5 mm Hg in MABP. Experimentally, there is some evidence that there may be a mismatch between oxygen delivery and consumption during rewarming.[26,27] A proxy marker for this observation is an increase in plasma lactate value, which should normally not increase during rewarming. In two newborns who were self-ventilating at the start of rewarming, the author and her colleagues have experienced intermittent apnea during the beginning of rewarming. Continuous positive airway pressure (CPAP) during the rest of the rewarming period was necessary, and within a few hours of normal temperature, these neonates were again self-ventilating.

AMPLITUDE-INTEGRATED ELECTROENCEPHALOGRAPHY AND TEMPERATURE DURING SELECTIVE HEAD COOLING OR TOTAL BODY COOLING

There is a linear relation between temperature and electroencephalography (EEG) amplitude. Cooling healthy halothane-anesthetized piglets from 39°C to 35°C reduces the background voltage of approximately 30 μV by 2.3 μV[28] (raw EEG); 0.6 μV/°C.

Because the temperature difference between normothermia and hypothermia in clinical cooling is 3.5°C, one would not expect a significant change in voltage in the temperature range of 37°C to 33.5°C. Horan found that cooling term newborns from 37°C to 34°C during extracorporeal membrane oxygenation (ECMO) did not significantly reduce aEEG.[29] **Fig. 9** shows aEEG in a 7-day-old rat pup that was cooled to 20°C and rewarmed.[30] The aEEG pattern does not change visually until the temperature has dropped to 30°C. Because SHC cools the cortex more than core temperature, one would be more likely to see a change in aEEG voltage when the cap is taken off the head as the cortex quickly rewarms to core temperature. In **Fig. 10**, the upper trace shows an aEEG when rewarming was begun by stopping SHC. There is a 1- to 1.5-μV increase in the lower margin voltage. The scalp (skin) temperature increased from 22.6°C to 33.4°C during the first 20 minutes, and the rectal temperature was unchanged. The lower panel indicates when cooling stops and rewarming starts after whole-body cooling. The rectal temperature increases from 33.5°C to 34.5°C, but there is no change in the aEEG.

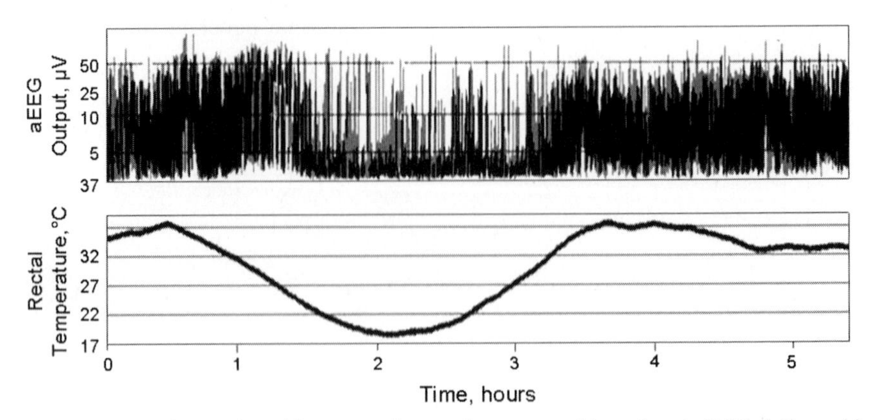

Fig. 9. aEEG trace in a 7-day-old rat pup that underwent rapid cooling to 20°C, followed by rewarming. The aEEG trace was visually unaffected by the low temperature until the rectal temperature was lower than 30°C.[30]

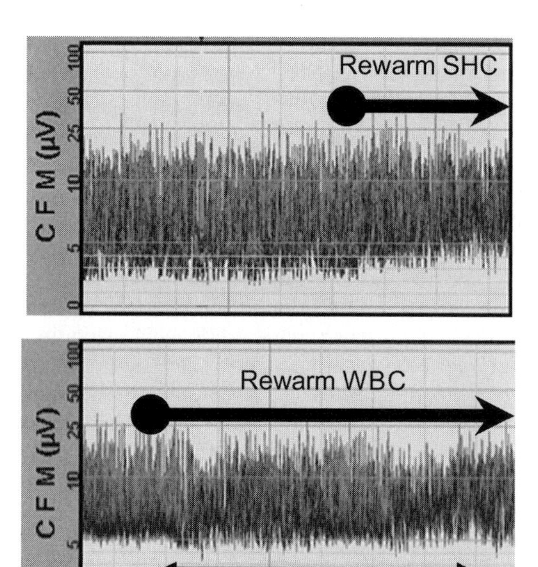

Fig. 10. aEEG trace at the start of rewarming in two infants. The upper trace shows rewarming after stopping SHC, and an accompanying small increase in the lower margin of the aEEG trace. When whole-body cooling (WBC) stops (*lower trace*), there is no change in aEEG voltage. CFM, cerebral function monitor.

BLOOD GASES AND COOLING

The partial pressure of gases depends on temperature. As such, all blood gas machines have the option of analyzing the blood at "actual" temperature. Because this is cumbersome, most clinicians have chosen not to correct for temperature. The author and her colleagues have changed the "normal" range for cooled infants, taking into account the temperature effect on P_{CO_2}. The partial pressure of CO_2 is reduced by approximately 4% per degree Centigrade reduction in core temperature[31] (and as more CO_2 is dissolved in the blood). It is the partial pressure of CO_2 that affects cerebral blood flow (CO_2 reactivity; with higher CO_2, there is higher cerebral blood flow). In ventilated infants who are cooled to a rectal temperature of 33.5°C, the author and her colleagues therefore adjust the normal P_{CO_2} range, which at 37°C is 36 to 44 mm Hg to 41 to 51 mm Hg. Interestingly, it has been suggested that the seizure threshold is lower with alkalosis attributable to hypocapnia.[32] This finding is yet another reason to keep CO_2 within the corrected normal range.

VENTILATION

A reduction in metabolism (5%–8% per degree Centigrade reduction in temperature) is the expected and desired effect of low temperature[33] and results in a decrease in CO_2 production is decreased. To keep CO_2 within the suggested normal range during cooling, the ventilator frequency or tidal volume must therefore be turned down to reduce minute ventilation. Often, it is not possible to achieve normocapnia, because the infant is driving his or her own ventilation, compensating for a metabolic acidosis. It is not known whether it would be better to paralyze and take control of the ventilation and maintain a higher CO_2 or to allow the low P_{CO_2} to occur. The evidence for a damaging effect of low CO_2 is mainly from ventilated premature infants,[34,35] but it also comes from term infants who were kept ventilated on extra corporeal membrane oxygenation (ECMO) with different CO_2 levels.[36]

From a practical point of view, secretions are stickier during hypothermia, and cooled infants therefore benefit from frequent turning, suctioning, and instillation of saline as needed.

In previous cooling guidelines, it was recommended not to cool if there was persistent pulmonary hypertension and a need for a high fraction of inspired oxygen (FiO_2). In published trials so far, however, the incidence of persistent pulmonary hypertension has been the same in the cooled and noncooled groups. When needed, the author and her colleagues administer inhaled nitric oxide (NO) using the standard protocol, and cooling does not seem to be contraindicated.

The author and her colleagues also think it is important that the infant does not become hyperoxic after asphyxia. They therefore follow FiO_2 and saturation closely to keep values within the normal range. The effect of temperature on PO_2 is different and smaller than for PCO_2 during hypothermia, such that the author and her colleagues do not use different PO_2 ranges.[37] The same applies for pH.

Most infants have been ventilated throughout the treatment period, although 20% breathe spontaneously the whole or part of the cooling period. **Fig. 11** shows simultaneous measurements of nasopharyngeal and rectal temperature during SHC. The two temperatures are identical as long as the infant is ventilated; however, after extubation, the nasopharyngeal temperature measures 1.5°C to 2.0°C lower than the rectal temperature.

CLOTTING AND COOLING

Blood flows mores slowly and is "stickier" during hypothermia, with a potentially increased risk for microembolism.[38] Human newborns have a relatively high hemoglobin level, which may result in poor microcirculation, but there is no evidence that infants undergoing therapeutic hypothermia suffer more emboli than during normothermic

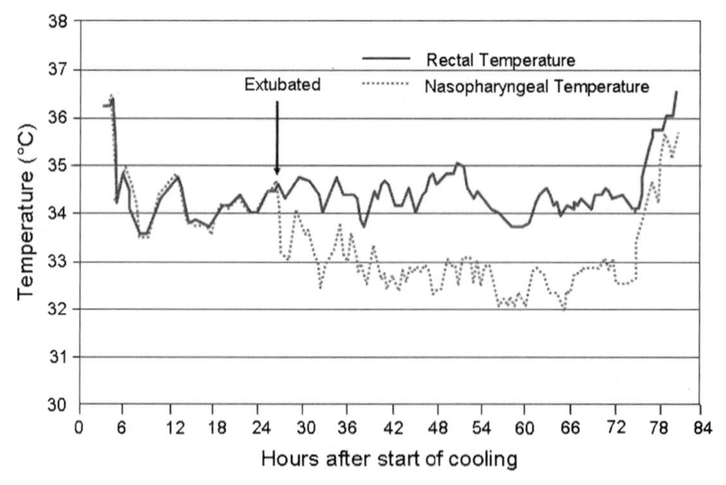

Fig. 11. Simultaneous recordings of nasopharyngeal and rectal temperature during SHC. While intubated, these core temperatures are identical. After extubation, the nasopharyngeal temperature drops nearly 2° because the sensor is influenced by the air temperature in the pharynx. Hence, nasopharyngeal temperature is only valid while the patient is intubated.

care or that hypothermia, per se, increases the hematocrit (hct). The author and her colleagues therefore maintain the same intervention level for normothermic and hypothermic children with regard to hemodilution.

It is physiologic that coagulation is prolonged during hypothermia, and animals that hibernate have a vastly prolonged bleeding time.[39] If coagulation is normal to start with, there are no problems with clotting attributable to therapeutic hypothermia per se. Sick asphyxiated newborns often have deranged clotting at birth, however, and it is not known whether cooling them may further derange their clotting function.

The most concerning infants are those with traumatic deliveries and ongoing bleeding, such as subgaleal hemorrhages. The author and her colleagues have treated three such cases with total body cooling and have been aggressive with fresh-frozen plasma, blood, cryoprecipitate, and volume infusion on clinical indication. They do not use SHC when there is trauma to the head, because one could fear deranged clotting attributable to low cortex/scalp temperature.

In piglets, the author and her colleagues examined activated partial thromboplastin time (APPT) at two temperatures: 39°C, which is normothermia for piglets, and 29°C, which is a typical brain cortex temperature during SHC. APPT increased from [mean (SD)] 20.8 (8.3) seconds to 26.7 (10.6) seconds ($P < .01$), a 10% prolongation, which is not clinically significant.[40] In infants and pigs, a 10% to 39% lower platelet count has been found,[41,42] although the author and her colleagues have not observed that this change has any clinical significance. They have not seen hemorrhagic lesions in the brain on pathologic examination of term piglets' brains instrumented with invasive probes, in which the cortex temperature has been as low as 26°C for 24 hours.[43]

HEART RATE AND HYPOTHERMIA: IS A LOW HEART RATE DANGEROUS?

As with ventilation, reduced metabolic rate reduces cardiac output and heart rate. The author and her colleagues have found that heart rate is reduced by 14 beats per degree Centigrade reduction in body temperature in the range of 39°C to 32°C for piglets and 37°C to 33°C for infants (given that they are not stressed, hypovolemic, anemic, or in pain). Despite many occasions with overcooling, the author and her colleagues have never experienced arrhythmias, only sinus bradycardia with heart rate, on one occasion, as low as 64 beats per minute in overcooled infants. In adults, it has been shown that the heart is more stable against arrhythmias at low temperatures.[44]

DRUG TREATMENT IN HYPOTHERMIC INFANTS

Currently, there is no general recommendation to treat hypothermic infants differently from normothermic infants with regard to the choice of drug or dose.

There are several groups of drugs that most infants receive: antibiotics, inotropic support, anticonvulsive treatment, and sedative treatment, and some are paralyzed.

Drugs that are excreted unchanged by way of the kidneys are less affected by temperature. Routine antibiotic treatment is often penicillin or ampicillin combined with an aminoglycoside. In piglets, gentamicin levels are the same in cooled and noncooled animals.[45] Recently, the author and her colleagues presented clinical data from 54 patients showing that there was no difference in gentamicin serum levels among 30 infants who were cooled as compared with those maintained at normothermia.[46]

Drugs that are metabolized by the liver, such as morphine and phenobarbital, have been shown to have higher levels in the cooled group.[47,48] Vecuronium, which is metabolized in the liver, has been shown in adults to have a prolonged half-life during hypothermia.[49] In practice, when hypothermic infants are started on continuous infusions, the author and her colleagues run the "normothermic" dose for 6 to 12 hours and then reduce the dose until clinical signs of less drug effect appear, such as lack of sedation (increased heart rate) or paralysis (movement). In their piglet studies, the author and her colleagues did not find that piglets needed less pancuronium to maintain paralysis (M. Thoresen, unpublished data, 2007).

The author and her colleagues have used the same drug regimen to treat hypotension in normothermic and hypothermic infants, and they have not experienced a difference in response to inotropic support in hypothermic infants compared with normothermic infants, although there could be differences in receptor activation at different temperatures.

NUTRITION AND FLUID MANAGEMENT

Large cooling trials,[2,3] as a part of the protocol, withheld enteral feeding during hypothermia. The rationale was to relieve the burden on a gastrointestinal tract made vulnerable by hypoxia-ischemia and the additional risk for hypothermia. There has been a low incidence of necrotizing enterocolitis in the trials, and this complication is similar in both groups (1%–2%).

The Scandinavian hypothermia protocols are different; they allow nonnutritive feeding (breast milk, 1 mL/kg given every 4 hours throughout the hypothermia period), and researchers report no cases of necrotizing enterocolitis (M. Blennow, personal communication, 2007).

The author and her colleagues start with clear fluids at 60 mL/kg/d, followed by total parenteral nutrition. Volume is increased as clinically indicated (cardiac and renal function). Often, asphyxiated infants receive volume in response to hypotension, and the average actual volume on day 1 has been 90 mL/kg. None of the 70 children in the author 's cohort who were cooled over the past 10 years developed permanent kidney failure or needed transient dialysis. In randomized piglet experiments, the author and her colleagues found that 24 hours of hypothermia delayed the postinsult increase in creatinine until after the cooling period.[50] In the same study, they also found that the need for glucose was slightly higher in the cooled group. In the clinical data set, however, the author and her colleagues do not have enough detail to be able to address this question.

LEVELS OF PLASMA ELECTROLYTES

Electrolytes should be kept within the normal range. There is conflicting experimental evidence as to whether magnesium is neuroprotective[51] on its own or only in combination with hypothermia.[52] In adults, increased magnesium levels reduce shivering (if only modestly)[53] and are advocated in cooled patients. The recommendation of the author and her colleagues is to maintain magnesium at a level greater than 1.0 mmol/L during hypothermic treatment (ie, within the high normal range).

INOTROPIC SUPPORT

The published trials did not find that hypothermic infants are more hypotensive than normothermic infants with the same severity of asphyxia.[2,3] The author and her colleagues use the same treatment principles for all asphyxiated infants: if hypotensive, first correct hypovolemia (best examined with echocardiography). If reduced myocardial contractility is found, they use dobutamine; if the infant is hypotensive and not hypovolemic or having poor contractility, they use dopamine or noradrenaline.

SUMMARY

Hypothermia as a neuroprotective treatment requires significant knowledge of how temperature affects all organ systems and interventions used in intensive care. The incidence of moderate and severe perinatal asphyxia is low, and such treatment is best undertaken in a large unit that would treat at least eight cases per year for staff to have the necessary experience and confidence. Education and training in resuscitation, including avoidance of hyperthermia, early diagnosis of eligible infants, and initiation of early cooling followed by safe transport of cooled infants to the cooling center is the way forward.

ACKNOWLEDGMENTS

The author is grateful to Dr. Catherine Hobbs for making the figures and commenting on the manuscript; to her clinical colleagues for their support in recruiting patients since 1998; to Olympic Medical (Seattle, Washington) for making available the CoolCap; to Inspiration (United Kingdom) for the cooling mattress; and to MTRE Medical (Israel) for the cooling wrap. The clinical trials were funded by Olympic Medical, United States (CoolCap trial) and the Medical Research Council, United Kingdom (TOBY trial); and equipment was provided by SPARKS (United Kingdom), Laerdal Foundation for Acute Medicine (Norway), and donations from parents.

REFERENCES

1. Eicher DJ, Wagner CL, Katikaneni LP, et al. Moderate hypothermia in neonatal encephalopathy: efficacy outcomes. Pediatr Neurol 2005;32(1):11–7.
2. Gluckman PD, Wyatt JS, Azzopardi D, et al. Selective head cooling with mild systemic hypothermia after neonatal encephalopathy: multicentre randomised trial. Lancet 2005;365(9460):663–70.
3. Shankaran S, Laptook AR, Ehrenkranz RA, et al. Whole-body hypothermia for neonates with hypoxic-ischemic encephalopathy. N Engl J Med 2005;353(15): 1574–84.
4. Hoehn T, Hansmann G, Bührer C, et al. Therapeutic hypothermia in neonates. Review of current clinical data, ILCOR recommendations and suggestions for implementation in neonatal intensive care units. Resuscitation 2008;78(1):7–12.
5. Gunn AJ, Gluckman PD, Gunn TR. Selective head cooling in newborn infants after perinatal asphyxia: a safety study. Pediatrics 1998;102(4 Pt 1):885–92.
6. Thoresen M, Whitelaw A. Therapeutic hypothermia for hypoxic-ischaemic encephalopathy in the newborn infant: review. Curr Opin Neurol 2005;18(2):111–6.
7. Azzopardi D, Brocklehurst P, Edwards D, et al. The TOBY study: whole body hypothermia for the treatment of perinatal asphyxial encephalopathy: a randomised controlled trial. BMC Pediatr 2008;8:17.
8. Available at: http://www.npeu.ox.ac.uk/tobyregister/contact.
9. Compagnoni G, Bottura C, Cavallaro G, et al. Safety of deep hypothermia in treating neonatal asphyxia. Neonatology 2008;93(4):230–5.
10. Dahm LS, James LS. Newborn temperature and calculated heat loss in the delivery room. Pediatrics 1972;49:504–13.
11. Burnard EE, Cross KW. Rectal temperature in the newborn after birth asphyxia. BMJ 1958;ii:1197–9.
12. Thoresen M, Whitelaw A. Cardiovascular changes during mild therapeutic hypothermia and rewarming in infants with hypoxic-ischemic encephalopathy. Pediatrics 2000;106(1 Pt 1):92–9.

13. Available at: http://www.natus.com/index.cfm?page=products_1&crid=115.
14. Hertzman AB, Roth LW. The absence of vasoconstriction reflexes in the forehead circulation. Effects of cold. J Physiol 1949;149:692–7.
15. Karlsson M TJ, Satas S, H, et al. Delayed hypothermia as selective head cooling or whole body cooling does not protect brain or body in newborn piglets. Pediatr Res 2008;64:74–8.
16. Thoresen M, Simmonds M, Satas S, et al. Effective selective head cooling during posthypoxic hypothermia in newborn piglets. Pediatr Res 2001;49(4):594–9.
17. Rutherford MA, Azzopardi D, Whitelaw A, et al. Mild hypothermia and the distribution of cerebral lesions in neonates with hypoxic-ischemic encephalopathy. Pediatrics 2005;116(4):1001–6.
18. Hobbs C, Brun C, Eagle R, et al. Post insult hyperthermia exacerbates hypoxic-ischaemic brain damage in the neonatal rat. Crit Care Med, Submitted for publication.
19. Kim Y, Busto R, Dietrich WD, et al. Delayed postischemic hyperthermia in awake rats worsens the histopathological outcome of transient focal cerebral ischemia. Stroke 1996;27(12):2274–80 [discussion: 81].
20. Kim Y, Truettner J, Zhao W, et al. The influence of delayed postischemic hyperthermia following transient focal ischemia: alterations of gene expression. J Neurol Sci 1998;159(1):1–10.
21. Yager JY, Armstrong EA, Jaharus C, et al. Preventing hyperthermia decreases brain damage following neonatal hypoxic-ischemic seizures. Brain Res 2004;1011(1):48–57.
22. Reith J, Jorgensen HS, Pedersen PM, et al. Body temperature in acute stroke: relation to stroke severity, infarct size, mortality, and outcome. Lancet 1996; 347(8999):422–5.
23. Wyatt JS, Gluckman PD, Liu PY, et al. Determinants of outcomes after head cooling for neonatal encephalopathy. Pediatrics 2007;119(5):912–21.
24. Battin M, Bennet L, Gunn AJ. Rebound seizures during rewarming. Pediatrics 2004;114(5):1369.
25. Wirrell EC, Armstrong EA, Osman LD, et al. Prolonged seizures exacerbate perinatal hypoxic-ischemic brain damage. Pediatr Res 2001;50(4):445–54.
26. Morray JP, Pavlin EG. Oxygen delivery and consumption during hypothermia and rewarming in the dog. Anesthesiology 1990;72(3):510–6.
27. van der Linden J, Ekroth R, Lincoln C, et al. Is cerebral blood flow/metabolic mismatch during rewarming a risk factor after profound hypothermic procedures in small children? Eur J Cardiothorac Surg 1989;3(3):209–15.
28. Haaland K, Loberg EM, Steen PA, et al. Posthypoxic hypothermia in newborn piglets. Pediatr Res 1997;41(4 Pt 1):505–12.
29. Horan M, Azzopardi D, Edwards AD, et al. Lack of influence of mild hypothermia on amplitude integrated-electroencephalography in neonates receiving extracorporeal membrane oxygenation. Early Hum Dev 2007;83(2):69–75.
30. Tucker A, Ferguson J, Thoresen M. The effect of core temperature on aEEG in 7-day-old rat pups. Pediatr Res 2006; PAS2006.59.3726.8.
31. Dill D. Respiratory and metabolic effects of hypothermia. Am J Physiol 1941;132:685.
32. Schuchmann S, Schmitz D, Rivera C, et al. Experimental febrile seizures are precipitated by a hyperthermia-induced respiratory alkalosis. Nat Med 2006;12(7):817–23.
33. Erecinska M, Thoresen M, Silver IA. Effects of hypothermia on energy metabolism in mammalian central nervous system. J Cereb Blood Flow Metab 2003;23(5):513–30.
34. Greisen G, Trojaborg W. Cerebral blood flow, $Paco_2$ changes, and visual evoked potentials in mechanically ventilated, preterm infants. Acta Paediatr Scand 1987; 76(3):394–400.

35. Pryds O, Greisen G. Effect of $Paco_2$ and haemoglobin concentration on day to day variation of CBF in preterm neonates. Acta Paediatr Scand Suppl 1989;360:33–6.
36. Bennett CC, Johnson A, Field DJ, et al. UK collaborative randomised trial of neonatal extracorporeal membrane oxygenation: follow-up to age 4 years. Lancet 2001;357(9262):1094–6.
37. Ashwood ER, Kost G, Kenny M. Temperature correction of blood-gas and pH measurements. Clin Chem 1983;29(11):1877–85.
38. Schreiner RS, Rider AR, Myers JW, et al. Microemboli detection and classification by innovative ultrasound technology during simulated neonatal cardiopulmonary bypass at different flow rates, perfusion modes, and perfusate temperatures. ASAIO J 2008;54(3):316–24.
39. Svihla A, Bowman HR, Ritenour R. Prolongation of clotting time in dormant estivating mammals. Science 1951;114(2960):298–9.
40. Ferguson J, Britton F, Simmonds M, et al. Selective head cooling is safe, cooling by 10°C only mildly prolongs coagulation time in the newborn pig. Early Hum Dev 2006;82:613.
41. Faustini M, Bronzo V, Maffeo G, et al. Reference intervals and age-related changes for platelet count, mean platelet volume and plateletcrit in healthy pre-weaning piglets in Italy. J Vet Med A Physiol Pathol Clin Med 2003;50(9):466–9.
42. McPherson RJ, Juul S. Patterns of thrombocytosis and thrombocytopenia in hospitalized neonates. J Perinatol 2005;25(3):166–72.
43. Tooley JR, Satas S, Porter H, et al. Head cooling with mild systemic hypothermia in anesthetized piglets is neuroprotective. Ann Neurol 2003;53(1):65–72.
44. Johansson BW. The hibernator heart—nature 's model of resistance to ventricular fibrillation. Cardiovasc Res 1994;31:826–32.
45. Satas S, Hoem NO, Melby K, et al. Influence of mild hypothermia after hypoxia-ischemia on the pharmacokinetics of gentamicin in newborn pigs. Biol Neonate 2000;77(1):50–7.
46. Liu X, Borooah M, Hoque N, et al. Does 72-hours of therapeutic hypothermia in encephalopathic infants affect plasma gentamicin levels? [abstract]. Pediatr Res 2008; E-PAS2008.63.3761.2.
47. Thoresen M SJ, Hoem NO, Brun C, et al. Hypothermia after perinatal asphyxia more than doubles the plasma half-life of Phenobarbitone. Ped Res 2003; [abstract].
48. Roka A, Melinda KT, Vasarhelyi B, et al. Elevated morphine concentrations in neonates treated with morphine and prolonged hypothermia for hypoxic ischemic encephalopathy. Pediatrics 2008;121(4):e844–9.
49. Withington D, Menard G, Harris J, et al. Vecuronium pharmacokinetics and pharmacodynamics during hypothermic cardiopulmonary bypass in infants and children. Can J Anaesth 2000;47(12):1188–95.
50. Satas S, Loberg EM, Porter H, et al. Effect of global hypoxia-ischaemia followed by 24 h of mild hypothermia on organ pathology and biochemistry in a newborn pig survival model. Biol Neonate 2003;83(2):146–56.
51. Penrice J, Amess PN, Punwani S, et al. Magnesium sulfate after transient hypoxia-ischemia fails to prevent delayed cerebral energy failure in the newborn piglet. Pediatr Res 1997;41(3):443–7.
52. Zhu H, Meloni BP, Moore SR, et al. Intravenous administration of magnesium is only neuroprotective following transient global ischemia when present with post-ischemic mild hypothermia. Brain Res 2004;1014(1–2):53–60.
53. Wadhwa A, Sengupta P, Durrani J, et al. Magnesium sulphate only slightly reduces the shivering threshold in humans. Br J Anaesth 2005;94(6):756–62.

Technical Aspects of Starting a Neonatal Cooling Program

John D.E. Barks, MD

KEYWORDS

- Hypothermia • Induced hypothermia • Newborn infant
- Brain hypoxia-ischemia • Asphyxia neonatorum

Clinicians who are convinced by the available evidence that cooling is a safe and effective treatment of hypoxic-ischemic encephalopathy (HIE) in the term or near-term infant are now faced with a series of decisions around implementation of therapeutic hypothermia in their neonatal ICU (NICU) or region. The evidence in support of the safety and efficacy of hypothermia is reviewed in several published meta-analyses[1–4] and is also discussed elsewhere in this issue. A statistical argument, using the concept of the "optimal information size," can be made that there is currently uncertainty about either the efficacy of cooling or at least the magnitude of the effect, and that precise estimates of the benefit of cooling must await the publication of the results of the several pending trials.[5] This article assumes loss of equipoise on the part of the center planning to implement a cooling program (ie, that clinicians are sufficiently convinced by the available evidence of safety and efficacy to proceed to the implementation step).

DECIDING TO OFFER THERAPEUTIC HYPOTHERMIA

HIE is a relatively rare occurrence, on the order of 1 to 4 per 1000 live births in the developed world, although it occurs more frequently in the developing world. Before embarking on the development of a cooling program, therefore, clinicians and their administrative support staff should first review their own data over a period of several years to determine whether their NICU has a sufficient volume of in-born or referred infants 36 weeks' gestation or more who have HIE each year to justify the effort and expense entailed. There are no clear guidelines on what constitutes a sufficient volume of cases to merit development of a neonatal cooling program. Two recent series from centers that have implemented regional cooling programs reported 21 patients cooled in 2 years[6] and 46 patients cooled in 42 months,[7] roughly 1 patient per month. It is likely that additional patients were evaluated but not cooled in both programs. Centers

Neonatal-Perinatal Medicine, F5790 C.S. Mott Children's Hospital, Box 5254, 1500 East Medical Center Drive, University of Michigan Health System, Ann Arbor, MI 48109-5254, USA
E-mail address: jbarks@med.umich.edu

Clin Perinatol 35 (2008) 765–775
doi:10.1016/j.clp.2008.07.009
perinatology.theclinics.com
0095-5108/08/$ – see front matter

participating in regional data sharing or benchmarking efforts (e.g., by way of the Vermont-Oxford Network) might consider coordinated implementation of a regional program in neonatal hypothermia, in which the expertise is concentrated in a subset of NICUs selected from a geographic distribution of cases and centers. A recent economic modeling analysis based on data from the state of Massachusetts indicated that, in that state, a regionally integrated program with cooling (two units per NICU) available in all level III or IV NICUs, and transport from level I and II hospitals, was cost effective.[8] Massachusetts is a relatively small but populous geographic area; it is not known whether that model would apply to larger regions with more dispersed populations. Centers that are more geographically isolated may find it justifiable to implement cooling even with a limited number of anticipated cases per year, because distance and unpredictability of weather may preclude timely, reliable, or safe transport of these critically ill infants.

In addition, it is important to determine whether your center has the resources necessary to handle the full range of multiorgan complications typically presented by infants who have HIE. These resources include consultant services, such as pediatric neurology, pediatric cardiology, pediatric nephrology, and pediatric surgery; the availability of advanced care modalities, such as inhaled nitric oxide, high-frequency ventilation, extra corporeal membrane oxygenation, and dialysis; and the availability of diagnostic modalities, including ultrasound, ECG, electroencephalography (EEG), and neuroimaging (CT or MRI). Before the advent of cooling, when there were no therapeutic options to decrease the devastating impact of HIE (60%–70% death or severe handicap), many NICUs had a relatively nihilistic approach to HIE, frequently resulting in withdrawal of support in the first few days of life or a nonaggressive approach to multiorgan failure. It is clear from the reports of the three larger randomized trials published to date that infants who have HIE are sick babies, with many well-known complications of multiorgan ischemia-reperfusion injury.[9–11] Management of these complications in the context of therapeutic hypothermia is covered elsewhere in this issue.

GROUP PROCESS FOR IMPLEMENTATION

Whichever cooling modality is chosen, hypothermia is not a treatment to be undertaken on the spur of the moment. It takes months of preparation before a unit is ready to cool its first patient. Our center's experience, and that of others,[6] suggests that successful implementation of a new program requires a multidisciplinary approach. This suggestion is consistent with the recommendation of the Vermont-Oxford neonatal intensive care quality program for quality assessment and improvement in NICUs.[12] Membership in this interdisciplinary team should include all parties likely to be affected by the implementation of a new program, including nursing (leadership, staff nurses, including "opinion-leaders," educators, and nurse practitioners), neonatologists and their subspecialty trainees, pediatric neurologists, respiratory therapists, social workers, hospital administrators, outreach coordinators, transport services, and parent representatives. This multidisciplinary group may have several tasks, which may change over time, including review of evidence in favor of cooling, evaluation of center need for cooling, identification of available resources and potential barriers or pitfalls, clarification of roles and expectations, delegation of tasks, and determination of an implementation schedule. It is likely that a few people (e.g., one neonatologist and one or two allied health professionals) may need to take on the role of championing and shepherding cooling in its initial implementation. Nevertheless it is important for the broader group to take the time to talk out the issues involved in cooling, so that there can be a broad consensus before rolling out a cooling program to the entire NICU and referral region.

POTENTIAL BARRIERS TO IMPLEMENTATION

One of the purposes of the multidisciplinary process is to identify potential psychologic barriers to implementation of hypothermia. One major barrier is the preference for the familiar; for some, any change can be threatening. Others may not be fully aware of the evidence in support of the safety and efficacy of hypothermia, or, alternatively, they may not find the published data sufficiently convincing. Experienced NICU staff may have cared for many babies who had HIE who either died in the neonatal period or had obvious profound impairment, and may have trouble believing that any treatment could have an impact. Another potential source of resistance could be a bad prior experience with hypothermia (e.g., caring for a baby who was critically ill as a result of being born in a toilet in a cold apartment in the middle of winter). Concerns about limited space, personnel, or financial resources may also lead to resistance.

At the time of writing, there are some more concrete barriers to the implementation of cooling. Availability of the US Food and Drug Administration (FDA)–approved selective head cooling (SHC) device (Olympic Cool Cap System, Natus, San Carlos, CA) was initially limited. In part this was because the FDA approval process required that this second-generation device was never used on a human infant until after FDA approval, and its initial roll-out was limited primarily to centers that had extensive experience with the prior clinical trial device. Although the device used in both published whole body cooling (WBC) trials (Blanketrol II, Cincinnati Sub-Zero, Cincinnati, OH) has been commercially available for many years, and is freely available in some large North American hospitals, it is less easy to find in other parts of the world. Because this WBC device was not FDA approved for cooling for HIE, it does not come with a detailed step-by-step cooling protocol. The current lack of FDA-approved labeling for cooling for neonatal HIE for the Blanketrol may be considered a barrier to implementation by some hospitals. Many of the treatments used in neonatology are off-label uses, however, and safety and efficacy of the Blanketrol was demonstrated in two peer-reviewed, randomized, controlled trials.

CHOICE OF PROTOCOLS

At this time, the admonitions of expert bodies to only implement cooling in the context of one of the protocols with established safety and efficacy (or in the context of an ongoing trial) are still the best advice.[13,14] The two larger trials with published efficacy and safety data, both cooling for 72 hours, are the National Institute of Child Health and Human Development (NICHD) Neonatal Research Network protocol,[11] using a commercially available circulating water heating/cooling system (protocol available online at https://neonatal.rti.org/studies_hypothermia2.cfm) or an SHC protocol[10] using the only device so far FDA approved for neonatal hypothermia for HIE. A third option would be the South Carolina body-cooling protocol (48 hours' duration) of Eicher and colleagues,[15] which also has demonstrated efficacy but in a smaller number of patients than the NICHD trial, and which uses the same cooling equipment as the NICHD protocol. The published meta-analyses all indicate that hypothermia decreases the combined outcome of death or disability, and some (but not all) indicate that hypothermia decreases both death and disability considered separately. The author's opinion is that any apparent differences in the results of the two larger published trials are the result of differences in trial design (primarily patient population and outcome measures), and that, at the time of writing, either approach (SHC or WBC) is acceptable.

For reasons explained elsewhere, the author's unit, which participated in the original selective head cooling trial, currently offers both selective head cooling and WBC depending on individual patient circumstances.[7] A NICU's choice of cooling modality may be constrained by cost or product availability. In the absence of such constraints, the advantages and disadvantages of the two major cooling protocols can be considered.

Advantages of the NICHD WBC protocol include servo-controlled temperature regulation, less expensive equipment that may already be available in many larger hospitals (e.g., in the patient equipment department, operating rooms, or other ICUs), and full access to the scalp for amplitude-EEG (aEEG), conventional EEG, or video-EEG. One might assume that it would not be possible for an infant's temperature to fall outside the target range of 33.5 $\pm$ 0.5°C with a servo-controlled system. This is not the case, however, in part because there are internal limits to water temperature for safety reasons. In addition, the circulating water mattress is ordinarily the only means of thermoregulation in these infants, who are cared for on a radiant warmer bed with the heat off. In 3 out of 36 infants cooled using WBC in our center at the time of writing, the maximum mattress temperature of the system (42°C) was not sufficient to keep the infant's esophageal temperature from falling below the target range. Some overhead radiant heat was required to bring the esophageal temperature up to the desired level, and a reflective shield was added over the head to protect it from the radiant heat source. Potential disadvantages include off-label use and that the device used in the original protocol is overpowered for neonates, requiring the work-around of an adult mattress hung in the air next to the bedside. A hidden cost is the time needed to locate or purchase and then test the necessary supplies and equipment, and to develop a local protocol sufficiently detailed to be useful when there is a long gap in time between patients.

Advantages of SHC using the FDA-approved commercial device include built-in step-by-step instructions in a touch-screen graphic user interface, inclusion of all equipment and supplies in a single-source "package," and user training provided by the manufacturer or distributor. Potential disadvantages include higher price, limited scalp access for more than bifrontal aEEG (a nonvalidated location), and the need for manual regulation of the cap temperature throughout the 72-hour protocol. Manual control of the cooling cap temperature was believed necessary when the clinical trial device was designed because there are two independent sources of thermoregulation. The cooling cap removes heat from the head at the same time as the radiant warmer, operating on servo-control to achieve 100% output, pours heat into the rest of the body. The desired result is an equilibrium between the cap and the warmer, with a rectal temperature of 34.5 $\pm$ 0.5°C Because the FDA approval process required that the commercial device work the same way as the trial device (the user interface being only a superficial difference), a servo-control mechanism could not have been added, at least at the initial step of commercial availability. It is not clear whether user demand could change this in the future.

Whichever you decide is your first-choice system for hypothermia, develop a backup plan in case your primary equipment breaks down or in case you have more than one infant in need of cooling simultaneously. If you opt for WBC, be sure there are at least two of the hypothermia units in your institution, preferably more if they are in frequent use in locations other than the NICU. If you opt for SHC, for which the equipment is used exclusively in neonates, acquire at least two systems or develop a body-cooling protocol to use as a backup.

There are other cooling protocols and devices that have been used in clinical trials that are closed to enrollment. The results of these trials are not yet available in the peer-reviewed literature, however, and some use devices that are not approved in all markets at the time of writing (April 2008). The author is aware that investigators in some centers that participated in these now-closed trials with efficacy results pending are offering cooling on a compassionate use basis, using their trial protocols. Considering the recommendations cited previously, this practice is best limited to those trial centers, with continuing informed parental consent, until such time as their safety and efficacy data are published in the peer-reviewed literature. There are other cooling devices available that have not been used in any clinical trial in neonates; their use cannot be recommended based on currently available evidence.

ROLE OF AMPLITUDE-ELECTROENCEPHALOGRAPHY

For units unfamiliar with aEEG, involvement of a trained electrophysiologist, at least for post-hoc educational review of tracings, is helpful. Although some pediatric neurologists or electrophysiologists are not familiar with the compressed aEEG tracings, they quickly grasp the principles because the raw EEG signal is included in the new generation of digital aEEGs. In addition to helping neonatologists learn to recognize basic patterns of raw EEG in neonates, electrophysiologists need to help neonatologists learn to recognize artifacts (electrocardiogram, muscle activity, electrical interference) that can falsely elevate the aEEG voltage band. Lack of recognition of these artifacts that cause upward drift of the baseline might result in an infant not being offered cooling if aEEG is part of the selection process.

ROLES AND RESPONSIBILITIES

Who will be responsible for evaluation of infant eligibility for cooling? Most likely this individual will be a neonatologist, at least in the beginning. Will it be the neonatologist on call, or will there be a core group selected specifically for cooling babies? In the early phase of implementation, or in a large group practice, it may make sense to have a core group develop the expertise in assessment of encephalopathy and possibly aEEG and the expertise in initiating hypothermia. Subsequently, the core group can disseminate this expertise to other neonatologists and to subspecialty trainees, advanced practice nurses, or physician assistants.

The two major cooling protocols have similar first and second selection steps, the first of which is straightforward but the second of which may be problematic. The first criteria describe birth depression (e.g., one of: Apgar score ≤ 5 at 10 minutes, continued need for positive pressure ventilation at 10 minutes after birth, pH$<$7.0, or base deficit ≥ 16 mmol/L in cord blood or any arterial or venous sample within the first hour of life). These criteria are objective enough to be evaluated by telephone. The second criteria, for detection of moderate or severe encephalopathy or seizures, are potentially more challenging to evaluate, especially by telephone. Obtunded or comatose infants are easily recognized. The major challenge lies in the evaluation of infants who have moderate encephalopathy. If they do not require ongoing ventilation, subtle reductions in level of consciousness or alterations in tone and reflexes may not be noticed immediately by the casual observer. If they are intubated and ventilated for reasons that are not overtly central nervous system–related, for example, meconium aspiration syndrome, the systemic illness may mistakenly be assumed to be responsible for decreased activity, or the caregivers may simply be preoccupied with the pulmonary or systemic illness. As neonatologists take on responsibility for evaluating infants for eligibility for cooling, neonatal neurologic examination skills may need to be honed or relearned. Furthermore, the attempt to evaluate encephalopathy by telephone discussion with referring professionals can be challenging; an abbreviated neurologic examination checklist focusing on encephalopathy evaluation could be faxed to the birth hospital, to assist in the pre-transport evaluation.

Although neonatologists might initiate cooling because they need to be present to evaluate eligibility, the duration of the cooling protocols makes it a necessity to include training of allied health professionals (nurses, respiratory therapists, nurse practitioners, or physician assistants) in the maintenance of cooling. Ideally, sufficient allied health professionals would be trained to permit at least one such individual to be on duty at all times. To promote consistent care, consideration should be given to creating a standard order set for whichever hypothermia protocol is chosen.

CONSENT VERSUS ASSENT

Units implementing therapeutic hypothermia should consider whether to obtain procedure-specific informed consent. Anecdotally, and based on public statements, the author is aware that not all centers obtain procedure-specific consent for cooling, but statements in *Pediatrics* and *Journal of Pediatrics* suggest doing so.[13,14] The argument in favor of obtaining separate informed consent is that cooling is, at the time of writing, a novel therapy, not a standard of care. The argument cited for not obtaining procedure-specific consent is that it will delay initiation of cooling; this may have been a concern in the era of randomized trials, but a less protracted discussion (and an abbreviated consent form) could suffice for centers that accept the current body of evidence in favor of cooling. In the author's experience, most parents understand the analogy of icing an injured joint, even though the brain is more complex. If you plan to obtain procedure-specific consent and your hospital does not already have a formal process for telephone/fax consent, develop one in conjunction with your hospital attorneys or risk management department. This procedure will be needed because many of the babies eligible for cooling will be out-born.

TRAINING AND PREPARING FOR YOUR FIRST PATIENT

If you decide to do WBC, using the NICHD protocol, gather together whatever equipment and supplies are available in your hospital and purchase the remainder. You may discover that all the necessary equipment and supplies are already in your hospital, in use in the operating room, pediatric or adult ICUs, or emergency department. In addition to the hypo/hyperthermia system, reusable supplies include a YSI-400–compliant temperature cable to connect a disposable temperature probe to the system, and an extra set of hoses to connect the second cooling blanket. We find it helpful to have a few extra temperature cables, because they are sometimes inadvertently discarded. The choice of infant- and adult-size mattresses and esophageal temperature probes should be made after consulting with the NICHD protocol online. There are other potential sources of YSI-400–compliant esophageal temperature probes and temperature cables in addition to the manufacturer of the cooling system, but be sure the plugs of the probes, cables, and cooling unit are compatible. If your hospital does not already stock all the necessary supplies, you need to initiate a process for regularly restocking them in your NICU. If you choose SHC with the commercial FDA-approved device, initial supplies are included, but as with WBC, a system for regular restocking needs to be established.

Whichever protocol and device is chosen, before cooling the first patient, be sure that you have a local protocol with sufficient detail that it can be readily learned and used, even when patients are infrequent (e.g., once a month or longer). For WBC, and for any unit-specific issues in SHC, a digital slide presentation, including digital photographs showing how to connect the equipment, may be helpful. Also, plan to revise the local protocol based on experience. Key representatives of the device users should test the entire system before cooling the first infant. A useful training exercise can be conducted by cooling a large foam or similar insulated cup of approximately 39°C hot water with the core temperature probe in the water and surface probes, if any, attached to the outside of the cup. This exercise should be conducted on the same type of radiant warmer that will be used for hypothermia patients.

For WBC, following the NICHD protocol, start in manual control and pre-cool the blankets to 5°C. Remember to attach the second, adult-size mattress hanging in the air from an IV pole, using a second set of hoses. That second mattress damps down temperature fluctuation in the system. Then place the cup of hot water on the pre-cooled infant mattress on the bed, turn off the radiant warmer heat (if not already done), switch to automatic control with a set point of 33.5°C, watch the cup cool, and then feel the blankets warm up as the temperature in the cup falls below 33.5°C.

For SHC, begin with the insulated cup of hot water on the radiant warmer, set at 100% output. Follow all cooling initiation steps in the on-screen guide, entering imaginary patient data and turning the radiant warmer off when prompted, but place the rectal probe into the hot water through the cup lid, and place the cooling system fontanelle and abdominal wall skin probes and the radiant warmer skin probe on the exterior of the cup. The touch screen guide includes digital "check-boxes" for the user to indicate completion of each step. When instructed to place the circulating water cap on the head, nestle the hot water cup within the cap. When the water temperature in the cup falls to 35.5°C you will be prompted to turn on the radiant warmer in servo-controlled mode to a target temperature of 37°C. With this commercial system, set aside, and do not discard, a cap set and probe set for recurrent training use, not to be used on patients. With the commercial SHC system it is also worthwhile to explore the help screens during the training process; they include reminders of the approved indications and examples of qualifying aEEG traces.

MONITOR YOUR EXPERIENCE

When embarking on a new therapy, ideally one ought to monitor various short- and long-term results for purposes of quality assessment and improvement (QA/QI). For example, how well are staff adhering to (or able to adhere to) cooling protocols? How much time are infants spending outside of the target temperature range? Are potential systemic complications of either birth depression or hypothermia being systematically monitored? Are there guidelines for regularly evaluating skin integrity and are they followed? Is developmental follow-up available and used? Have you joined a national or international data collection and benchmarking registry?

TEMPERATURE REGULATION QUALITY ASSESSMENT AND IMPROVEMENT

The WBC equipment (Blanketrol II) lacks the ability to record temperature data. Although the SHC system records and displays temperatures graphically during the 72 hours of cooling and 4 hours of rewarming, the FDA (shortsightedly, in the author's view) mandated that this information not be downloadable. It is hoped that this barrier to QA/QI will be overcome in time. In any case, the SHC graphical user interface, which also shows when the set temperature was adjusted, may be helpful in real-time QA/QI by demonstrating the excessive temperature fluctuations that can result from staff waiting too long to adjust the cap set temperature in response to changes in core temperature. Bedside flow sheets specifically designed for neonatal hypothermia patients are one approach to data collection for purposes of quality assessment or improvement. The argument for dedicated data collection for QA/QI of therapeutic hypothermia is that the extra temperatures to be gathered, which might help trouble-shoot, would not normally have a place on a typical NICU nursing flow sheet. Data might be collected every 15 minutes for the first 2 hours and hourly thereafter for the first few patients. As experience grows, temperature recording might be reduced to hourly until 8 to 12 hours of cooling, then every 3 or 4 hours. Records should include all temperatures being monitored (for WBC: blanket actual, blanket set-point, skin, and esophageal temperatures; for SHC: cap actual, cap set-point, skin, fontanel, and rectal temperatures), along with heart rate and blood pressure. In addition to data collection for retrospective QA/QI, the reality of starting a cooling program is that some temperature-control problems will arise that need to be dealt with in real time by the neonatologist on call. Experience gained from QA/QI ought to be quickly incorporated into unit-specific protocols available to all staff. Hypothermia management, including updates, should be incorporated into recurring staff education schedules.

SYSTEMIC AND SKIN COMPLICATIONS OF COOLING AND OF BIRTH ASPHYXIA

Systemic complications and their management are discussed elsewhere in this issue. A NICU establishing a cooling program needs to consider development of protocols to systematically monitor these complications (e.g., as part of a hypothermia order set). Sclerema neonatorum is a known complication of either inadvertent hypothermia or of birth asphyxia, and rare cases have been reported in infants treated with SHC (Cool Cap Continued Access Protocol, as reported in http://www.fda.gov/ohrms/dockets/ac/05/minutes/2005-4162m1_Summary%20minutes.pdf) or WBC.[11] Sclerema eventually resolved as the infants recovered. Exaggerated scalp swelling, generally in infants who had total body fluid overload, has been reported in infants treated with SHC, and in rare cases this has been complicated by bruising or compromised skin integrity in critically ill infants who had coagulopathy or refractory hypotension.[10] Minimum guidelines for performing scalp checks (every 12 hours) are included in the on-screen prompts in the commercial SHC system. Other skin complications reported in cooled infants in the NICHD WBC trial included subcutaneous fat necrosis (a known complication of asphyxia neonatorum in the pre-cooling era), erythema, and cyanosis. In the author's experience with WBC, exaggerated acrocyanosis may be seen, especially when cooling is initiated on a pre-cooled mattress, or at other times when the mattress water temperature is cold. At a minimum it seems prudent to evaluate dependent skin integrity in infants treated with WBC at a frequency similar to the SHC recommendations.

ANTICIPATING AND MONITORING NEUROLOGIC COMPLICATIONS AND RECOVERY

Seizures are a common complication of HIE, and HIE is the most common cause of seizures in term neonates. Although there is one single-center human trial reporting improved long-term outcome in term infants treated prophylactically with phenobarbital during the first 6 hours of life,[16] this result has not been replicated and there is currently no human evidence that prophylactic anticonvulsant administration improves outcome in cooled infants. Treatment of seizures in infants treated with hypothermia should be undertaken with the knowledge that metabolism of phenobarbital is reportedly slowed by hypothermia treatment in infants who have HIE.[17] This finding, and the frequent complication of HIE by hepatocellular injury,[18] suggests that close monitoring of anticonvulsant levels is merited in infants treated with hypothermia. Emergence or re-emergence of seizures has been observed during or after rewarming in infants and fetal sheep treated with hypothermia.[19,20]

Do not expect infants who have HIE treated with hypothermia to rapidly "wake up" after rewarming. Delayed clearance of anticonvulsants[17] or morphine[21] (commonly used for sedation in some NICUs) may contribute to slow recovery. It takes time to recover from encephalopathy even in the babies that ultimately do well. For example, a secondary analysis from the Cool Cap trial demonstrated that among infants who had moderate (modified Sarnat stage II) encephalopathy after rewarming, most eventually did well.[22] Secondary analyses from the SHC trial and the Cochrane meta-analysis suggest that infants who have either moderate or severe clinical encephalopathy can benefit from hypothermia.[4,23] There is no evidence to support withholding of cooling from infants who present with severe encephalopathy, or even with a so-called "flat tracing" on aEEG. The number needed to treat for the combined outcome of death or disability is approximately seven (ie, for every seven infants cooled there will be one more intact survivor[4]) so a new program's first several cases might not do well.

Two common concerns about hypothermic therapy are that death is only "traded" for severe disability, and that somehow cooling deprives families and clinicians of a window of opportunity for withdrawal of support. The Cochrane meta-analysis suggests that these concerns are not borne out by the evidence to date, and that hypothermia decreases both death and disability in survivors,[4] although there are several large trials yet to report. Trial results and the Cochrane meta-analysis clearly indicate that there will be handicapped survivors, some of whom will have severe handicaps. Secondary analyses have so far not yielded a reliable means of early identification of those patients who will not respond to cooling, however.[24]

Infants who have HIE are at high risk for permanent neurodevelopmental disabilities. Hypothermia reduces but does not eliminate the risk for disability in survivors[4] and these infants merit developmental follow-up to facilitate early detection and referral for management of disabilities. Any center embarking on a cooling program should thus have a plan for neurodevelopmental follow-up during the first 18 to 24 months of life. Another resource that may be required is a pediatric palliative care or hospice program.

INFORM YOUR REFERRING HOSPITALS

When you are ready to begin cooling infants, let your usual referring hospitals know the criteria in simple terms (e.g., with posters or laminated pocket cards), and emphasize the importance of the 6-hour eligibility window. Because of the 6-hour window, you may have to encourage some referring hospitals to transport an eligible baby to your center (if they are capable), which generally saves time if a significant distance is involved. If you are the first center to introduce cooling program in your region, you may need to work to break habits of nihilistic thinking about HIE.

You may also wish to develop a protocol for your own hospital and referring hospitals to use to avoid hyperthermia in babies who seem to be cooling candidates while they are being transported or evaluated. Core hyperthermia is associated with worse outcome in infants who have HIE.[25] One option is to take the skin temperature probe (if it is a plastic-covered wire, but not if it is a metal disc) and insert it about 3 to 4 cm into the rectum, and then either servo-control the warmer to keep the rectal temperature in the 36 to 37°C range, or manually adjust the warmer output with the same goal. Some units, when they become experienced with hypothermia, but only when their transport team has the capability of measuring core temperature lower than 33°C, may consider adapting a protocol for cooling on transport. For example, the South Carolina (Eicher) protocol may be modified to their own unit's target temperature for hypothermia.[6,9,15] The latter protocol relies primarily on turning off external heat sources and if necessary, brief (minutes) application of small bags of ice covered in a cloth to the side of the head or upper trunk. Additional information on protocols for and safety and efficacy of passive cooling before and during neonatal transport to a cooling center will be available when the results of the infant cooling evaluation and total body hypothermia trials are published.

SUMMARY

Hypothermia is an emerging therapy for neonatal hypoxic-ischemic encephalopathy. Many former clinical trial sites are now offering this therapy, and a growing number of NICUs that did not participate in the original trials are adopting one or more of the already-published regimens for use in their NICU. Units offering hypothermia should strongly consider joining a registry (e.g., the Vermont-Oxford Neonatal Encephalopathy Registry or the TOBY Register) that facilitates benchmarking of short- and long-term outcomes and supports local quality enhancement efforts. Results of the three randomized controlled trials that have closed to enrollment and are currently following infants to their primary outcome will likely provide additional information to inform decision making about several issues raised in this review. Centers already using hypothermia or considering it should thus closely monitor the medical literature.

REFERENCES

1. Edwards AD, Azzopardi DV. Therapeutic hypothermia following perinatal asphyxia. Arch Dis Child Fetal Neonatal Ed 2006;91(2):F127–31.
2. Schulzke SM, Rao S, Patole SK. A systematic review of cooling for neuroprotection in neonates with hypoxic ischemic encephalopathy—are we there yet? BMC Pediatr 2007;7:30.
3. Shah PS, Ohlsson A, Perlman M. Hypothermia to treat neonatal hypoxic ischemic encephalopathy: systematic review. Arch Pediatr Adolesc Med 2007;161(10): 951–8.
4. Jacobs S, Hunt R, Tarnow-Mordi W, et al. Cooling for newborns with hypoxic ischaemic encephalopathy. Cochrane Database Syst Rev 2007;(4): CD003311.
5. Kirpalani H, Barks J, Thorlund K, et al. Cooling for neonatal hypoxic ischemic encephalopathy—is the answer in? Pediatrics 2007;120:1126–30.
6. Zanelli SA, Naylor M, Dobbins N, et al. Implementation of a "hypothermia for HIE" program: 2-year experience in a single NICU. J Perinatol, 2008;28:171–5.
7. Sarkar S, Barks JD, Donn SM. Should amplitude-integrated electroencephalography be used to identify infants suitable for hypothermic neuroprotection? J Perinatol 2008;28:117–22.
8. Gray J, Geva A, Zheng Z, et al. CoolSim: using industrial modeling techniques to examine the impact of selective head cooling in a model of perinatal regionalization. Pediatrics 2008;121(1):28–36.
9. Eicher DJ, Wagner CL, Katikaneni LP, et al. Moderate hypothermia in neonatal encephalopathy: safety outcomes. Pediatr Neurol 2005;32(1):18–24.
10. Gluckman PD, Wyatt JS, Azzopardi D, et al. Selective head cooling with mild systemic hypothermia after neonatal encephalopathy: multicentre randomised trial. Lancet 2005;365(9460):663–70.
11. Shankaran S, Laptook AR, Ehrenkranz RA, et al. Whole-body hypothermia for neonates with hypoxic-ischemic encephalopathy. N Engl J Med 2005;353(15): 1574–84.

12. Horbar JD, Plsek PE, Leahy K. NIC/Q 2000: establishing habits for improvement in neonatal intensive care units. Pediatrics 2003;111(4 Pt 2):e397–410.
13. Higgins RD, Raju TN, Perlman J, et al. Hypothermia and perinatal asphyxia: executive summary of the National Institute of Child Health and Human Development workshop. J Pediatr 2006;148(2):170–5.
14. Blackmon LR, Stark AR. Hypothermia: a neuroprotective therapy for neonatal hypoxic-ischemic encephalopathy. Pediatrics 2006;117(3):942–8.
15. Eicher DJ, Wagner CL, Katikaneni LP, et al. Moderate hypothermia in neonatal encephalopathy: efficacy outcomes. Pediatr Neurol 2005;32(1):11–7.
16. Hall RT, Hall FK, Daily DK. High-dose phenobarbital therapy in term newborn infants with severe perinatal asphyxia: a randomized, prospective study with three-year follow-up. J Pediatr 1998;132(2):345–8.
17. Thoresen M, Stone J, Hoem NO, et al. Hypothermia after perinatal asphyxia more than doubles the plasma half-life of phenobarbitone. Pediatr Res 2003;53(4):24A.
18. Shah P, Riphagen S, Beyene J, et al. Multiorgan dysfunction in infants with post-asphyxial hypoxic-ischaemic encephalopathy. Arch Dis Child Fetal Neonatal Ed 2004;89(2):F152–5.
19. Battin M, Bennet L, Gunn AJ. Rebound seizures during rewarming. Pediatrics 2004;114(5):1369.
20. Gerrits LC, Battin MR, Bennet L, et al. Epileptiform activity during rewarming from moderate cerebral hypothermia in the near-term fetal sheep. Pediatr Res 2005; 57(3):342–6.
21. Roka A, Melinda KT, Vasarhelyi B, et al. Elevated morphine concentrations in neonates treated with morphine and prolonged hypothermia for hypoxic ischemic encephalopathy. Pediatrics 2008;121(4):e844–9.
22. Gunn AJ, Wyatt JS, Whitelaw A, et al. Therapeutic hypothermia changes the prognostic value of clinical evaluation of neonatal encephalopathy. J Pediatr 2008;152:55–8.
23. Wyatt JS, Gluckman PD, Liu PY, et al. Determinants of outcomes after head cooling for neonatal encephalopathy. Pediatrics 2007;119(5):912–21.
24. Ambalavanan N, Carlo WA, Shankaran S, et al. Predicting outcomes of neonates diagnosed with hypoxemic-ischemic encephalopathy. Pediatrics 2006;118(5): 2084–93.
25. Laptook A, Tyson J, Shankaran S, et al. Elevated temperature after hypoxic-ishemic encephalopathy: risk factor for adverse outcomes. Pediatrics 2008;122: 491–9.

The Diagnosis, Management, and Postnatal Prevention of Intraventricular Hemorrhage in the Preterm Neonate

Heather J. McCrea, PhD[a,b], Laura R. Ment, MD[c,d,*]

KEYWORDS

- Intraventricular hemorrhage • Preterm • Prevention
- Indomethacin • Ibuprofen • Phenobarbital

Preterm birth can result in significant developmental disability, and many studies have identified intraventricular hemorrhage (IVH) as a major cause of adverse outcome for very low birthweight (VLBW) preterm neonates. IVH, or hemorrhage into the germinal matrix tissues of the developing brain, has been attributed to changes in cerebral blood flow to the immature germinal matrix microvasculature and secondary periventricular venous infarction. The more severe grades of IVH are characterized by the acute distension of the cerebral ventricular system with blood and hemorrhage with parenchymal venous infarction and are associated with high degrees of morbidity and mortality.

Nationally, 20% to 25% of all VLBW infants suffer IVH. Among neonates of less than 1500 g birthweight, 10% to 15% suffer the more severe grades of hemorrhage, and more than three quarters of these develop mental retardation or cerebral palsy (CP). Based on data from the United States Census Bureau, the National Institute of Child Health and Human Development Neonatal Network, and the Centers for Disease

This work was supported by grants number NS 27116 and NS 53865 from the National Institutes of Health.

[a] Yale University School of Medicine, 333 Cedar Street, New Haven, CT 06510, USA
[b] Department of Cell Biology, BCMM 235, Yale University, 295 Congress Avenue, New Haven, CT 06520, USA
[c] Department of Pediatrics, 3089 LMP, Yale University School of Medicine, 333 Cedar Street, New Haven, CT 06520, USA
[d] Department of Neurology, Yale University School of Medicine, 333 Cedar Street, New Haven, CT 06510, USA
* Corresponding author. Department of Pediatrics, 3089 LMP, Yale University School of Medicine, 333 Cedar Street, New Haven, CT 06520.
E-mail address: laura.ment@yale.edu (L.R. Ment).

Clin Perinatol 35 (2008) 777–792
doi:10.1016/j.clp.2008.07.014 **perinatology.theclinics.com**
0095-5108/08/$ – see front matter

Control, there are more than 3600 new cases of mental retardation attributable to IVH in the United States each year, and the lifetime care costs for these children exceed $3.6 billion.

Preterm birth represents a unique environment for the developing brain, and many important environmental factors, including inflammation, hypotension, and hypoxemia, that contribute to IVH are identified. To address the enormous societal and financial burden of IVH, pharmacologic and care-oriented prevention strategies have been implemented. These studies have led to significant reductions in the incidence of IVH by changing practices in newborn resuscitation and perinatal care.

Nonetheless, the incidence of grades (Gr) 3–4 IVH has not changed over the past 10 years, and the role of genetics factors in the pathophysiology of IVH is just beginning to be explored. These data suggest that, for VLBW infants, IVH is a complex disorder. To further lower the incidence of IVH and thus neurodevelopmental handicap in the preterm population, prevention strategies must target environmental and genetic factors.

INTRAVENTRICULAR HEMORRHAGE IS AN IMPORTANT PREDICTOR OF ADVERSE NEURODEVELOPMENTAL OUTCOME

Although several early studies reported that cognitive outcome may be directly related to gestational age at birth,[1,2] recent data suggest that medical risk factors may be equally important predictors of neurologic outcome.[3–9] Chief among these is Gr 3–4 IVH.[7]

IVH occurs in infants of 32 weeks' gestation or less, and the overall incidence of IVH is inversely related to gestational age. For the purposes of this article, IVH is described by the following classification: grade 1—germinal matrix hemorrhage; grade 2—intraventricular blood without distension of the ventricular system; grade 3—blood filling and distending the ventricular system; and grade 4—parenchymal involvement of hemorrhage, also known as periventricular venous infarction.[10–12]

In the newborn period, 5% to 10% of preterm infants who have Gr 3–4 IVH suffer seizures and as many as 50% experience posthemorrhagic hydrocephalus. Finally, mortality is higher in infants who have Gr 3–4 IVH than in gestational age–matched subjects who do not have Gr 3–4 IVH.[12]

Although prematurely born children who have Gr 3–4 IVH are at high risk for CP and mental retardation,[2,13–20] children who have Gr 1–2 IVH also are at risk for developmental disability. One half to three quarters of infants who have Gr 3–4 IVH develop disabling CP in childhood, and in the large and well characterized cohort of Pinto-Martin and colleagues, Gr 3–4 IVH was associated with CP with an odds ratio (OR) of 15.4 (95% CI, 7.6–31.1).[17] Furthermore, 45% to 86% of preterm children who have Gr 3–4 IVH are reported to suffer major cognitive handicaps; approximately 75% of them are in special education classrooms or receive extensive special education services in school, and a recent review found that the presence of Gr 3–4 IVH is significantly associated with mental retardation at 2 to 9 years, with OR values ranging from 9.97 to 19.0.[16,20]

PATHOPHYSIOLOGY: INTRAVENTRICULAR HEMORRHAGE IS A COMPLEX DISORDER

Risk Factor Studies

Studies addressing the etiology of Gr 3–4 IVH have identified many environmental and medical risk factors, including low gestational age, absence of antenatal steroid exposure, antenatal maternal hemorrhage, maternal chorioamnionitis/infection/inflammation, maternal fertility treatment, outborn status (ie, neonatal transport), early sepsis, hypotension requiring therapeutic intervention, hypoxemia, hypercapnia, pneumothorax, pulmonary hemorrhage, respiratory distress syndrome, severity of illness score, seizures, small for gestational age status, treatment for acidosis, and treatment with pressors.[12,21–27]

Role of Cerebral Blood Flow and the Germinal Matrix Microvasculature

IVH generally has been attributed to alterations in cerebral blood flow to the immature germinal matrix microvasculature. During the risk period for IVH, this region is richly supplied with microvessels lacking basement membrane deposition, tight junctions, and glial endfoot investiture, all components of a competent blood-brain barrier. In response to hypotension, hypoxemia, hypercapnia, or acidosis, cerebral blood flow rises, hemorrhage begins within the germinal matrix, and blood may rupture into the ventricular system. After ventricular distension by an acute hemorrhagic event, blood flow falls. Venous stasis occurs within the periventricular white matter, and parenchymal venous infarction may follow.

Significant modulators of cerebral blood flow in the developing brain include the cyclooxygenase 2 (COX-2) system and prostaglandins.[28–30] COX-2 expression is induced by hypoxia; hypotension; growth factors, such as epidermal growth factor receptor and transforming growth factor-beta; and inflammatory modulators, including interleukin (IL)-6, IL-1β, tumor necrosis factor α (TNF-α), and nuclear factor κB.[31–42] The resultant prostanoids promote the production and release of vascular endothelial growth factor (VEGF), a potent angiogenic factor.[35,43]

Those same triggers that initiate hemorrhage into the germinal matrix set in motion a cascade leading to the disruption of tight junctions, increased blood-brain barrier permeability, and microglial activation within the developing periventricular white matter. These events are mediated by cytokines, VEGF, and nitric oxide. In vitro, endothelial cells and astrocytes release the pro-inflammatory cytokines, IL-1β and TNF-α, and both of these promote transmigration of leukocytes across the endothelium and developing blood-brain barrier. Furthermore, hypoxia alone has been shown to alter the blood-brain barrier proteins, ZO-1, occludin, and ZO-2. Finally, reactive microglia release reactive oxygen species (ROS), which in turn not only contribute to endothelial damage but also alter hemostasis and increase anaerobic metabolism.[44–47]

The preterm brain is more susceptible to ROS than the adult brain because of the immaturity of those enzyme systems designed to detoxify them. In addition to their release by activated microglia, ROS also are generated after the activation of the COX-2 system.[48] Because of their multifaceted effects on the developing vasculature, ROS are believed to play a significant role in periventricular parenchymal infarction.[49]

Genetic Factors May Play a Role

The relatively recent description of the thrombophilias associated with the factor V Leiden and prothrombin G20210A mutations and the implication of both in perinatal stroke suggest these also might be candidate genes for IVH (**Table 1**).[50–53] Likewise, mutations in collagen IVA1 result in IVH in neonatal mice and porencephaly in human infants, and adults who have intracerebral hemorrhage have a high incidence of the apolipoprotein E4 or E2 allele.[54–58]

Polymorphisms in the proinflammatory cytokine IL-6 also are proposed as possible genetic modifiers of the risk for IVH, although the results are somewhat contradictory.[59,60] Position 174 can be a G or a C, and IL-6 production is believed greater in neonates who have a CC genotype.[60] Harding and colleagues[60] demonstrated that preterm infants (≤32 weeks' gestation) who had the CC genotype at amino acid 174 had a statistically significant increase in the rate of IVH, white matter disease,

Table 1
Candidate genes for intraventricular hemorrhage

Gene	Allele	Effect
Inflammation		
IL-6	174 G or C, 572 G or C	CC has increased IL-6 production, question of increased risk for IVH, white matter disease, and CP
TNF-α		Possible candidate gene for IVH
Hemostasis		
Factor V Leiden		Increased thrombosis, increased risk for perinatal stroke, possible candidate gene for IVH
Prothrombin	G20210A	Increased thrombosis, increased risk for perinatal stroke, possible candidate gene for IVH
Apolipoprotein E4 or E2		Increased incidence in adults who have intracerebral hemorrhage, candidate gene for IVH
Vascular stability		
COL4A1		Mutations result in IVH in neonatal mice and porencephaly in human infants, candidate gene for IVH

and disability compared with neonates who had the GC or GG genotype. CP also was seen at twice the rate in infants who had the CC genotype compared with GC or GG genotype, but this did not reach statistical significance. Despite the increase in IVH and white matter disease, long-term developmental outcome as measured by the Griffiths development quotient at 2 years and the British Ability Scales II (BAS) and Movement Assessment Battery for Children at age 5.5 years was not statistically different between the two groups. In contrast, using a considerably larger sample size, Gopel and colleagues[59] noted no effects of the CC genotype on cerebral injury, including IVH, periventricular leukomalacia (PVL), or the need for placement of a ventriculoperitoneal shunt.

A polymorphism at position 572 in the IL-6 gene also has been studied.[61] Similar to the 174 position, the 572 position can be a G or more rarely a C and the C allele is associated with higher levels of IL-6. Preterm neonates (born at ≤32 weeks' gestation) who had the C allele showed decreased performance on the Griffiths developmental quotient at 2 years and the general cognitive ability portion of the BAS at 5.5 years; they did not have an increased rate of IVH or PVL. The rate of the C allele is very low, however; thus, the number of patients included in this study was small, and results must be interpreted with caution.

Finally, recent studies suggest that the interaction of thrombophilia mutations, inflammatory factors, and ROS may contribute to IVH. Infants who have IVH may suffer mutations of TNF-α and IL-6. In addition, thrombin can induce ROS in microglia. Studies of preterm infant have shown that neonates at risk for CP are more likely than their peers to have evidence of activation of systemic inflammatory factors and elevated levels of coagulation factors.[32,62–64]

In summary, available epidemiologic, laboratory, and clinical studies suggest that multiple environmental and genetic factors may affect the risk for IVH independently or interactively via at least five different and yet overlapping pathways: angiogenesis and vascular pathology, control of cerebral blood flow in the developing brain, inflammation/infection, oxidative pathways, and coagulation and thrombophilia mutations. Therapies to prevention IVH must address the complexity of this disease.

THE RISK PERIOD FOR INTRAVENTRICULAR HEMORRHAGE IS INDEPENDENT OF GESTATIONAL AGE

To prevent injury, knowledge of the risk period is critical for success. IVH is encountered most commonly within the first 24 hours after birth, and hemorrhages can progress over 48 hours or more. By the end of the first postnatal week, 90% of the hemorrhages can be detected at their full extent, and this risk period for IVH is independent of gestational age.

MANAGEMENT OF INTRAVENTRICULAR HEMORRHAGE

Screening for Intraventricular Hemorrhage in Very Low Birthweight Preterm Neonates

Management of IVH typically is confined to screening for sequelae of IVH and managing systemic issues of the neonate, such as blood pressure and respiratory status, which might influence progression of IVH. The American Academy of Neurology "Practice parameter: neuroimaging of the neonate" suggests that screening ultrasonography should be performed on all preterm neonates of less than 30 weeks' gestation at two time points.[16] The first ultrasound is recommended between 7 and 14 days of age to detect signs of IVH, and the second ultrasound is recommended at 36 and 40 weeks' postmenstrual age to look for CNS lesions, such as periventricular leukomalacia and ventriculomegaly, which affect long-term outcome. MRI is better than ultrasound at detecting white matter abnormalities, hemorrhagic lesions, and cysts, and emerging data are providing preliminary evidence for the importance of this imaging modality at term equivalent as a predictor of outcome at 2 to 3 years of age in VLBW preterm infants.

Radiologic Assessment of Risk for Intraventricular Hemorrhage

If preventing injury is hoped for in a patient population, markers of impending injury must be sought. In particular, therefore, diffusion-weighted imaging studies in the acute perinatal period are shown predictive of cystic PVL. To the best of the authors' knowledge, however, no antenatal or postnatal MRI findings have been reported that are predictive of IVH.

Short-Term Sequelae of Intraventricular Hemorrhage

Posthemorrhagic hydrocephalus (PHH) and PVL are two significant sequelae of IVH. Patients who have PHH usually present with rapidly increasing head circumferences, enlarging ventricles on radiologic examination, and signs of increased intracranial pressure, but the signs and symptoms of hydrocephalus may not be evident for several weeks post hemorrhage because of the compliance of neonatal brain.[65] The majority of cases of PHH are communicating, as shown in **Fig. 1**, and are believed secondary to the impaired cerebrospinal fluid (CSF) reabsorption, which accompanies the chemical arachnoiditis commonly found after blood is introduced into the CSF. Neonates also can exhibit a noncommunicating hydrocephalus secondary to the acute obstruction of the foramen of Monro or the aqueduct by clot or to subependymal scarring. Randomized controlled trials performed to evaluate several potential treatments to prevent or reduce the extent of PHH include intraventricular streptokinase, repeated lumbar or ventricular punctures, and DRIFT (drainage, irrigation, and fibrinolytic therapy), but these interventions have proved ineffective.[12,66,67]

Further, although Whitelaw[12] has recommended ventricular puncture with removal of between 10 and 20 mL/kg of CSF for cases of rapid ventricular enlargement and increased intracranial pressure, others have explored temporizing measures, such

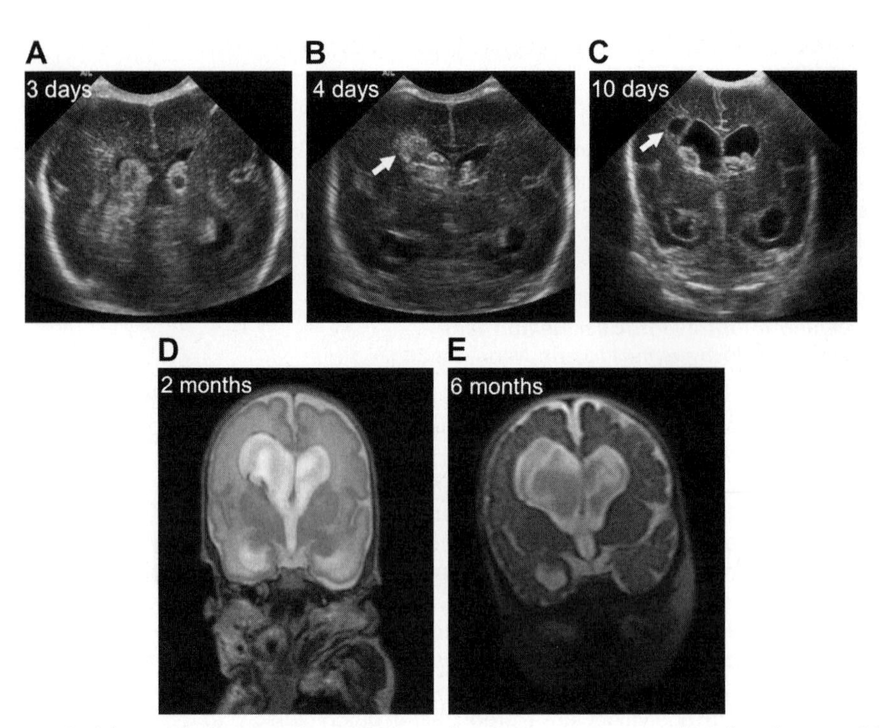

Fig. 1. Serial cranial ultrasounds and MRI studies from a preterm male infant born at 24 weeks of gestation. The initial diagnosis of grade 3 IVH at age 3 days (*A*) was followed by parenchymal involvement of hemorrhage, or grade 4 IVH, on postnatal day 4 (*arrow*) (*B*). A cranial ultrasound performed on day 10 because of increasing occipitofrontal head circumference and full fontanelle revealed bilateral ventriculomegay, residual intraventricular blood and a developing porencephaly (*arrow*) (*C*). MRI study at 2 months demonstrated ventriculomegaly (*D*). Because of excessive increase in head circumference and increasing spasticity, the patient underwent third ventriculostomy after MRI scan at age 6 months (*E*).

as subgaleal shunt placement or ventricular reservoir placement for intermittent tapping (RES), with the hope of avoiding permanent VP shunt placement. A small retrospective review of these interventions in IVH patients recently determined that 91% of patients who had subgaleal shunt placement and 62% of patients who had RES required subsequent permanent shunt placement.[68] Infection rates were similar in the two populations. Future randomized trials are required to confirm this information and determine the appropriate time and manner of intervention.

IVH also can result in white matter abnormalities, including PVL. PVL, shown in **Fig. 2**, is classically defined as multiple cystic foci in the periventricular cerebral white matter,[69] which on histology demonstrate coagulation necrosis and loss of cellular architecture.[70] When PVL follows IVH, it has been attributed to the sometimes profound and long-lasting decreases in cerebral blood flow that accompany the introduction of blood into the CSF. Some of these cases of PVL after IVH also have progressed to porencephaly (Greek for "hole in the brain"),[71] so it is important to distinguish enlarged ventricles caused by white matter destruction from those under increased pressure as in PHH.

Depending on the severity and location of the PVL lesions, the clinical presentation of affected children may range from spastic diplegia to decreased visual fields and

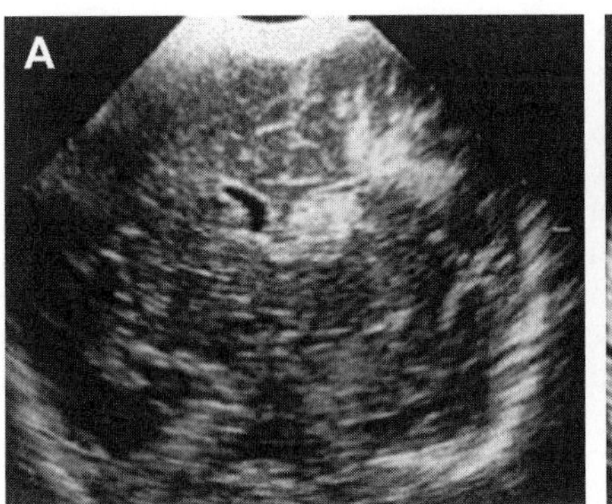

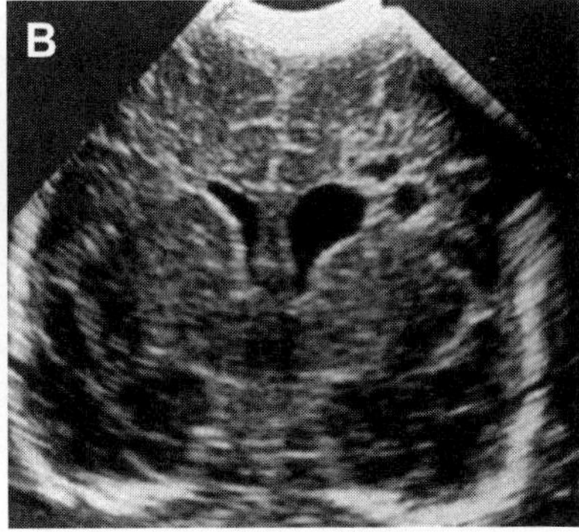

Fig. 2. Serial cranial ultrasounds of a 30-week preterm male infant who had grade 3 IVH and hemorrhagic PVL at age 10 days (*A*). Repeat ultrasound 3 weeks later demonstrated unilateral ventriculomegaly and periventricular cystic cavities consistent with PVL (*B*).

cognitive impairment,[72,73] and many investigators believe that the white matter injury that accompanies IVH represents the major cause of the neurodevelopmental impairments suffered by these neonates.

Finally, a grade 4 IVH also may result in porencephaly independent of PVL or PHH.[74] These hemispheric cavitary lesions generally are freely communicating with the ventricular system, although rarely a porencephaly may present as a fluid-filled cyst that obstructs the ventricular system and may present with symptoms of increased intracranial pressure.

RATIONALE FOR PREVENTION STRATEGIES

As support in the neonatal period has improved, more low birthweight infants are surviving, and it has become increasingly clear that certain newborns seem to do better than their similarly premature counterparts. Differences even are noted in rates of IVH at different neonatal intensive care units, with those treating higher patient volumes and with a higher neonatologist-to-housestaff ratio having lower rates of IVH.[75] It is uncertain what accounts for this difference, but there is speculatation on environmental, genetic, and pharmacologic effects. Environmental and pharmacologic strategies to prevent IVH have increasingly been tried with varying degrees of success, although it is not the mandate of this review to discuss environmental manipulations or antenatal pharmacologic agents for the prevention of IVH.

Furthermore, as pharmacologic treatments have emerged, it also has become apparent that some children respond better to treatment than others. As a result, an understanding of the role that gender and genetics play in the natural course of IVH and in response to IVH prevention strategies is critical, as it will enable better allocation of resources to those infants at greatest risk for IVH and those most likely to benefit from the intervention.

Finally, newborn follow-up is critical to the successful evaluation of any proposed intervention. Therapeutic strategies designed to modulate cerebral blood flow to the preterm brain may alter perfusion to other developing organs and result in adverse renal or gastrointestinal sequelae. Similarly, agents believed to modulate blood pressure may impair neurogenesis and, thus, cognition in the developing nervous system.

POSTNATAL PHARMACOLOGIC PREVENTIONS STRATEGIES FOR INTRAVENTRICULAR HEMORRHAGE

The well-known sequelae of IVH have prompted the development of pharmacologic prevention strategies for this injury to developing brain for almost 4 decades (**Table 2**). These interventions have included phenobarbital, pavulon, vitamin E, ethamsylate, indomethacin, ibuprofen, and recombinant activated factor VIIa. Because the preclinical and clinical trials for pavulon, vitamin E, and ethamsylate took place many years ago and these agents currently are not in wide use, these studies are reviewed only briefly in this article. Mechanisms of action and study results for the other four agents are discussed.

Phenobarbital

Phenobarbital is believed to stabilize blood pressure and potentially offer protection from free radicals. Because variations in blood pressure, subsequent changes in cerebral blood flow, and oxygen free radical damage during reperfusion are believed to contribute to IVH, phenobarbital was proposed as a possible prevention strategy. Whitelaw and Odd[76] reviewed the literature regarding phenobarbital in the prevention of IVH. Overall, eight of the ten trials reviewed showed no statistically significant difference in risk for IVH in phenobarbital- versus control-treated patients. One trial showed an increased risk for IVH in the phenobarbital-treated group, but in this study, the phenobarbital group was younger in age and smaller in size than the control group.[77] These factors would have increased the risk for IVH in this patient group, independent of treatment with phenobarbital. One study showed a decreased risk for IVH in the phenobarbital-treated group, but patients in this study were not checked for IVH before instituting treatment.[78] Rates of severe IVH, studied in all 10 trials, and ventricular dilation or hydrocephalus, studied in four trials, also did not differ significantly between phenobarbital- and control-treated infants. Whitelaw and Odd concluded that in the ten trials examined, patients treated with phenobarbital did not have a significant decrease in IVH or severity of IVH, but they did have an increased risk for requiring mechanical ventilation.

Table 2
Postnatal prevention strategies for intraventricular hemorrhage

Pharmacologic Agent	Proposed Mechanism
Phenobarbital	Stabilize blood pressure and free radical production
Pavulon	Prevent asynchronous breathing in ventilated newborns with secondary BP stabilization
Ethamsylate	Promote platelet adhesion; increase capillary basement membrane stability
Vitamin E	Free radical protection
Indomethacin	Promote microvascular maturation; blunt fluctuations in BP and cerebral blood flow
Ibuprofen	Improve autoregulation of cerebral blood flow
Factor VIIa[a]	Promote clot formation

[a] Rescue therapy to prevent extension of IVH.

Indomethacin

Indomethacin is used in preterm neonates to close patent ductus arteriosus and for prevention of IVH. Indomethacin acts via nonspecific inhibition of the constitutive and inducible isoforms of cyclooxygenase, COX-1, and COX-2, respectively, which subsequently decreases prostaglandin synthesis. Indomethacin is believed to prevent IVH through effects on blood flow and on basement membrane maturation. Insults, such as hypertension, asphyxia, or hypercapnia, typically lead to hyperemia in experimental animals, but intravenous delivery of indomethacin blunts this response and improves cerebral autoregulation.[29,79,80] Indomethacin also is shown to promote microvessel maturation of the germinal matrix in beagle pups[81] and in a pig model to inhibit the alterations in blood-brain barrier permeability that result from ischemia.[29] Consistent with this experimental data, infants treated with indomethacin have been shown to have a decrease in the incidence and severity of IVH.[82,83]

Despite the obvious effect in preventing IVH, the long-term cognitive benefit of indomethacin treatment has been more controversial, and recent scientific work has attempted to understand the effect of indomethacin on developing brain. Some groups have proposed that indomethacin should be neuropathologic because it blocks COX activity with a resulting inhibition in production of the neuroprotective prostaglandin E2,[84] whereas others have proposed that this agent may confer neuroprotection by preventing the up-regulation of genes linked to oxidative stress[85] and down-regulating those inflammatory factors, such as IL-6 and TNF-α, which inhibit neurogenesis.[86] In addition, the COX-2 gene has two polymorphic variants, a G or a C at position 765.[84] Patients who have the C allele have reduced COX-2 activity and thus may exhibit different responses to indomethacin than those who have the alternative allele.

Neurodevelopmental outcome has been reported for three of the indomethacin trials. Age at subject assessment and cognitive measures used differed considerably among the studies, and the meta-analysis of Fowlie and Davis[87] concluded that treatment with indomethacin did not affect rates of severe developmental delay or neurosensory impairment. Several investigators have questioned why, if indomethacin decreases the incidence and lowers the severity of IVH, it does not seem to globally improve outcome.[82–84] Harding and colleagues[84] have reported that prematurely born subjects with the COX-2 C765 allele had decreased cognitive performance at age 2 and 5.5 years when compared with their G allele peers.

Furthermore, Ment and colleagues[88] analyzed their indomethacin data on the basis of gender. The rate of IVH was found significantly decreased with indomethacin treatment in male infants, but there was no corresponding decrease in IVH rate after indomethacin treatment in female neonates. IVH grade also was significantly reduced in males treated with indomethacin. In addition, boys treated with indomethacin performed significantly better on the Peabody Picture Vocabulary Test—Revised at 3, 4.5, 6, and 8 years' corrected age when compared with placebo-treated boys. This increased performance was independent of the decrease in IVH and was not seen in girls. These data suggest that gender may play an important role in injury to the developing brain and long-term cognitive outcome and that gender must be considered when evaluating new treatments.

Ibuprofen

Intravenous ibuprofen was tested in newborns as a result of evidence in newborn animals that it improved cerebral blood flow autoregulation.[89] Aranda and Thomas[90] reviewed the use of ibuprofen in neonates and found that although ibuprofen has a similar effect to indomethacin on closure of patent ductus arteriosus, it was ineffective with respect to IVH prevention.

Activated Factor VII

Recombinant activated factor VII (rFVIIa) originally was developed in preclinical trials as a hemostatic agent for use in patients who have hemophilia.[91,92] rFVIIa is believed to act in the clotting cascade through tissue factor–dependent and –independent mechanisms.[93] Tissue factor normally is exposed only at sites of endothelial damage. The enzymatic activity of endogenous factor VIIa is weak unless bound to tissue factor. Upon binding to tissue factor, downstream factors in the coagulation cascade are activated, leading to conversion of prothrombin to thrombin with subsequent conversion of fibrinogen to fibrin. When rFVIIa is used, the plasma concentration is approximately 10 times that seen with endogenous factor VIIa. As a result of this increased concentration, rFVIIa is able to bind to activated platelets leading to a "thrombin burst," a major increase in the amount of thrombin generated, which is independent of tissue factor. This leads to the formation of a thrombin clot, and factors that prevent fibrinolysis and prevent dissolution of this clot are activated. Factor VII was proved safe and effective in treating the hemophiliac patient population and since then, its off-label use has widened to include nonhemophiliac patients who have uncontrolled bleeding resulting from oral anticoagulation, trauma, thrombocytopenia, platelet dysfunction, and liver dysfunction.[94] Placebo-controlled, randomized clinical trials looking at safety and efficacy, however, are lacking for the off-label use of factor VII. In neonates, Greisen and Andreasen conducted a small study on preterm infants (gestational age less than 33 weeks) who had prolonged PT. Ten babies were evaluated for side effects of factor VII administration and to compare different doses of factor VII, and then two babies were randomized to rFVIIa with four randomized to fresh frozen plasma.[95] Factor VII was demonstrated to decrease PT more than fresh frozen plasma, but the investigators note that the PT may not be representative of clotting function, as the test they used is particularly sensitive to factor VII concentration in the sample. The results suggest that the half-life of rFVIIa in preterm babies was similar to that of adults, ranging between 2 and 3 hours. The neonates included in this study had no adverse events. Although there have not been other randomized clinical trials of factor VII in the neonatal population, two case series, one involving nine patients less than 4 months of age[96] and one nine patients that included 6 preterm infants,[97] have further suggested that factor VII may be safe and effective as a rescue therapy to control bleeding the in the newborn population after conventional treatments are exhausted.

Because evidence suggests that factor VII may be an effective agent in prevention of bleeding in a diverse array of situations, it has also been proposed as a potential treatment for IVH.[98] Because factor VII is believed to require exposed tissue factor or activated platelets in order for it to promote coagulation, it is believed that the prothrombotic effects of factor VII should be restricted to the site of injury, thus contributing to its safety. Administration just after onset of IVH would be expected to promote clotting in the periventricular region without promoting a hypercoagulable state.[98] Although results with factor VII in nonhemophiliac patients are preliminary and further study is necessary, its proposed mechanism of action, positive results in some patient populations with major bleeding, and the observed safety so far in the admittedly small number of neonates in which it has been assessed suggest that this is an intervention which deserves further study in the setting of IVH.

Other Prevention Trials

Additional postnatal treatments evaluated have included ethamsylate, vitamin E, and pavulon. Ethamsylate promotes platelet adhesion and increases stability of the capillary basement membrane by causing hyaluronic acid polymerization. In clinical trials, ethamsylate decreased the rates of IVH in VLBW infants without altering rates of severe IVH, death, or neurologic abnormality.[12] Similarly, vitamin E, an antioxidant, also has been shown to decrease the rate of IVH although the effect on high grade IVH was not specifically examined and overall mortality was unaffected.[99] Finally, pavulon (pancuronium) also has been tested as an intervention to decrease IVH in mechanically ventilated newborns. By inducing muscular paralysis, pavulon is believed to prevent asynchronous breathing and the alterations in oxygenation and secondary changes in cerebral blood associated with this phenomenon in preterm neonates.[100]

SUMMARY

IVH remains a common problem of VLBW preterm neonates and may be associated with significant neurodevelopmental disability. Prevention strategies must address the environmental and genetic causes of this injury to developing brain. The effect of gender on the efficacy of indomethacin treatment and of genetics on the cognitive outcome of preterm neonates argues that as new interventions are developed, their effect on specific subgroups of neonates must be considered in addition to their overall population effect. Studying all preterm neonates as a single group, although an important first strategy, risks missing treatments that potentially could benefit subgroups of this population. The authors suggest that when studies are performed in the future, in addition to evaluating safety and efficacy in the entire study group, researchers should analyze their data with respect to gender and, ideally, genetic polymorphisms. This strategy for assessing interventions should allow for a more thorough analysis of potential benefits.

ACKNOWLEDGMENTS

The authors thank Deborah Hirtz, MD, and Charles C. Duncan, MD, for scientific advice and Ms. Marjorene Ainley for administrative assistance.

REFERENCES

1. McCormick MC, Gortmaker SL, Sobel AM. Very low birth weight children: behavior problems and school difficulty in a national sample. J Pediatr 1990; 117:687–93.
2. Whitaker AG, Feldman JF, Rossem RV, et al. Neonatal cranial ultrasound abnormalities in low birth weight infants: Relation to cognitive outcomes at six years of age. Pediatrics 1996;98:719–29.
3. Anderson A, Swank P, Wildin S. Modeling analysis of change of neurologic abnormalities in children born prematurely: a novel approach. J Child Neurol 1999;14:502–8.
4. Hansen BM, Dinesen J, Hoff B, et al. Intelligence in preterm children at four years of age as a predictor of school function: a longitudinal controlled study. Dev Med Child Neurol 2002;44:517–21.
5. Koller H, Lawson K, Rose SA. Patterns of cognitive development in very low birth weight children during the first six years of life. Pediatrics 1997;99:383–9.
6. Ment LR, Vohr BR, Allan WA, et al. Change in cognitive function over time in very low-birth-weight infants. JAMA 2003;289:705–11.
7. Morris BH, Smith KE, Swank PR, et al. Patterns of physical and neurologic development in preterm children. J Perinatol 2002;22:31–6.

8. Tommiska V, Heinonen K, Kero P, et al. A national two year follow up of extremely low birthweight infants born in 1996-1997. Arch Dis Child Fetal Neonatal Ed 2003;88:F29–35.
9. Vollmer B, Roth S, Baudin J, et al. Predictors of long-term outcome in very preterm infants: gestational age versus neonatal cranial ultrasound. Pediatrics 2003;112:1108–14.
10. Papile LS, Burstein J, Burstein Rea. Incidence and evolution of the subependymal intraventricular hemorrhage: a study of infants with weights less than 1500 grams. J Pediatr 1978;92:529–34.
11. Volpe JJ. Neurology of the newborn. 4th edition. Philadelphia: W.B.Saunders; 2001.
12. Whitelaw A. Intraventricular haemorrhage and posthaemorrhagic hydrocephalus: pathogenesis, prevention and future interventions. Semin Neonatol 2001; 6:135–46.
13. Arzoumanian Y, Mirmiran M, Barnes PD, et al. Diffusion tensor brain imaging findings at term-equivalent age may predict neurologic abnormalities in low birth weight preterm infants. AJNR Am J Neuroradiol 2003;24:1646–53.
14. de Vries LS, Roelants-van Rijn AM, Rademaker KJ, et al. Unilateral parenchymal haemorrhagic infarction in the preterm infant. Eur J Paediatr Neurol 2001;5: 139–49.
15. Krishnamoorthy KS, Shannon DC, DeLong GE, et al. Neurologic sequelae in the survivors of neonatal intraventricular hemorrhage. Pediatrics 1979;64:233–7.
16. Ment LR, Bada HS, Barnes PD, et al. Practice parameter: neuroimaging of the neonate. Neurology 2002;58:1726–38.
17. Pinto-Martin JA, Whitaker AH, Feldman J, et al. Relation of cranial ultrasound abnormalities in low-birthweight infants to motor or cognitive performance at ages 2, 6 and 9 years. Dev Med Child Neurol 1999;41:826–33.
18. Szymonowicz W, Yu VYH, Bajuk B, et al. Neurodevelopmental outcome of periventricular hemorrhage and leukomalacia in infants. Early Hum Dev 1986;14:1–7.
19. Vohr B, Garcia-Coll C, Flanagan P, et al. Effects of intraventricular hemorrhage and socioeconomic status of perceptual cognitive and neurologic status of low birth weight infants at 5 years of age. J Pediatr 1992;121:280–5.
20. Vohr BR, Allan WA, Westerveld M, et al. School age outcomes of very low birth weight infants in the indomethacin intraventricular hemorrhage prevention trial. Pediatrics 2003;111:e340–6.
21. Ancel P-Y, Marret S, Larroque B, et al. Are maternal hypertension and small-for-gestational age risk factors for severe intraventricular hemorrhage and cystic periventricular leukomalacia? Results of the EPIPAGE cohort study. Am J Obstet Gynecol 2005;193:178–84.
22. Hall RW, Kronsberg SS, Barton BA, et al. Morphine, hypotension, and adverse outcomes among preterm neonates: who's to blame? Secondary results from the NEOPAIN Trial. Pediatrics 2005;115:1351–9.
23. Kaiser JR, Gauss CH, Pont MM, et al. Hypercapnia during the first 3 days of life is associated with severe intraventricular hemorrhage in very low birth weight infants. J Perinatol 2006;26(5):279–85. Epub.
24. Kluckow M. Low systemic blood flow and pathophysiology of the preterm transitional circulation. Early Hum Dev 2005;81:429–37.
25. Linder N, Haskin O, Levit O, et al. Risk factors for intraventricular hemorrhage in very low birth weight premature infants: a retrospective case-control study. Pediatrics 2003;111:e590–5.

26. Osborne DA, Evans N. Early volume expansion for prevention of morbidity and mortality in very preterm infants. Cochrane Database Syst Rev 2004;2: CD002055.pub2.
27. Synnes AR, Chien L-Y, Peliowski A, et al. Variations in intraventricular hemorrhage incidence rates among Canadian neonatal intensive care units. J Pediatr 2001;138:525–31.
28. Leffler CW, Busija DW, Beasley DG. Effects of Indomethacin on cardiac outcome distribution in normal and asphyxiated piglets. Prostaglandins 1986;31:183–90.
29. Leffler CW, Busija DW, Fletcher AM, et al. Effects of indomethacin upon cerebral hemodynamics of newborn pigs. Pediatr Res 1985;19:1160–4.
30. Ment LR, Stewert WB, Duncan CC, et al. Beagle puppy model of intraventicular hemorrhage. Effect of indomethacin on cerebral blood flow. J Neurosurg 1983; 58:857–62.
31. Ackerman WE IV, Rovin BH, Kniss DA. Epidermal growth factor and interleukin-1 (beta) utilize divergent signaling pathways to synergistically upregulate cyclooxygenase-2 gene expression in human amnion-derived WISH cells. Biol Reprod 2004;71:2079–86.
32. Dammann O, Leviton A. Inflammatory brain damage in preterm newborns - dry numbers, wet lab, and causal inferences. Early Hum Dev 2004;79:1–15.
33. Hedtjarn M, Mallard C, Eklind S, et al. Global gene expression in the immature brain after hypoxia-ischemia. J Cereb Blood Flow Metab 2004;24:1317–32.
34. Heep A, Behrendt D, Nitsch P, et al. Increased serum levels of interleukin 6 are associated with severe intraventricular haemorrhage in extremely premature infants. Arch Dis Child Fetal Neonatal Ed 2003;88:F501–4.
35. Kuwano T, Nakao S, Yamamoto H, et al. Cyclooxygenase 2 is a key enzyme for inflammatory cytokine-induced angiogenesis. FASEB J 2004;18:300–10.
36. Pan JZ, Jornsten R, Hart RP. Screening anti-inflammatory compounds in injured spinal cord with microarrays: a comparison of bioinformatics analysis approaches. Physiol Genomics 2004;17:201–14.
37. Parfenova H, Levine V, Gunther WM, et al. COX-1 and COX-2 contributions to basal and IL-1 beta-stimulated prostanoid synthesis in human neonatal microvascular endothelial cells. Pediatr Res 2002;52:342–8.
38. Ribeiro ML, Ogando D, Farina M, et al. Epidermal growth factor modulation of prostaglandins and nitrite biosynthesis in rat fetal membranes. Prostaglandins Leukot Essent Fatty Acids 2004;70:33–40.
39. Richardson CM, Sharma RA, Cox G, et al. Epidermal growth factor receptors and cyclooxygenase-2 in the pathogenesis of non-small cell lung cancer: potential targets for chemoprevention and systemic therapy. Lung Cancer 2003;39: 1–13.
40. Seibert K, Masferrer J, Zhang Y, et al. Mediation of inflammation by cyclooxygenase-2. Agents Actions Suppl 1995;46:41–50.
41. Stanimirovic D, Satoh K. Inflammatory mediators of cerebral endothelium. Brain Pathol 2000;10:113–26.
42. Takada Y, Bhardwaj A, Paotdar P, et al. Nonsteroidal anti-inflammatory agents differ in their ability to suppress NF-kappaB activation, inhibition of expresion cyclooxygenase-2 and cyclin D1, and abrogation of tumor cell proliferation. Oncogene 2004;23:9247–58.
43. Smith WL, Meade EA, DeWitte DL. Interactions of PGH synthase isozymes-1 and -2 with NSAIDs. Ann N Y Acad Sci 1994;774:50–7.
44. Chao CC, Hu S, Molitor TW, et al. Activated microglia mediate neuronal cell injury via a nitric oxide mechanism. J Immunol 1992;149:2736–41.

45. Colton CA, Gilbert DL. Microglia, an in vivo source of reactive oxygen species in the brain. Adv Neurol 1993;59:321–6.
46. Possel H, Noack H, Putzke J, et al. Selective upregulation of inducible nitric oxide synthase (INOS) by lipopolysaccharide (LPS) and cytokines in microglia: in vitro and in vivo studies. Glia 2000;32:51–9.
47. Rezaie P, Dean A, Male D, et al. Microglia in the cerebral wall of the human telencephalon at second trimester. Cereb Cortex 2005;15(7):938–49.
48. Akundi RS, Candelario-Jalil E, Hess S, et al. Signal transduction pathways regulating cyclooxygenase-2 in lipopolysaccharide-actived primary rat microglia. Glia 2005;51:199–208.
49. Folkert RD, Haynes RL, Borenstein NS, et al. Developmental lag in superoxide dismutases relative to other antioxidant enzymes in premyelinated telencephalic white matter. J Neuropathol Exp Neurol 2004;63:990–9.
50. Debus O, Koch HG, Kurlemann G, et al. Factor V Leiden and genetic defects of thrombophilia in childhoold porencephaly. Arch Dis Child Fetal Neonatal Ed 1998;78:121–4.
51. Gopel W, Gortner L, Kohlmann T, et al. Low prevalence of large intraventricular haemorrhage in very low birthweight infants carrying the factor V Leiden or prothrombin G20210A mutation. Acta paediatr 2001;90:1021–4.
52. Gopel W, Kattner E, Seidenberg J, et al. The effect of the Val37Leu polymorphism in the factor XIII gene in infants with a birth weight below 1500 g. J Pediatr 2002;140:688–92.
53. Petaaja J, Hiltunen L, Fellman V. Increased risk of intraventricular hemorrhage in preterm infants with thrombophilia. Pediatr Res 2001;49:643–6.
54. Adcock K, Hedberg C, Loggins J, et al. The TNF-alpha - 308, MCP - 1-2518 and TGF - beta 1 + 915 polymorphisms are not associated with the development of chronic lung disease in very low birth weight infants. Genes Immun 2003;4:420–6.
55. Alberts MJ, Tournier-Lasserve E. Update on the genetics of stroke and cerebrovascular disease 2005. Stroke 2005;36:179–81.
56. Gould DB, Phalan C, Breedveld GJ, et al. Mutations in Col4a1 cause perinatal cerebral hemorrhage and porencephaly. Science 2005;308:1167–71.
57. Gould DB, Phalan C, van Mil SE, et al. Role of COL4A1 in small-vessel disease and hemorrhagic stroke. N Engl J Med 2006;354:1489–96.
58. Woo D, Sauerbeck LR, Kissela BM, et al. Genetic and environmental risk factors for intracerebral hemorrhage: preliminary results of a population-based study. Stroke 2002;33:1190–5.
59. Gopel W, Hartel C, Ahrens P, et al. Interleukin-6-174-genotype, sepsis and cerebral injury in very low birth weight infants. Genes Immun 2006;7:65–8.
60. Harding DR, Dhamrait S, Whitelaw A, et al. Does interleukin-6 genotype influence cerebral injury or developmental progress after preterm birth? Pediatrics 2004;114:941–7.
61. Harding D, Brull D, Humphries SE, et al. Variation in the interleukin-6 gene is associated with impaired cognitive development in children born prematurely: a preliminary study. Pediatr Res 2005;58:117–20.
62. Choi S-H, Lee DY, SKim SU, et al. Thrombin-induced oxidative stress contributes to the death of hippocampal neurons in viv: role of microglial NADPH oxidase. J Neurosci 2005;25:4082–90.
63. Dammann O, Leviton A, Gappa M, et al. Lung and brain damage in preterm newborns and their association with gestational age, prematurity subgroup, infection/inflammation and longterm outcome. BJOG 2005;112(Suppl 1):4–9.

64. Leviton A, Dammann O. Coagulation, inflammation, and risk of neonatal white matter disease. Pediatr Res 2004;55:541–5.
65. Volpe JJ. Brain injury in the premature infant. Clin Perinatol 1997;24:567–87.
66. Whitelaw A, Evans D, Carter M, et al. Randomized clinical trial of prevention of hydrocephalus after intraventricular hemorrhage in preterm infants: brain-washing versus tapping fluid. Pediatrics 2007;119:e1071–8.
67. Whitelaw A, Odd DE. Intraventricular streptokinase after intraventricular hemorrhage in newborn infants. Cochrane Database Syst Rev 2007;4:CD000498.
68. Wellons J, Shannon C, Oakes W, et al. Comparison of conversion rates from temporary CSF management to permanent shunting in premature IVH infants. Presented at the 36th Annual Meeting of the AANS/CNS Section on Pediatric Neurological Surgery. South Beach (Miami), Florida, November 26–December 1, 2007. p. 35.
69. Banker BQ, Larroche JC. Periventricular leukomalacia of infancy: a form of neonatal anoxic encephalopathy. Arch Neurol 1962;7:32–50.
70. Deguchi K, Oguchi K, Takashima S. Characteristic neuropathology of leukomalacia in extremely low birth weight infants. Pediatr Neurol 1997;16:296–300.
71. Grant EG, Schellinger D, Smith Y, et al. Periventricular leukomalacia in combination with intraventricular hemorrhage: sonographic features and sequelae. AJNR Am J Neuroradiol 1986;7:443–7.
72. Bax M, Tydeman C, Flodmark O. Clinical and MRI correlates of cerebral palsy: the European Cerebral Palsy Study. JAMA 2006;296:1602–8.
73. Graham M, Levene MI, Trounce JQ, et al. Prediction of cerebral palsy in very low birthweight infants: prospective ultrasound study. Lancet 1987;2:593–6.
74. Ment LR. Intraventricular hemorrhage of the preterm neonate. In: Swaiman KF, Ashwal S, Ferriero DM, editors. 4th edition, Pediatric neurology; principles and practice, Vol I. Philadelphia: Mosby; 2006. p. 309–28.
75. Synnes AR, Macnab YC, Qiu Z, et al. Neonatal intensive care unit characteristics affect the incidence of severe intraventricular hemorrhage. Med Care 2006;44:754–9.
76. Whitelaw A, Odd D. Postnatal phenobarbital for the prevention of intraventricular hemorrhage in preterm infants. Cochrane Database Syst Rev 2007;4: CD001691.
77. Kuban KC, Leviton A, Krishnamoorthy KS, et al. Neonatal intracranial hemorrhage and phenobarbital. Pediatrics 1986;77:443–50.
78. Donn SM, Roloff DW, Goldstein GW. Prevention of intraventricular hemorrhage in preterm infants by phenobarbitone: a controlled trial. Lancet 1981;2:215–7.
79. Pourcyrous M, Busija DW, Shibata M, et al. Cerebrovascular responses to therapeutic dose of indomethacin in newborn pigs. Pediatr Res 1999;45:582–7.
80. Van Bel F, Klautz JM, Steenduk P, et al. The influence of indomethacin on the autoregulatory ability of the cerebral vascular bed in the newborn lamb. Pediatr Res 1993;34:278–81.
81. Ment LR, Stewert WB, Ardito TA, et al. Indomethacin promotes germinal matrix microvessel maturation in the newborn beagle pup. Stroke 1992;23:1132–7.
82. Ment LR, Oh W, Ehrenkranz RA, et al. Low dose indomethacin and prevention of intraventicular hemorrhage: A multicenter randomized trial. Pediatrics 1994;93: 543–50.
83. Schmidt B, David P. Long-term effects of indomethacin prophylaxis in extremely-low-birth-weight infants. N Engl J Med 2001;344:1966–72.
84. Harding DR, Humphries SE, Whitelaw A, et al. Cognitive outcome and cyclo-oxygenase-2 gene (-765 G/C) variation in the preterm infant. Arch Dis Child Fetal Neonatal Ed 2007;92:F108–12.

85. Scheel JR, Ray J, Gage FH, et al. Quantitative analysis of gene expression in living adult neural stem cells by gene trapping. Nat Methods 2005;2:363–70.
86. Monje ML, Toda H, Palmer TD. Inflammatory blockade restores adult hippocampal neurogenesis. Science 2003;302:1760–5.
87. Fowlie PW, Davis PG. Prophylactic indomethacin for preterm infants: a systematic review and meta-analysis. Arch Dis Child Fetal Neonatal Ed 2003;88: F464–6.
88. Ment LR, Vohr BR, Makuch RW, et al. Indomethacin for the prevention of intraventricular hemorrhage is effective only in boys. J Pediatr 2004;145:832–4.
89. Chemtob S, Beharry K, Barna T, et al. Differences in the effects in the newborn piglet of various nonsteroidal anti-inflamatory drugs on cerebral blood flow but not on cerebrovascular protaglandin. Pediatr Res 1991;30:106–11.
90. Aranda JV, Thomas R. Systematic review: intravenous Ibuprofen in preterm newborns. Semin Perinatol 2006;30:114–20.
91. Brinkhous KM, Hedner U, Garris JB, et al. Effect of recombinant factor VIIa on the hemostatic defect in dogs with hemophilia A, hemophilia B, and von Willebrand disease. Proc Natl Acad Sci U S A 1989;86:1382–6.
92. Macik BG, Lindley CM, Lusher J, et al. Safety and initial clinical efficacy of three dose levels of recombinant activated factor VII (rFVIIa): results of a phase I study. Blood Coagul Fibrinolysis 1993;4:521–7.
93. Labattaglia MP, Ihle B. Recombinant activated factor VII: current perspectives and Epworth experience. Heart Lung Circ 2007;16(Suppl 3):S96–101.
94. Ghorashian S, Hunt BJ. “Off-license” use of recombinant activated factor VII. Blood Rev 2004;18:245–59.
95. Greisen G, Andreasen RB. Recombinant factor VIIa in preterm neonates with prolonged prothrombin time. Blood Coagul Fibrinolysis 2003;14:117–20.
96. Brady KM, Easley RB, Tobias JD. Recombinant activated factor VII (rFVIIa) treatment in infants with hemorrhage. Paediatr Anaesth 2006;16:1042–6.
97. Mitsiakos G, Papaioannou G, Giougi E, et al. Is the use of rFVIIa safe and effective in bleeding neonates? A retrospective series of 8 cases. J Pediatr Hematol Oncol 2007;29:145–50.
98. Robertson JD. Prevention of intraventricular haemorrhage: a role for recombinant activated factor VII? J Paediatr Child Health 2006;42:325–31.
99. Chiswick M, Gladman G, Sinha S, et al. Vitamin E supplementation and periventricular hemorrhage in the newborn. Am J Clin Nutr 1991;53:370S–2S.
100. Cools F, Offringa M. Neuromuscular paralysis for newborn infants receiving mechanical ventilation. Cochrane Database Syst Rev 2005;2:CD002773.

Inhaled Nitric Oxide and Neuroprotection in Preterm Infants

Jeremy D. Marks, PhD, MD[a,*], Michael D. Schreiber, MD[b]

KEYWORDS

• Chronic lung disease • Periventricular leukomalacia
• Intraventricular hemorrhage • Neurodevelopment • Bayley

Infants born very prematurely (<32 weeks gestation) are well documented to be at risk for neurodevelopmental impairments, including blindness, deafness, cerebral palsy, and global cognitive delay, as well as more subtle cognitive deficits, such as language delay, learning disabilities, and attention and executive function abnormalities. Longitudinal studies of several large cohorts of extremely premature (<28 weeks gestation) infants including the Victorian Infant Collaborative Study Group (VICS) in Australia[1] (<28 weeks gestation), the EPICure study group in the United Kingdom[2,3] (<26 weeks gestation), and the National Institute for Child Health and Development (NICHD) in the United States, have provided a rough consensus regarding the incidence of abnormal neurobehavioral outcomes at 18 to 30 months for these smallest infants born during the 1990s (for recent reviews, see Anderson and Doyle[4] and Aylward[5]). Reported rates of cerebral palsy vary between 8% for infants less than 28 weeks[2] to as high as 21% for infants less than 25 weeks,[6] whereas rates of severe cognitive delay (scores on the Bayley Scales of Infant Development[7] [BSD-II, Bayley] < 70) are reported to vary between 18% and 30%.[3] Blindness and deafness are relatively uncommon, with an incidence for each around 2%. The percentages of children of these gestational ages reported as having no neurodevelopmental impairment is disturbingly small: fewer than half the children in the VICS 1997 cohort and 21% for children less than 25 weeks gestation in the NICHD cohort.

This work was supported by NS056313 from the National Institute of Neurologic Disorders and Stroke to JDM and a grant from the Gerber Foundation to MDS. Dr Schreiber has received grant support from Ikaria for investigator-initiated clinical research studies. Drs. Schreiber and Marks report receiving speakers' honoraria from Ikaria.

[a] Department of Pediatrics, Neurology, and The College Committees on Cell Physiology and Molecular Medicine, MC 6060, University of Chicago, 5841 S. Maryland Avenue, Chicago, IL 60637, USA

[b] Department of Pediatrics and the College Committees on Cell Physiology and Molecular Medicine, MC8000, University of Chicago, 5841 S. Maryland Avenue, Chicago, IL 60637, USA

* Corresponding author.

E-mail address: jmarks@uchicago.edu (J.D. Marks).

Clin Perinatol 35 (2008) 793–807
doi:10.1016/j.clp.2008.07.015 **perinatology.theclinics.com**

RISK FACTORS FOR ABNORMAL NEURODEVELOPMENTAL OUTCOMES IN PRETERM INFANTS

The risk of abnormal neurodevelopmental outcome is well documented to increase at progressively earlier gestational ages; neurologic morbidity becomes a significant concern with infants with birth weights less than 1000 g. Those infants born at less than 27 weeks gestation are at high risk, and this risk progressively increases with each 1-week decrease in gestational age to 24 weeks. Biological risks factors contributing to an abnormal neurodevelopmental outcome can be partitioned into (a) those occurring before birth; (b) direct brain injury sustained at or after birth; (c) co-morbidities sustained during maturation to term; (d) ongoing challenges to brain development encountered following discharge from the intensive care nursery.

Chronic placental insufficiency leading to ongoing hypoxia, acute placental insufficiency and asphyxia, as well as chorioamnionitis constitute important risks before birth.[8,9] Intraventricular hemorrhage and periventricular leukomalacia are the two primary signs of acute brain injury in the premature infant contributing significantly to abnormal neurodevelopmental outcome. Infants who have suffered major complications of prematurity, including hypotension, sepsis, and necrotizing enterocolitis have a greater overall illness severity and are at greater risk of abnormal neurodevelopmental outcomes.[10] The presence of chronic lung disease at discharge is an independent risk factor for abnormal neurodevelopmental outcome,[11–13] as is exposure to prolonged postnatal courses of corticosteroids.[14,15] Infants discharged home on oxygen or with apnea are at risk for continuing episodes of hypoxia and subsequent brain injury.[16] Discharge to families challenged by low socioeconomic class, with the attendant lack of appropriate, supportive home environments, educational supports, and decreased access to health care constitutes socioeconomic risk for abnormal neurodevelopmental outcome.[17]

Despite increasing understanding of the risk factors leading to abnormal neurodevelopmental outcomes, and despite intensive investigation,[18,19] until recently little progress had been made in the development of interventions during the initial hospitalization to improve neurodevelopmental outcomes. Recently, however, evidence has been accruing that inhaled nitric oxide (iNO) may provide an unanticipated therapy to improve neurodevelopment in preterm infants.

INHALED NITRIC OXIDE IN PRETERM INFANTS: A TREATMENT TO IMPROVE CARDIOPULMONARY OUTCOMES

Inhaled NO is currently approved for use for the treatment of hypoxic respiratory failure and persistent pulmonary hypertension in the full- and near-term newborn. Inhaled NO promotes pulmonary vasodilatation, decreases pulmonary artery pressure, decreases right-to-left extra- and intra-cardiac shunting and intrapulmonary shunting, and improves arterial oxygenation.[20–22] In preterm infants, trials of iNO therapy were undertaken initially to test the overall hypothesis that iNO, by improving ventilation–perfusion matching in the immature lung, would allow infants to be supported with lower levels of mechanical ventilation than would be necessary in the absence of iNO. This potentially decreased support was hypothesized to reduce the incidence of chronic lung disease and death. Thus, trials of iNO therapy in preterm infants were initiated to improve cardiopulmonary outcomes.

INITIAL TRIALS OF INHALED NITRIC OXIDE THERAPY IN PRETERM INFANTS: LACK OF INCREASED CENTRAL NERVOUS SYSTEM COMPLICATIONS

Trials of iNO have been undertaken in the preterm infant amid theoretic concerns regarding its safety in this population, particularly with respect to bleeding, methemoglobinemia, and oxidative stress. Inhaled NO increases bleeding times in adults[23] and full-term infants,[24] and an early, uncontrolled study of iNO in premature infants showed a concerning incidence of intraventricular hemorrhage (IVH).[25] Methemoglobinemia has been reported in full-term infants treated with high concentrations of inhaled nitric oxide (80 ppm) but not in infants receiving less than 20 ppm,[20,22,26] the maximum concentration used in the best-run studies discussed here.[27–29] A recent study of infants weighing less than 1250 g who were randomly assigned to receive iNO (20 ppm, weaned to 2 ppm) or placebo for 24 days found no significant differences between control and treated infants for concentrations of 3-nitrotyrosines or protein carbonylation, markers of oxidative stress.[30] As will be reviewed below, studies have ranged in sophistication from retrospective, uncontrolled studies to prospective, double-blind, randomized controlled trials. We focus here on the impact of iNO therapy on markers of neurologic injury during hospitalization and, where possible, the effect of iNO therapy on neurodevelopmental outcomes during early childhood.

An early study in the United Kingdom enrolled premature infants less than 32 weeks gestation into a four-armed open trial of iNO therapy and early dexamethasone.[31] Mechanically ventilated infants treated with surfactant were eligible if they were calculated to have a high risk for the development of chronic lung disease, using a previously published metric validated by logistic regression.[32] Infants were randomly assigned to receive either iNO (20 ppm weaned to 5 ppm, if possible, for 72 hours), dexamethasone (0.5-1 mg/kg/day x 6 days), both treatments, or neither. Mean birth weights across the groups varied from 750 g (iNO) to 870 g (dexamethasone). Neither iNO nor dexamethasone treatment decreased the primary outcome of chronic lung disease or death before hospital discharge. In this small study of 42 babies, only 60% of infants survived to discharge, suggesting that these infants were very ill. This conclusion is supported by the entry criterion of having a high risk for chronic lung disease. There are few data provided regarding acute neurologic outcomes in these patients; although rates of IVH did not differ between groups, the group sizes were small. Only grades I and II IVH were reported; periventricular leukomalacia (PVL) was not reported.

At 30 months corrected age, surviving infants (N = 25) underwent formal, blinded developmental assessments.[33] Children were classified as having mild, moderate, or severe neurodevelopmental delay based on mental or physical developmental indices (MDI or PDI) of the Bayley[7] (mild: 71–85 [1–2 standard deviations below the mean], moderate: 50–75 [>2 standard deviations below the mean]; severe < 50). Children with "significant" abnormalities of tone or movement received a diagnosis of cerebral palsy. There was a nonsignificant trend toward less neurodevelopmental delay in the iNO group, and no children in the iNO group received a diagnosis of cerebral palsy compared with two of 14 children in the control group. The very small numbers of this study, the selection bias toward very ill children, and the open nature of the study conspire to render the results unhelpful in determining the safety of iNO in preterm infants, let alone any effects on neurodevelopmental outcome.

The first double-blind, randomized controlled trial of iNO therapy in preterm infants[26] enrolled 80 infants less than 34 weeks gestation from 12 centers in the United States. Infants had a mean birth weight of about 1000 g and a mean gestational age of about 27 weeks. The primary entry criterion was severe hypoxic respiratory failure unresponsive to standard therapies (alveolar to arterial ratio <0.1 on two sequential blood gas measurements). Infants were randomly selected to receive iNO (5 ppm) or placebo for 7 days. The primary outcome was survival to discharge. The trial was stopped after a planned interim analysis showed no significant difference in the primary outcome between the groups, and that with the enrollment rate at the time, detection of a difference was unlikely in a reasonable time frame. Infants in the two groups did not vary in the rates of grades II to IV IVH at study entry. Relevant to this review is the observation that, after detailed analyses, there were no differences in the rates of IVH, mild or severe, in survivors and nonsurvivors, between the iNO and placebo groups at study end. Using a worst-case scenario analysis, in which infants without cranial ultrasound or pathologic data regarding IVH were assigned grade IV IVH in the iNO group and no IVH in the control group, the authors determined that a clinical trial designed to detect a difference in grade IV IVH in this population of infants with this high level of illness severity would require enrollment of a minimum of 15,000 infants.

At the time this trial was designed, concerns regarding the safety of iNO in preterm infants had not been addressed. Consequently, patient selection for this randomized, controlled trial was necessarily restricted to extremely ill infants whose respiratory disease was refractory to conventional methods. The observation, therefore, that IVH rates were not significantly higher in iNO-treated infants compared with control infants, although far from definitive proof that iNO did not increase the risk of IVH, nonetheless provided an indication that it might be safe in this population. A lack of increase in IVH after iNO treatment in preterm infants was also found in several other studies.[34–36] Finally, a small (N = 34) randomized, placebo-controlled trial of iNO treatment[37] was performed to ascertain safety of iNO in preterm infants. In this study, infants with birth weights between 500 and 2000 g were enrolled within 72 hours of birth. Infants (mean birth weight approximately 900 g and mean gestational age 27 weeks) were randomly assigned to receive iNO (20 ppm, weaned to 5 ppm over 24–48 hours) or placebo. In this study, mean oxygen indices were about 12. No significant difference in the rates of severe IVH between iNO and placebo-treated groups was observed. Similarly, the incidences of other acute complications of prematurity, as well as early neonatal death, were comparable between the iNO and placebo-treated groups. This pilot study provided reassurance that iNO did not increase severe IVH in at-risk preterm infants and allowed further study of the efficacy of iNO in this population.

INHALED NITRIC OXIDE THERAPY DECREASES CENTRAL NERVOUS SYSTEM COMPLICATIONS OF PREMATURITY: RANDOMIZED TRIALS

The first study to assess the role of iNO in less sick preterm infants was performed by Schreiber and colleagues.[29] In this single-center, double-blinded, randomized, controlled trial performed at the University of Chicago, 207 preterm infants less than 34 weeks gestation who were receiving mechanical ventilation for respiratory distress syndrome and who had received surfactant were, within 3 days of birth, randomly assigned to receive iNO (10 ppm on day 1, followed by 5 ppm) or placebo for the shorter of 7 days or until extubation. The primary hypothesis was that iNO would decrease the incidence of death and chronic lung disease among surviving infants. Mean birth weight of this cohort was approximately 1000 g, and mean gestational age was 27 weeks. Inhaled NO treatment conferred a significant 0.76 relative risk of death or chronic lung disease compared with treatment with placebo gas.

A key difference between this study and previously performed trials was the illness severity of the population. In contrast to previous studies, in which patient enrollment was restricted to infants with severe respiratory disease,[26,32] the median initial oxygenation index (OI) of the enrolled population was about 7. In fact, iNO therapy decreased significantly the risk of the primary outcome (by 47%) for infants having an initial OI below the median but not for the remainder of the infants. While suggesting that iNO reduced chronic lung disease and death only in a less-ill subset of infants, this observation was derived from a post hoc analysis and should be interpreted cautiously.

Among the secondary outcomes evaluated for this study, the overall incidence of IVH and PVL did not differ between iNO- and placebo-treated infants. Unexpected, however, was a marked, significant reduction in severe (grades III or IV) IVH and PVL in iNO-treated infants compared with placebo-treated infants (risk reduction 47%).

Previously, only antenatal corticosteroids have been shown to reduce IVH in preterm infants.[38–40] Indeed, phenobarbital,[41,42] indomethacin,[43,44] and vitamin E[45] have all, at one time, appeared to be promising therapies. Therefore, although this unanticipated finding from a post hoc analysis was intriguing, these data could hardly be taken as clear evidence of iNO being a neuroprotective agent, especially before information regarding long-term neurodevelopmental outcomes of this cohort of infants became available.

Similar reductions in central nervous system (CNS) complications by iNO therapy, however, have been recently reported by Kinsella and colleagues,[27] at the University of Colorado, in a large (N = 793), 16-center, randomized, double blind, placebo-controlled trial performed in the United States. Infants less than 34 weeks gestation were randomly assigned within 48 hours of birth to receive iNO (5 ppm) or placebo for 21 days. Similar to the Chicago study, the primary outcome was the incidence of death or chronic lung disease in survivors. Mean birth weight of this population was about 800 g, and mean gestational age 25.6 weeks gestation, about 2 weeks more premature than those in the Chicago study. More than 70% of infants had mothers who received antenatal steroids (higher than the 50% in the Chicago study). There were no differences between iNO- and placebo-treated groups in baseline ventilator requirements. Overall, there was no difference between the two groups in the incidence of the primary outcome. However, prespecified subgroup analyses by birth weight strata showed that iNO-treated infants weighing 1000 to 1250 g had a significantly lower incidence of the primary outcome as well as a lower incidence of chronic lung disease alone, compared with placebo-treated infants. Most importantly, iNO-treated infants, across all weight strata, had a significantly decreased incidence of PVL, the primary ischemic lesion of the preterm brain. The combined outcome of severe IVH, ventriculomegaly, and PVL was also significantly and markedly reduced among infants weighing 750 to 999 g. Bolstering the findings from the Chicago study, these observations from the Colorado study strongly suggest that low-dose iNO therapy can safely improve short-term neurologic outcomes in preterm infants. The OI in this cohort of less than six, combined with a mean birth weight that was approximately 200 g smaller than that in the Chicago cohort, makes direct comparison of this population's risk for complications of prematurity with that of the Chicago study more difficult. Nonetheless, these two, well-designed studies, encompassing 1000 infants in total, have shown that low-dose iNO therapy, begun within the first 72 hours of birth, decreases the incidence of CNS complications, particularly severe IVH and PVL, by 40% to 50%.

Infants with severe IVH are at risk for abnormal neurodevelopmental outcome,[46–48] as are infants with PVL.[49–52] Similarly, the presence of chronic lung disease adversely affects long-term neurodevelopmental outcome.[11] Reductions in severe IVH and chronic lung disease in preterm infants by low-dose iNO therapy, therefore, would be predicted to result in improved neurodevelopmental outcomes. This prediction has been borne out in the only follow-up study to date of a double-blind, randomized, placebo-controlled trial of iNO treatment in which infants received iNO for more than several days.

Children enrolled in the Chicago trial (10 ppm day 1, 5 ppm days 2–7 vs. placebo)[29] were studied in a prospective, longitudinal follow-up study at 2 years corrected age.[53] The primary outcome variable—abnormal neuro developmental outcome—was defined as either disability (cerebral palsy, blindness, or hearing loss) or delay (a Bayley score more then two standard deviations below the mean, ie, below 70). Eighty-two percent of surviving infants enrolled in the initial study were captured for assessment at two years of age by means of close contact with their families after discharge from the intensive care nursery. Children were examined by a pediatrician and a neurologist, and infant development was assessed by a single, certified, neonatal occupational therapist. Importantly, all assessors (and families) were unaware of the children's assignments to iNO or placebo. In the follow-up cohort, the percentage of iNO- to placebo-treated children was similar to that in the initial report (53% versus 51%, respectively).

Inhaled NO–treated survivors had approximately half the risk of abnormal neurodevelopmental outcome than did placebo-treated survivors. After adjustment of the primary outcome individually for each of the factors potentially associated with abnormal neurodevelopmental outcomes, including birth weight, sex, socioeconomic status, type of ventilation (high frequency or conventional), and postnatal exposure to corticosteroids, the decreased risk of an abnormal neurodevelopmental outcome remained unchanged. Furthermore, simultaneous adjustment for the two most powerful epidemiologic confounders, ie, birth weight and sex, did not alter the magnitude of the risk reduction by iNO. These statistical analyses demonstrate that iNO treatment cut the incidence of abnormal neurodevelopmental outcome by about half, independent of the effects of confounding variables. Therefore, in this cohort, iNO treatment provided powerful neuroprotection from the multifactorial causes of abnormal neurodevelopmental outcome. Comparative follow-up data from the Colorado study are not yet available.

What aspects of abnormal neurodevelopmental outcome did iNO treatment impact in the Chicago follow-up study? The incidence of disability (cerebral palsy, blindness, hearing loss) was not significantly different between iNO- and placebo-treated infants. Children with these conditions constituted less than 10% of the cohort. Although these numbers are certainly too low to detect a significant difference, no trend toward decrease on disability is apparent. It is clear, then, that iNO exerted its neuroprotective effect on behaviors measured by the Bayley scales: children in the iNO-treated group had half the incidence of having either MDI or PDI scores below 70 compared with placebo-treated children. Furthermore, this same magnitude of decrease was apparent in the incidence of isolated MDI less than 70, whereas the incidences of isolated PDI less than 70 were not different between the groups. Of note is the observation that there was no significant difference (or even a trend) in the incidence of both MDI and PDI below 70—the worst affected children—in the iNO-treated group. Thus, the primary effect of iNO treatment in this follow-up study was to decrease the number of children with mental delay.

If iNO treatment during the first week of postnatal life improves long-term neurodevelopmental outcomes in preterm infants, by what mechanisms does this neuroprotection occur? Further statistical analysis of the Chicago follow-up data sheds some light on the role played by key neonatal conditions in altering neurodevelopmental outcome. Because iNO treatment decreased the incidences of chronic lung disease and severe IVH/PVL, conditions known to adversely affect neurodevelopmental outcome,[11,46–52] it is possible that improved neurodevelopmental outcome occurs because of an iNO-induced decrease in the incidence of these conditions. Indeed, as anticipated, the incidences of severe IVH/PVL and chronic lung disease were decreased significantly in the cohort of iNO-treated survivors compared with placebo-treated survivors. However, adjustment for the presence, individually or collectively, of severe IVH/PVL and chronic lung disease did not appreciably alter the relative risk of the incidence of abnormal neurodevelopmental outcome.

Without adjustment for any factors, the relative risk for abnormal neurodevelopmental outcome in the iNO-treated group was 0.53 (95% confidence interval: 0.33–0.87, $P = .01$). With simultaneous adjustment for chronic lung disease and severe IVH/PVL, the relative risk was 0.60 (0.38–0.96, $P = .03$). Thus, the substantial neuroprotective effect of iNO treatment in this follow-up study appears to be independent of known CNS complications of prematurity. If these findings are corroborated by other studies that follow graduates of low-dose NO trials, iNO will constitute the only postnatal intervention to date that improves neurodevelopmental outcome in preterm infants.

Two additional randomized, placebo-controlled studies of iNO treatment in preterm infants deserve examination. Ballard and colleagues,[28] at the Children's Hospital of Philadelphia performed a multicenter, placebo-controlled, double-blind trial of iNO versus placebo in infants weighing <1250 g. In this 21-center trial, 582 infants requiring ventilatory support were enrolled at 7 to 21 days of age and treated with iNO (beginning at 20 ppm) or placebo for a minimum of 24 days. The overall hypothesis was that prolonged therapy, ie, 24 days, might be needed to prevent increased airway resistance and muscularity, conditions associated with chronic lung disease, as well as to improve alveolarization and lung growth. The primary outcome variable was survival without chronic lung disease at 36 weeks postconceptional age. There was a significant increase in survival without chronic lung disease in the iNO-treated patients (relative benefit, 1.23 [95% confidence interval 1.01–1.51, $P = 0.04$]).

Enrollment was delayed until 7 days of age because of concerns of an interaction between iNO treatment and brain injury. Importantly, the investigators found no evidence of increased evolution of brain injury in iNO-treated infants, either during or after gas delivery. The incidences of PVL or severe IVH in the iNO- and placebo-treated groups were not reported. Information on long-term neurodevelopmental outcomes has not yet been reported.

The NICHD performed a moderately sized (N = 420), double-blind, placebo-controlled, randomized, multicenter trial of iNO (5–10 ppm) in preterm infants with severe respiratory failure.[54] The primary outcome was the incidence of death or chronic lung disease. Children weighing less than 1500 g who had an OI of 10 twice in succession were eligible. However, the infants in this study had, in fact, very severe respiratory disease: the mean OI in enrolled patients was 23 in the iNO-treated group and 22 in the placebo-treated group. In this study, only infants who responded to study gas with an immediate improvement in oxygenation continued to receive treatment. The median duration of therapy for the iNO-treated and responsive group was 76 hours.

In this trial, iNO treatment did not reduce the incidence of the primary outcome across the study population. Post hoc analysis showed a decrease in the primary outcome among children with birth weights more than 1000 g. More concerning, though, is the finding that infants in the iNO group having birth weights less than 1000 g had higher mortality rates and increased rates of severe IVH. The relative risk for severe IVH in the iNO-treated infants was 1.40 (95% confidence interval 1.03–1.88, $P = .03$). It is important to note that the rates of death or chronic lung disease in both groups (80% iNO and 82% placebo) were far higher than those reported in the Chicago study (51% and 65%) or the Philadelphia study (56% and 64%). Furthermore, the OIs in the NICHD trial were far higher than those of the cohorts in Chicago and Denver studies, and indicate how ill the infants were in this NICHD study. More importantly, because the protocol required that oxygenation improve in order for study gas to be continued, infants received study gas for variable times, some for as little as 30 minutes. Even infants who responded to study gas with an improvement in oxygenation were weaned from study gas after 10 to 14 hours, if tolerated. Thus, the duration of study gas therapy was highly variable and far shorter than any of the other reports. Although the increases in mortality and severe intraventricular hemorrhage rates in infants with birth weights less than 1000 g are concerning, it should be noted that these infants had extremely severe respiratory disease, quite a different population from those studied by the Chicago or Philadelphia group.

When the survivors of this trial were studied at 18 to 22 months corrected age,[55] investigators reported that iNO did not reduce the combined rate of death or neurodevelopmental impairment (defined as moderate to severe cerebral palsy, blindness, deafness, or a Bayley scale [MDI or PDI] less than 70). In infants weighing less than 1000 g at birth, the combined incidence of death or cerebral palsy was reported to be higher in the iNO-treated group. However, because the study investigators believed that it was crucial to encompass patient outcomes from the time of randomization rather than focus on patients who survived to discharge,[55] all deaths that occurred during the initial hospitalization were included in the follow-up data set. Evaluation only of children who survived the initial hospitalization, an analysis that can be directly compared with other follow-up studies, shows no significant increase in neurodevelopmental impairment or isolated delay either across the study population or in those children who weighed less than 1000 g at birth. Thus, although it is likely prudent to withhold iNO therapy from desperately ill infants weighing less than 1000 g, there remains no evidence that long-term neurodevelopmental outcome is worsened by iNO therapy in any weight group. In fact, in children who are not desperately ill, the evidence for a marked improvement in neurodevelopmental outcome is hopeful.

A relatively small (N = 108), nonblinded, randomized, placebo-controlled, 34-center trial performed in the United Kingdom and Europe[56] provides little additional data on whether iNO improves neurodevelopmental outcome in preterm infants. The mean gestational age was 27 weeks. Because an infant was enrolled only if the attending physician was unsure whether the infant would benefit from iNO, enrollment was highly skewed toward infants thought likely to die. (Presumably, infants believed by the physician to likely benefit from iNO were treated with open-label iNO and thus not enrolled.) Enrolled infants had extremely severe respiratory disease, with a median OI of 32. Half of the infants received iNO for less than 48 hours, and half received iNO for more than 3 days. At one-year corrected age, there was no difference in the incidence of death or severe neurologic disability (defined as minimal head control or inability to sit or developmental quotient less than 50) between iNO- and placebo-treated groups.

Recently, Tanaka and colleagues,[57] compared the incidence of cerebral palsy in 61 consecutive preterm infants with documented persistent pulmonary hypertension (PPHN) over two periods—1988 to 1993 (pre-iNO) and 1993 to 1999 (iNO era). After 1992, iNO was given to all infants with PPHN. Inhaled NO was started initially at 10 ppm and titrated to clinical (oxygenation) response to a maximum of 30 ppm. Median duration of iNO treatment was 19.8 hours (interquartile range: 29.5–56.0 hours). Mean gestational age was 25.5 weeks, with mean birth weight about 820 g. Follow-up examinations were performed at 3 years of age, at which time infants exhibiting abnormal muscle tone in more than one extremity as well as abnormal movement or posture were diagnosed with cerebral palsy. In the period after iNO treatment was initiated, the incidence of cerebral palsy was 12.5%, significantly lower than the 46.7% observed during the pre-iNO period. This retrospective study suffers from the drawbacks inherent in any historical retrospective study. First, it is impossible to differentiate between effects stemming from changes in neonatal care other than iNO during the two periods and iNO itself; the absence of a contemporaneous control group makes direct comparisons difficult. Second, there was a death rate of more than 50% within 3 years of birth. Third, neurologic assessments were performed by multiple nonneurologist pediatricians without prespecification of criteria for cerebral palsy. Finally, the study is quite small, so that generalization of results to other populations is difficult.

MECHANISMS OF NEUROPROTECTION FROM INHALED NITRIC OXIDE

What are the mechanisms underlying abnormal neurodevelopmental outcomes in preterm infants, and how might iNO alter these mechanisms? White matter injury is the hallmark of preterm brain injury. Evidence is accumulating in rodent models that a primary mechanism of white matter injury involves maturation-dependent vulnerability to ischemic injury of progenitors of oligodendrocytes.[58,59] Such white matter injury can lead to PVL and cerebral palsy. Rodent models have also implicated ischemic injury to subplate neurons that occurs during development, such that pervasive abnormalities of cortical development occur, leading to cognitive and sensory deficits.[60]

Nitric oxide is a ubiquitous, endogenous, intercellular signaling molecule with autocrine and paracrine activities (reviewed in[61]). Nitric oxide regulates vascular tone in the pulmonary and systemic circulation and mediates neurotransmission and neurosecretion.[61] Nitric oxide is produced by nitric oxide synthase (NOS); in the presence of oxygen, NOS catalyzes the conversion of L-arginine to L-citrulline plus NO. Three primary isoforms of NOS have been identified: neuronal NOS (nNOS), endothelial NOS (eNOS), and inducible NOS (iNOS). Neuronal and eNOS are constitutively expressed and depend on Ca^{2+}-calmodulin for activation. In the central nervous system, nNOS is localized to neurons in multiple brain regions, as well as in astrocytes and cerebral blood vessels.[62] Endothelial NOS is expressed in cerebral endothelial cells. Nitric oxide interacts with soluble guanylyl cyclase to increase levels of cyclic guanosine monophosphate and has also been reported to interact with heme oxygenase 1[63] and cyclooxygenase.[64]

Inhaled NO may decrease lung-derived inflammatory mediators leading to brain injury.[65–67] However, if iNO provides neuroprotection at sites distal to the lung, it is unlikely that neuroprotection occurs through direct activity on neurons or preoligodendrocytes. There is considerable uncertainty regarding whether NO, even at pharmacologic doses, can be transported to distal vascular beds, let alone across multiple diffusion barriers to leave the capillary.

Although clinical evidence suggests that exogenous iNO provides neuroprotection in preterm infants, many studies using models of hypoxic–ischemic injury indicate that endogenous cytosolic NO produced in neurons results in neuronal death.[68–72] A key mechanism underlying hypoxic–ischemic neuronal death is the induction of an increase in cytosolic calcium concentration[73,74] mediated by overactivation of *N*-methyl-D-aspartate receptors.[75–77] This calcium increase activates calmodulin, which activates NOS.[78,79] The resultant NO increase, combined with an increase in reactive oxygen species production, leads to formation of peroxynitrite and subsequent neuronal injury and death.[69,80,81] Accordingly, if iNO were to reach immature subplate neurons and oligodendrocytes, the likely effect would be an increase in reactive nitrogen stress and peroxidative injury.

Clinical use of NO as a pulmonary vasodilator has been predicated on the fact that the action of NO on vascular smooth muscle is restricted to the pulmonary vasculature. This local restriction occurs because inhaled NO, once having crossed into the pulmonary circulation, reacts with molecules in plasma and erythrocytic hemoglobin.[82] As reviewed by Schechter and Gladwin,[82] NO is destroyed rapidly by its reaction with iron-containing heme groups of oxyhemoglobin. The reaction of NO with hemoglobin occurs at diffusion-limited rates, resulting in methemoglobin and nitrate (from reaction with oxyhemoglobin) and iron-nitrosyl hemoglobin (from reaction with deoxyhemoglobin).[83] Accordingly, exogenous iNO decreases pulmonary vascular resistance with out altering systemic blood pressure and, presumably, systemic vascular tone.

Importantly, some reactions of NO with hemoglobin do not destroy NO. The presence of iron-nitrosyl-hemoglobin (produced from NO-deoxyhemoglobin interaction) and S-nitrosyl-hemoglobin (produced by reaction of NO with the cysteine at position 93 of the hemoglobin beta chain), while at low concentrations, raises the possibility that hemoglobin in red cells may act as a carrier of gas in circulation.[82] Indeed, one hypothesis states that S-nitrosohemoglobin, produced in tissues at high O_2 tensions, decomposes at low O_2 tensions, releasing NO and increasing blood flow to relatively hypoxic tissues.[84] Competing studies argue that S-nitrosohemoglobin is at much lower concentrations in plasma than previously believed, and quite unstable.[85,86] Other molecules that may conserve NO activity in the plasma for delivery to distant vascular beds include nitrite ion (from reaction with oxygen) and iron-nitrosyl hemoglobin.[83] Nitrite ions can be converted to NO enzymatically, via xanthine oxidoreductase and heme proteins.[83] Although many of these pathways are likely to have negligible effects at physiologic levels of endogenous NO, they may serve as NO reservoirs under such pharmacologic NO levels as exist during iNO delivery.[83]

If iNO treatment does result in increased delivery of NO to the brain, how might this NO mediate neuroprotection during postnatal life in preterm infants? Animal and in vitro studies using isoform-specific NOS inhibitors, as well as mice in which single NOS-isoforms have been genetically knocked out, have found a differential role for NO, depending on which isoforms produce it and the tissue to which the isoforms are localized.[87,88] Thus, global inhibition of all NOS isoforms in an animal model of brain hypoxia-ischemia results in decreased infarct size, whereas eNOS blockade increases infarct size, indicating that eNOS is protective. Neuronal NOS–specific blockade also decreases infarct size, indicating that nNOS over-activity is neurotoxic.[87] Similar results are seen using eNOS- and nNOS-knockout mice.[88] Providing additional NO with iNO to cerebrovascular beds supplying vulnerable pre-oligodendrocytes and neurons, therefore, could result in improved blood flow during hypoxic episodes and neuroprotection.

A closely related hypothesis to explain a potential role for increased NO delivery to the cerebrovascular bed focuses on the inhibition of eNOS activity during hypoxia. Hypoxia-induced inhibition of eNOS is mediated by decreases in eNOS mRNA half-life and occurs within several hours after hypoxia.[89] Implicated in this mRNA down-regulation is Rho-kinase, a serine-threonine kinase. Rho-kinase also decreases eNOS activity via posttranslational mechanisms within minutes of activation.[90] Rho-kinase is activated in animal models of cerebral ischemia.[91] Thus, under conditions of hypoxia, eNOS can be down-regulated, leading to dysregulation of cerebral blood flow and worsening injury. Delivery of NO via iNO treatment to cerebral vasculature could, therefore, overcome down-regulated eNOS and improve cerebral blood flow and reducing ischemic injury.

SUMMARY

Preterm infants are at high risk for neurodevelopmental impairment, including blindness, deafness, cerebral palsy, and global cognitive delay. Despite an increasing understanding of the risk factors leading to abnormal neurodevelopmental outcomes, little progress has been made in treatment. Recent data suggest that for preterm infants with moderately severe respiratory distress syndrome, iNO decreases the incidence of severe acute brain injury and improves long-term neurodevelopmental outcomes. Although iNO-mediated decreases in chronic lung disease and severe intraventricular hemorrhage/periventricular leukomalacia undoubtedly contribute to improved neurodevelopmental outcomes, iNO may have an independent neuroprotective effect. Although these data are encouraging, additional studies are required before recommending the routine use of iNO for neuroprotection in preterm infants.

REFERENCES

1. Doyle LW. Neonatal intensive care at borderline viability–is it worth it? Early Hum Dev 2004;80(2):103–13.
2. Wood NS, Costeloe K, Gibson AT, et al. The EPICure study: associations and antecedents of neurological and developmental disability at 30 months of age following extremely preterm birth. Arch Dis Child Fetal Neonatal Ed 2005;90(2): F134–40.
3. Wood NS, Marlow N, Costeloe K, et al. Neurologic and developmental disability after extremely preterm birth. N Engl J Med 2000;343(6):378–84.
4. Anderson PJ, Doyle LW. Cognitive and educational deficits in children born extremely preterm. Semin Perinatol 2008;32(1):51–8.
5. Aylward GP. Neurodevelopmental outcomes of infants born prematurely. J Dev Behav Pediatr 2005;26(6):427–40.
6. Hintz SR, Kendrick DE, Vohr BR, et al. Changes in neurodevelopmental outcomes at 18 to 22 months' corrected age among infants of less than 25 weeks' gestational age born in 1993–1999. Pediatrics 2005;115(6):1645–51.
7. Bayley N. Bayley scales of infant development. 2nd edition. San Antonio (TX): Harcourt Brace; 1993.
8. Wu Y, Colford JJ. Chorioamnionitis as a risk factor for cerebral palsy: a meta-analysis. JAMA 2000;290:2677–84.
9. Ferriero DM. Neonatal brain injury. N Engl J Med 2004;351(19):1985–95.
10. Neubauer AP, Voss W, Kattner E. Outcome of extremely low birth weight survivors at school age: the influence of perinatal parameters on neurodevelopment. Eur J Pediatr 2008;167(1):87–95.
11. Jeng SF, Hsu CH, Tsao PN, et al. Bronchopulmonary dysplasia predicts adverse developmental and clinical outcomes in very-low-birthweight infants. Dev Med Child Neurol 2008;50(1):51–7.
12. Short EJ, Kirchner HL, Asaad GR, et al. Developmental sequelae in preterm infants having a diagnosis of bronchopulmonary dysplasia: analysis using a severity-based classification system. Arch Pediatr Adolesc Med 2007;161(11):1082–7.
13. Short EJ, Klein NK, Lewis BA, et al. Cognitive and academic consequences of bronchopulmonary dysplasia and very low birth weight: 8-year-old outcomes. Pediatrics 2003;112(5):e359.
14. O'Shea TM, Kothadia JM, Klinepeter KL, et al. Randomized placebo-controlled trial of a 42-day tapering course of dexamethasone to reduce the duration of ventilator dependency in very low birth weight infants: outcome of study participants at 1-year adjusted age. Pediatrics 1999;104(1 Pt 1):15–21.
15. Shinwell ES, Karplus M, Reich D, et al. Early postnatal dexamethasone treatment and increased incidence of cerebral palsy. Arch Dis Child Fetal Neonatal Ed 2000;83(3):F177–81.
16. Pillekamp F, Hermann C, Keller T, et al. Factors influencing apnea and bradycardia of prematurity - implications for neurodevelopment. Neonatology 2007;91(3): 155–61.

17. Msall M, Buck G, Rogers B, et al. Kindergarten readiness after extreme prematurity. AM J Dis Child 1992;146:1371–5.
18. Osborn DA, Hunt RW. Postnatal thyroid hormones for respiratory distress syndrome in preterm infants. Cochrane Database Syst Rev 2007;(1):CD005946.
19. Vohr BR, Allan WC, Westerveld M, et al. School-age outcomes of very low birth weight infants in the indomethacin intraventricular hemorrhage prevention trial. Pediatrics 2003;111(4 Pt 1):e340–6.
20. Roberts JD, Fineman JR, Morin FC, et al. Inhaled nitric oxide and persistent pulmonary hypertension of the newborn. N Engl J Med 1997;336(9):605–10.
21. The Neonatal Inhaled Nitric Oxide Study G. Inhaled nitric oxide in full-term and nearly full-term infants with hypoxic respiratory failure. N Engl J Med 1997; 336(9):597–604.
22. Clark RH, Kueser TJ, Walker MW, et al. Low-dose nitric oxide therapy for persistent pulmonary hypertension of the newborn. Clinical Inhaled Nitric Oxide Research Group. N Engl J Med 2000;342(7):469–74.
23. Hogman M, Frostell C, Arnberg H, et al. Bleeding time prolongation and NO inhalation. Lancet 1993;341(8861):1664–5.
24. Cheung PY, Salas E, Etches PC, et al. Inhaled nitric oxide and inhibition of platelet aggregation in critically ill neonates. Lancet 1998;351(9110):1181–2.
25. Van Meurs KP, Rhine WD, Asselin JM, et al. Response of premature infants with severe respiratory failure to inhaled nitric oxide. Preemie NO Collaborative Group. Pediatr Pulmonol 1997;24(5):319–23.
26. Kinsella JP, Walsh WF, Bose CL, et al. Inhaled nitric oxide in premature neonates with severe hypoxaemic respiratory failure: a randomised controlled trial. Lancet 1999;354(9184):1061–5.
27. Kinsella JP, Cutter GR, Walsh WF, et al. Early inhaled nitric oxide therapy in premature newborns with respiratory failure. N Engl J Med 2006;355(4):354–64.
28. Ballard RA, Truog WE, Cnaan A, et al. Inhaled nitric oxide in preterm infants undergoing mechanical ventilation. N Engl J Med 2006;355(4):343–53.
29. Schreiber MD, Gin-Mestan K, Marks JD, et al. Inhaled nitric oxide in premature infants with the respiratory distress syndrome. N Engl J Med 2003;349:2099–107.
30. Ballard PL, Truog WE, Merrill JD, et al. Plasma biomarkers of oxidative stress: relationship to lung disease and inhaled nitric oxide therapy in premature infants. Pediatrics 2008;121(3):555–61.
31. Subhedar NV, Ryan SW, Shaw NJ. Open randomised controlled trial of inhaled nitric oxide and early dexamethasone in high risk preterm infants. Arch Dis Child Fetal Neonatal Ed 1997;77(3):F185–90.
32. Ryan SW, Nycyk J, Shaw BN. Prediction of chronic neonatal lung disease on day 4 of life. Eur J Pediatr 1996;155(8):668–71.
33. Bennett AJ, Shaw NJ, Gregg JE, et al. Neurodevelopmental outcome in high-risk preterm infants treated with inhaled nitric oxide. Acta Paediatr 2001;90(5):573–6.
34. Group TF-BCNT. Early compared with delayed nitric oxide in moderately hypoxaemic neonates with respiratory failure: a randomised controlled study. Lancet 1999;354:1066–71 [Erratum, Lancet 1999; 354:1826].
35. Skimming J, Bender K, Hutchinson A, et al. Nitric oxide inhalation in infants with respiratory distress syndrome. J Pediatr 1997;130:225–30.
36. Srisuparp P, Marks JD, Dixit R, et al. Inhaled nitric oxide improves oxygenation index without increasing intraventricular hemorrhage in premature infants with respiratory distress syndrome. J Invest Med 1998;46:263A.

37. Srisuparp P, Heitschmidt M, Schreiber MD. Inhaled nitric oxide therapy in premature infants with mild to moderate respiratory distress syndrome. J Med Assoc Thai 2002;85(Suppl 2):S469–78.
38. Garland JS, Buck R, Leviton A. Effect of maternal glucocorticoid exposure on risk of severe intraventricular hemorrhage in surfactant-treated preterm infants. J Pediatr 1995;126(2):272–9.
39. Silver RK, Vyskocil C, Solomon SL, et al. Randomized trial of antenatal dexamethasone in surfactant-treated infants delivered before 30 weeks' gestation. Obstetrics & Gynecology 1996;87(5 Pt 1):683–91.
40. Crowley P, Chalmers I, Keirse MJ. The effects of corticosteroid administration before preterm delivery: an overview of the evidence from controlled trials. [see comments]. Br J Obstet Gynaecol 1990;97(1):11–25.
41. Donn SM, Roloff DW, Goldstein GW. Prevention of intraventricular haemorrhage in preterm infants by phenobarbitone. A controlled trial. Lancet 1981;2(8240): 215–7.
42. Crowther C, Henderson-Smart D. Phenobarbital prior to preterm birth for preventing neonatal periventricular haemorrhage. Cochrane Database Syst Rev 2003; Issue 3:Art. No.:CD000164.
43. Bada HS, Green RS, Pourcyrous M, et al. Indomethacin reduces the risks of severe intraventricular hemorrhage. [see comments]. J Pediatr 1989;115(4):631–7.
44. Ment LR, Ehrenkranz RA, Duncan CC, et al. Low-dose indomethacin and prevention of intraventricular hemorrhage: a multicenter randomized trial. Pediatrics 1994;93(4):543–50.
45. Chiswick M, Gladman G, Sinha S, et al. Vitamin E supplementation and periventricular hemorrhage in the newborn. Am J Clin Nutr 1991;53(1 Suppl):370S–2S.
46. Jarvenpaa AL, VIrtanen M, Pohjavuori M. The outcome of extremely low birthweight infants. Ann Med 1991;23(6):699–704.
47. Patel CA, Klein JM. Outcome of infants with birth weights less than 1000 g with respiratory distress syndrome treated with high-frequency ventilation and surfactant replacement therapy. Arch Pediatr Adolesc Med 1995;149(3):317–21.
48. Vohr BR, Wright LL, Dusick AM, et al. Neurodevelopmental and functional outcomes of extremely low birth weight infants in the National Institute of Child Health and Human Development Neonatal Research Network, 1993–1994. Pediatrics 2000;105(6):1216–26.
49. Hintz SR, O'Shea M. Neuroimaging and Neurodevelopmental Outcomes in Preterm Infants. Semin Perinatol 2008;32(1):11–9.
50. De Vries L, Groenendaal F, van Haastert I. Asymmetrical myelination of the posterior limb of the internal capsule in infants with periventricular haemorrhagic infarction: an early predictor of hemiplegia. Neuropediatrics 1999;30:314–9.
51. Nanba Y, Matsui K, Aida N. Magnetic resonance imaging regional T1 abnormalities at term accurately predict motor outcome in preterm infants. Pediatrics 2007; 120:e10–9.
52. Sie L, Hart A, van Hof J. Predictive value of neonatal MRI with respect to late MRI findings and clinical outcome. A study in infants with periventricular densities on neonatal ultrasound. Neuropediatrics 2005;36:78–89.
53. Mestan KL, Marks JD, Hecox K, et al. Neurodevelopmental outcomes of premature infants treated with inhaled nitric oxide. N Engl J Med 2005;353(1):23–32.
54. Van Meurs KP, Wright LL, Ehrenkranz RA, et al. Inhaled nitric oxide for premature infants with severe respiratory failure. N Engl J Med 2005;353(1):13–22.

55. Hintz SR, Van Meurs K, Perritt R, et al. Neurodevelopmental outcomes of premature infants with severe respiratory failure enrolled in a randomized controlled trial of inhaled nitric oxide. J Pediatr 2007;151(1):16–22.
56. Field D, Elbourne D, Truesdale A, et al. Neonatal ventilation with inhaled nitric oxide versus ventilatory support without inhaled nitric oxide for preterm infants with severe respiratory failure: the innovo multicentre randomised controlled trial (ISRCTN 17821339). Pediatrics 2005;115(4):926–36.
57. Tanaka Y, Hayashi T, Kitajima H, et al. Inhaled nitric oxide therapy decreases the risk of cerebral palsy in preterm infants with persistent pulmonary hypertension of the newborn. Pediatrics 2007;119(6):1159–64.
58. Back SA, Han BH, Luo NL, et al. Selective vulnerability of late oligodendrocyte progenitors to hypoxia- ischemia. J Neurosci 2002;22(2):455–63.
59. Drobyshevsky A, Song S-K, Gamkrelidze G, et al. Developmental changes in diffusion anisotropy coincide with immature oligodendrocyte progression and maturation of compound action potential. J Neurosci 2005;25(25):5988–97.
60. McQuillen PS, Sheldon RA, Shatz CJ, et al. Selective vulnerability of subplate neurons after early neonatal hypoxia-ischemia. J Neurosci 2003;23(8):3308–15.
61. Calabrese V, Mancuso C, Calvani M, et al. Nitric oxide in the central nervous system: neuroprotection versus neurotoxicity. Nat Rev Neurosci 1997;8:766–75.
62. Guix Fu I, Coma M, Munoz F. The physiology and pathophysiology of nitric oxide in the brain. Prog Neurobiol 2005;76:126–52.
63. Motterlini R, green C, Foresti R. Regulation of heme oxygenase-1 by redox signals involving nitric oxide. Antioxid Redox Signal 2002;4:615–24.
64. Mollace V, Muscoli C, Masini E, et al. Modulation of prostaglandin biosynthesis by nitric oxide and nitric oxide donors. Pharmacol Rev 2005;57:217–52.
65. Viscardi R, Muhumuza C, Rodriquez A. Inflammatory markers in intrauterine and fetal blood and cerebrospinal fluid compartments are associated with adverse pulmonary and neurologic outcomes in preterm infants. Pediatr Res 2004;55: 1009–17.
66. Haynes R, Baud O, Li J. Oxidative and nitrative injury in periventricular leukomalacia. Brain Pathol 2005;15:225–33.
67. Aaltonen M, Soukka H, Halkola R. Inhaled nitric oxide treatment inhibits neuronal injury after meconium aspiration in piglets. Early Hum Dev 2007;83:77–85.
68. Dawson VL, Dawson TM, London ED, et al. Nitric oxide mediates glutamate neurotoxicity in primary cortical cultures. PNAS 1991;88(14):6368–71. 91296822.
69. Gunasekar PG, Kanthasamy AG, Borowitz JL, et al. NMDA receptor activation produces concurrent generation of nitric oxide and reactive oxygen species: implication for cell death. J Neurochem 1995;65(5):2016–21.
70. Strijbos PJ. Nitric oxide in cerebral ischemic neurodegeneration and excitotoxicity. Crit Rev Neurobiol 1998;12(3):223–43.
71. Lipton SA. Neuronal protection and destruction by NO. Cell Death Differ 1999; 6(10):943–51.
72. Brown GC, Borutaite V. Nitric oxide, mitochondria, and cell death. IUBMB Life. 2001;52(3–5):189–95.
73. Goldberg MP, Weiss JH, Pham PC, et al. N-methyl-D-aspartate receptors mediate hypoxic neuronal injury in cortical culture. J Pharmacol Exp Ther 1987;243(2): 784–91.
74. Choi DW. Glutamate neurotoxicity and disease of the central nervous system. Neuron 1988;1:623–34. 39.
75. MacDermott AB, Mayer ML, Westbrook GL, et al. NMDA-receptor activation increases cytoplasmic calcium concentration in cultured spinal cord neurones.

[published erratum appears in Nature 1986 Jun 26–Jul 2;321(6073):888]. Nature 1986;321(6069):519–22.
76. Regehr WG, Tank DW. Postsynaptic NMDA receptor-mediated calcium accumulation in hippocampal CA1 pyramidal cell dendrites. Nature 1990;345(6278): 807–10.
77. Hartley DM, Kurth MC, Bjerkness L, et al. Glutamate receptor-induced 45Ca2+ accumulation in cortical cell culture correlates with subsequent neuronal degeneration. J Neurosci 1993;13(5):1993–2000. 93240223.
78. Sattler R, Charlton MP, Hafner M, et al. Distinct influx pathways, not calcium load, determine neuronal vulnerability to calcium neurotoxicity. J Neurochem 1998; 71(6):2349–64.
79. Sattler R, Xiong Z, Lu WY, et al. Specific coupling of NMDA receptor activation to nitric oxide neurotoxicity by PSD-95 protein. Science 1999;284(5421):1845–8. 99294869.
80. Schulz JB, Matthews RT, Klockgether T, et al. The role of mitochondrial dysfunction and neuronal nitric oxide in animal models of neurodegenerative diseases. Mol Cell Biochem 1997;174(1–2):193–7.
81. Misko TP, Highkin MK, Veenhuizen AW, et al. Characterization of the cytoprotective action of peroxynitrite decomposition catalysts. J Biolumin Chemilumin 1998; 273(25):15646–53.
82. Schechter AN, Gladwin MT. Hemoglobin and the paracrine and endocrine functions of nitric oxide. N Engl J Med 2003;348(15):1483–5.
83. Gladwin MT, Lancaster JR Jr, Freeman BA, et al. Nitric oxide's reactions with hemoglobin: a view through the SNO-storm. Nat Med 2003;9(5):496–500.
84. McMahon T, Moon R, Luschinger B. Nitric oxide in the human respiratory cycle. Nat Med 2002;8:711–7.
85. Joshi M, Ferguson TJ, Han T. Nitric oxide is consumed, rather than conserved, by reaction with oxyhemoglobin under physiological conditions. PNAS 2002;99: 10341–6.
86. Gladwin MT, Wang X, Reiter CD. S-nitrosylhemoglobin is unstable in the reductive erythrocyte environment and lacks O_2/NO-linked allosteric function. J Biolumin Chemilumin 2002;277:27818–28.
87. Dalkara T, Yoshida T, Irikura K, et al. Dual role of nitric oxide in focal cerebral ischemia. Neuropharmacology 1994;33(11):1447–52.
88. Huang Z, Huang PL, Panahian N, et al. Effects of cerebral ischemia in mice deficient in neuronal nitric oxide synthase. Science 1994;265(5180):1883–5.
89. Takemoto M, Sun J, Hiroki J, et al. Rho-kinase mediates hypoxia-induced downregulation of endothelial nitric oxide synthase. Circulation 2002;106:57–62.
90. Wolfrum S, Dendorfer A, Rikitake Y, et al. Inhibition of Rho-kinase leads to rapid activation of phosphatidylinositol 3-kinase/protein kinase Akt and cardiovascular protection. Arterioscler Thromb Vasc Biol 2004;24:1842–7.
91. Rikitake Y, Kim H, Huang Z, et al. Inhibition of Rho kinase (ROCK) leads to increased cerebral blood flow and stroke protection. Stroke 2005;36:2251–7.

Neuroprotection in Infant Heart Surgery

Robert Ryan Clancy, MD[a,b,c,*]

KEYWORDS

- Neuroprotection • Congenital heart defects
- Neonatal seizures • Periventricular leukomalacia
- Topiramate

Birth marks a time of joy and wonder for most newborn infants, but for some it harbors great danger that threatens their lives and clouds their future. Neonatal hypoxic-ischemic encephalopathy (HIE),[1,2] prematurity, sepsis-meningitis, and serious forms of complex congenital heart disease (CHD)[3] requiring infant heart surgery are just a few examples of disorders that share high mortality and morbidity rates.

The CHD population is worthy to consider for neuroprotection studies in its own right. Approximately 30,000 infants who have CHD are born in the United States each year, with at least a third needing surgical intervention in early infancy. About 11,000 heart operations are conducted annually. Advances in cardiothoracic surgical and anesthetic techniques, including cardiopulmonary bypass (CPB) and deep hypothermic circulatory arrest (DHCA), have substantially decreased mortality, expanding the horizon to address functional neurologic and cardiac outcomes in long-term survivors.[4–8] Acute neurocardiac morbidities in infants who have CHD undergoing newborn heart surgery (NBHS) are well described, including seizures, stroke, choreoathetosis, and cardiac arrest.[9–11] Interest in the functional status of survivors now stretches beyond the newborn period to childhood, adolescence, and adulthood.[12] Neurodevelopmental consequences in survivors include a distinctive profile of disturbances of cognition, behavior, attention deficit hyperactivity disorder, executive planning, feeding, speech and language, socialization, and fine and gross motor coordination. About half of school-aged survivors of infant heart surgery receive some type of special education assistance.[3,13,14] In this setting, new interventions to improve neurocardiac outcome are clearly needed.

There are other compelling reasons to study neuroprotection in infant heart surgery. It serves as a model to understand related neonatal neurologic conditions, including HIE[15,16] and the white matter injury that occurs with prematurity. The "blueprint" of

[a] Department of Neurology, The University of Pennsylvania School of Medicine, PA, USA
[b] Department of Pediatrics, The University of Pennsylvania School of Medicine, PA, USA
[c] Pediatric Regional Epilepsy Program, Division of Neurology, The Children's Hospital of Philadelphia, 34th Street and Civic Center Boulevard, Philadelphia, PA 19104, USA
* Corresponding author. The Children's Hospital of Philadelphia, Division of Neurology, 34th Street and Civic Center Boulevard, Philadelphia, PA 19104.
E-mail address: clancy@email.chop.edu

Clin Perinatol 35 (2008) 809–821
doi:10.1016/j.clp.2008.07.008 perinatology.theclinics.com
0095-5108/08/$ – see front matter

HIE is similar to the sequence of events during the conduct of NBHS and neuroprotection strategies may be complementary (**Table 1**):[17] (i) For both conditions, antecedent factors play important roles in outcome: patient-specific factors are major determinants of outcome after NBHS and birth asphyxia;[18] (ii) both conditions represent ischemia-reperfusion scenarios in which periods of reduced or absent cerebral blood flow are followed by restoration of the cerebral circulation; and (iii) following both HIE and NBHS, patients experience "multisystem malfunction" with reduced cardiac output from myocardial depression, abnormal lung mechanics, and impaired function of the GI tract, liver, and kidneys.

Infants who have undergone heart surgery and prematurity share similarities in their neurodevelopmental profile and a common form of white matter neuropathology called periventricular leukomalacia (PVL). Because prematurity accounts for a large percentage of chronic disability in the United States, lessons learned from preventing white matter injury in infant heart surgery might be readily applicable to the larger group of prematurely born infants.

Newborn heart surgery represents a period of planned and deliberate ischemia-reperfusion injury, which is obliged to occur to cure or palliate complex forms of congenital heart disease. In the past, there was a simple concept of brain injury from heart surgery (**Fig. 1**). The model considered the preoperative brain to be totally healthy and that the "insult" was conferred by surgery alone. In the wake of newborn heart surgery, acute neurologic signs could arise, such as stroke, seizures, altered consciousness, or choreoathetosis, and the evidence of their chronic effects would eventually surface in some. That simple, traditional concept is no longer valid.

THE CONDUCT OF SURGERY FOR CONGENITAL HEART DEFECTS

Infant heart surgery may be regarded in four stages: (i) the period before surgery, (ii) during the actual operation, (iii) the immediate postoperative period, and (iv) long-term survival.

Preoperatively, it has generally been assumed that the brains of children who have congenital heart disease are otherwise well (with the exception of those who have obvious genetic disorders, such as trisomy 21). It is now realized that even before heart surgery, pre-existing neurologic abnormalities are common: hypotonia,[19] small head circumferences, delays in brain maturation, and PVL. The CHD neonates have a much higher percentage of smaller head circumferences than the general population.[20] Furthermore, the size of the ascending aorta is significantly associated with microcephaly, implying that constricted cerebral blood flow from reduced cardiac output delays brain maturation and growth.[21] Signs of brain immaturity are also apparent.[22] The cerebral opercula, bilateral areas defined by the confluence of the frontal, temporal, and parietal lobes, are normally "open" in early development, but are

Table 1
Hypoxic-ischemic encephalopathy compared with infant heart surgery

HIE	Prepartum period	Intrapartum (labor & delivery) period	Postpartum period	Long-term survival and outcome
Infant heart surgery	Preoperative period	Intraoperative period	Postoperative period	Long-term survival and outcome

There are compelling parallels between neonatal HIE and infant heart surgery. Both represent premier examples of an ischemia-reperfusion injury and the status of the infant before the insult plays an important role in subsequent outcome in both conditions.

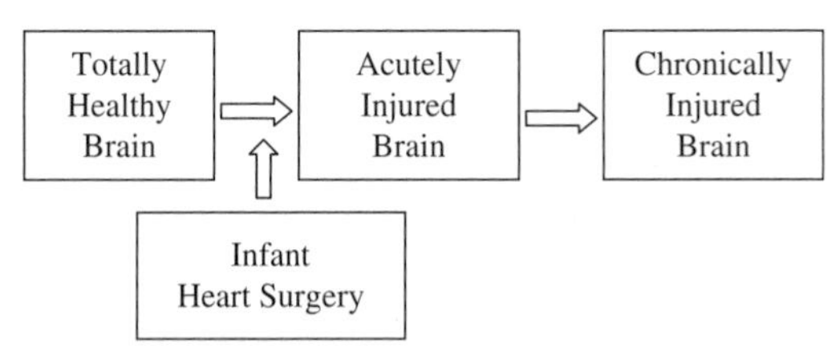

Fig. 1. The traditional model of acute and chronic brain injury after infant heart surgery assumes that the brain is previously normal and that the injury and adverse outcome are conferred by the stress of the operation. It is now believed that some brain injury precedes surgery and that many patient-specific factors significantly influence long-term outcome.

reduced to small, potential spaces by term. Neuropathologic and brain imaging studies show that many CHD neonates have open opercula, suggesting a delay in their maturation (**Fig. 2**). Anatomic scoring systems, based on semiquantitative MRI metrics such as the total maturation score,[23,24] show that the brains of term infants who have complex CHDs are simplified and younger appearing than expected. MRI spectroscopy and diffusion tensor imaging studies recently showed biochemical evidence of brain immaturity in term infants studied just before infant heart surgery.[25]

As in the premature infant, brain immaturity in CHD confers enhanced vulnerability to PVL. The vulnerability of white matter to hypoxia-ischemia depends heavily on brain maturity and the density of late oligodendrocyte progenitors, a vulnerable cell population.[26,27] The density of these delicate premyelinating oligodendrocyte progenitors peaks at a gestational age of 23 to 32 weeks but persists through 35 to 36 weeks. The high prevalence of PVL detected in term infants who have CHD in the pre- and postoperative periods suggests that they have similar susceptibilities to injury as

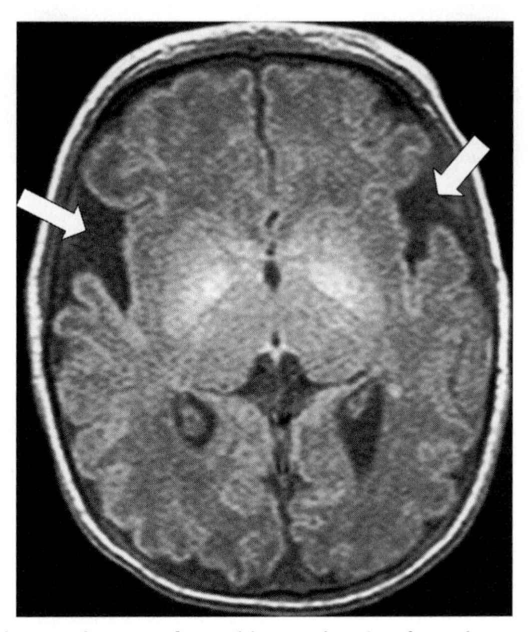

Fig. 2. The cerebral opercula, areas formed by overlapping frontal, temporal, and parietal cortices, remain exposed or open bilaterally (*arrows*). This structural simplicity is typical for a premature brain but the opercula are usually closed at term.

premature infants. Preoperative studies of cerebral blood flow have shown low values of brain perfusion by arterial spin label perfusion MRI examinations.[11] PVL is seen in about 20% in the preoperative period and is associated with low CBF values.[9,28] The distribution of PVL is in a vascular watershed along the walls of the lateral ventricles (**Fig. 3**). Clearly, the central nervous system in the infant heart surgery population is not normal before surgery.

The intraoperative period has historically been the spotlight to examine the causes of brain injury and has inspired several trials to lower those risks with surgical innovations. This period is an obvious starting point to begin studies of neuroprotection, considering the complexity of this impressive biotechnological feat. During heart surgery, the patient is anesthetized and then surface cooled, including ice packs to the head. Cannulas are inserted into the great vessels and core body and brain temperatures are reduced to 18 to 19°C by CPB. In addition to concerns regarding impaired cerebral perfusion, there are other considerations, such as microemboli from particulate matter or air in the circuit and inflammation from exposure of the infant's blood to the foreign materials of the pump tubing, membranes, and oxygenators. For some especially complex forms of CHDs, a motionless, bloodless operative field is needed for surgery: CPB is stopped, the aorta is cross-clamped, and DHCA occurs. During DHCA there is absolutely no blood flow to the brain or body. The duration of DHCA can vary from a few minutes to more than an hour, depending on the requirements of the surgical

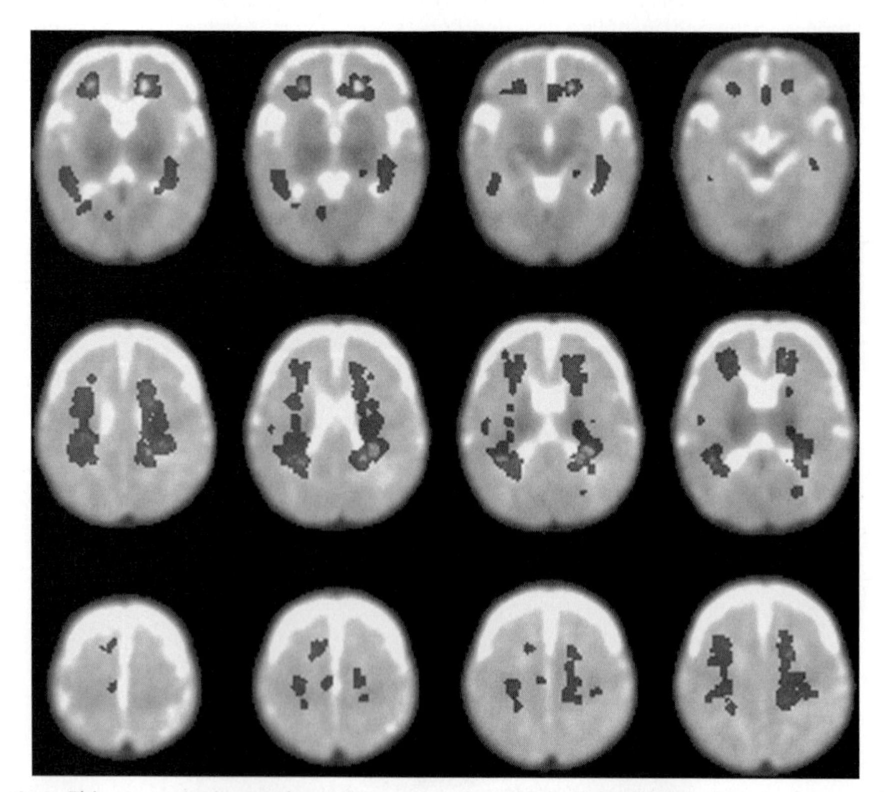

Fig. 3. This composite image shows the overlapping distribution of PVL in 34 infants imaged preoperatively. In these axial views, superimposed MRIs show that PVL distributes to a vascular watershed around the walls of the lateral ventricles. (*Courtesy of* D. Licht, MD, Philadelphia, PA.)

repair. On completion of the surgery, the cardiopulmonary bypass is reinstituted and warming occurs until the child can be removed from the bypass circuit. In a sense, infant heart surgery is a more controlled and milder version of HIE.

The postoperative period has its own hazards. The myocardium may be stunned from its own ischemia-reperfusion injury during surgery and there is commonly a period of transient low cardiac output peaking around 12 hours postoperatively,[29] resulting in low perfusion of the brain and body. A systemic inflammatory response from the CPB and ischemia-reperfusion also occurs, which functionally impairs the mechanics of heart, lung, gut, and kidney function.

FACTORS THAT INFLUENCE OUTCOME AFTER INFANT HEART SURGERY

Intra-Operative Variables

Intraoperative factors have received the most attention for relevance to short- and long-term outcome after infant heart surgery. In view of its complexity, many variables have been considered: the use and duration of DHCA, the total time of exposure to the CPB circuitry, the need in some infants for immediate reoperation if excessive bleeding occurs from a failed suture line or another surgical problem arises, the depth of hypothermia, the specific value of hemodilution (measured by the hematocrit in the CPB circuit), and even the style of acid-base management (because low temperature per se alters the pH). There is much interest in all of these variables because they are potentially modifiable and open the door to possible neuroprotective strategies within the control of the surgeons, anesthetists, and perfusionists. Although these technical variables are not unimportant, other factors play significant roles in shaping outcome. These patient-specific variables will be crucial to design future neuroprotection studies, because properly designed efficacy studies must understand how to stratify patients into similar risk categories, so that potential therapeutic intervention can have a fair chance of being proved beneficial or not.

Patient-Specific Variables

A large number of patient characteristics can be considered for relevance to short- and long-term outcome. The specific nature of the CHD, pattern of fetal growth (for example, intrauterine growth retardation), and other confounding variables, such as maternal illness or infection, may all conspire to influence fetal well-being long before labor, delivery, and heart surgery. Because these infants have CHD and pre-existing neurologic issues, it is not surprising that some may falter during their transition to extrauterine life. Compared with healthy full-term neonates, they have lower Apgar scores, need more newborn resuscitation, and may require endotracheal intubation even before heart surgery.[30]

There is a growing appreciation of the role of genetic syndromes, proved or suspected, and genetic polymorphisms in understanding the outcomes after infant heart surgery.

Congenital heart defects are themselves midline defects that sometimes imply an underlying genetic condition or syndrome. Some genetic conditions are subtle but others are not. Even the presence of a lateral cleft lip has significance in this context. Deletions of 22q11 are common in the CHD population, may be easily overlooked in the newborn period, and independently produce neurologic dysfunction.[31] Even in the absence of overt clinical dysmorphism, there may be underlying brain malformation in some babies who have CHD, such as agenesis of the corpus callosum.[32]

The genetic influences that shape the brain's resiliency or vulnerability to various acquired injuries are just beginning to be understood. Our group has studied polymorphisms of the apolipoprotein E (APOE) gene, which are significantly associated with neurodevelopmental outcome.[33,34] APOE-containing lipoproteins are the primary lipid transport vehicles in the brain and an important regulator of cholesterol metabolism. APOE is important for neuronal repair and the *APOE* genotype influences brain recovery after ischemia, hemorrhage, and trauma. *APOE* genotype is associated with neurocognitive status after adult cardiac surgery. APOE polymorphisms account for part of the variability in outcome following infant heart surgery after adjustment for other factors, such as the nature of the congenital heart defect, gender, race, and intraoperative variables. An unexplored area in this population is the contribution of variations in other genes, such as those that regulate oxidative stress,[35–37] apoptosis,[38] inflammatory response, coagulation cascades, and even the ability of children to metabolize fat in breast milk, which affects IQ in healthy children.[39]

INTERACTIONS BETWEEN PATIENT AND INTRAOPERATIVE CHARACTERISTICS

It is clear that short- and long-term outcomes after infant surgery are associated with both patient-specific and operative characteristics. These can be modeled to observe their interactions. For example, a risk-of-death model was constructed to identify the predictors of mortality after heart surgery in a population of mixed forms of CHD.[40] Knowledge of patient characteristics alone (eg, the type of cardiac defect, Apgar scores, age at surgery, and genetic conditions) allowed death to be predicted with 80% accuracy. By adding all of the descriptors of the intraoperative period to the model (such as the duration of DHCA, length of total CPB time, lowest body temperature, and so forth), the prediction sensitivity of the model was significantly increased, but only to 82%.

In a subset of the same population, a model was constructed to predict postoperative clinical seizures.[41] Aortic arch obstruction and genetic conditions significantly increased seizure risk. Adjusted for these factors, prolonged DHCA time also increased the risk. In the Boston Circulatory Arrest Study (BCAS), which examined neurodevelopmental outcomes in a population with exclusively transposition of the great arteries (TGA), postoperative seizures were predicted by variants of cardiac anatomy (the presence or absence of a ventricular septal defect along with the TGA), and the use and duration of DHCA.[4] More recently, Gaynor and colleagues[42] also reported that long DHCA time predicted seizures in a different CHD population. In a different subset of the APOE polymorphisms study, neurologic outcome was measured using the Bayley Scales of Infant Development (BSID). The subjects were "clean" children who had two-ventricle hearts that were repaired in a single operation in infancy using CPB and at most one period of DHCA.[34] There were 103 males and 85 females. Their median gestational age was 39 weeks and birth weight was 3.175 kg. Twenty percent of the variability in the mental developmental index (MDI) of the BSID was accounted for by patient factors, but only 9.5% by intraoperative factors. Similarly, 27% of the variability of the psychomotor developmental index (PDI) was related to patient factors but only 12.6% to intraoperative factors (**Table 2**).

PRIOR OPERATIVE NEUROPROTECTION TRIALS IN INFANT HEART SURGERY

The obvious place to begin exploring neuroprotection strategies for infant heart surgery is in the operating room. This topic has riveted our attention for the past 2 decades. The first question asked was whether there were short- and long-term outcome differences between surgeries performed exclusively on low-flow CPB versus DHCA. The target population of the BCAS was transposition of the great arteries. This specific lesion can be corrected in a single operation during the newborn period using either

Table 2
Variance in mental and psychomotor indices of the Bayley Scales of Infant Development

	MDI		PDI	
	r^2	*P*	r^2	*P*
Patient factors[a]	0.2006	.0008	0.2713	<.0001
Intraoperative factors[b]	0.0951	.011	0.1264	.0009
DHCA (yes/no)	0.0281	.0213	0.0178	.0679
Postoperative length of stay	0.0425	.0045	0.0829	<.0001

In this "clean" group of infants who had two-ventricle heart lesions repaired in a single operation using CPB and at most one period of DHCA, the variability of MDI and PDI scores was more associated with patient-specific than operative-specific factors.

[a] Patient factors: gender, ethnicity, birth weight, birth head circumference, APGAR 1, APGAR 5, genetic exclusion, APOE genotype.

[b] Intraoperative factors: weight at surgery, cooling time, DHCA time, CPB time, lowest nasopharyngeal temperature, hematocrit.

Data from Gaynor JW, Wernovsky G, Jarvik GP, et al. Patient characteristics are important determinants of neurodevelopmental outcome at one year of age after neonatal and infant cardiac surgery. J Thorac Cardiovasc Surg 2007;133(5):1344–53.

DHCA or low-flow CPB. The children were classified according to the presence or absence of a ventricular septal defect and then randomly assigned to a predominant strategy of either low-flow CPB or DHCA. There were clear differences in these groups of children in the immediate postoperative period.[4] With the passage of time, however, the differences between these two groups largely evaporated. By 8 years of age, the DHCA and low-flow CPB groups performed similarly on neurocognitive testing but both scored significantly worse than normal children.[5,6] The same neurodevelopmental disability profile has been documented in other forms of congenital heart defects, such as total anomalous pulmonary venous connection[43] and single ventricle heart lesions. Additional operating room–based studies were subsequently performed to compare neurodevelopmental outcomes after alpha stat versus pH stat blood gas management strategies[44] and high hematocrit versus low hematocrit.[45,46] There has been no consistent and meaningful improvement in their neurodevelopmental outcomes in more than 2 decades. Wernovsky compared the BSID scores obtained across different eras over the course of multiple studies in more than 400 infants who had TGA (**Fig. 4**). The well-intended modifications in intraoperative philosophies and strategies have had little impact on outcome, consistent with the perspective that patient-specific variables that exist before surgery exert a major influence on outcome.

An important caveat is to note that the lack of improvement of outcome by manipulating intraoperative factors does not mean there is no brain injury during surgery. Consider that about 20% of children have PVL preoperatively, and this increases to more than 50% in the postoperative period.[47] Localized structural lesions (stroke) detected by MRI also sharply increase postoperatively. We recently observed that 93% of electroencephalographic (EEG) examinations were normal in the immediate preoperative period, but only 49% were normal postoperatively.[48] It is clear that there are important stresses that occur during the conduct of infant heart surgery, but these may not yet be amenable to technological intervention.

PHARMACOLOGIC STUDIES OF NEUROPROTECTION IN INFANT HEART SURGERY

Infant heart surgery is an attractive model for pharmacologic neuroprotection trials because the insult of the surgery is scheduled ahead of time and patients can be

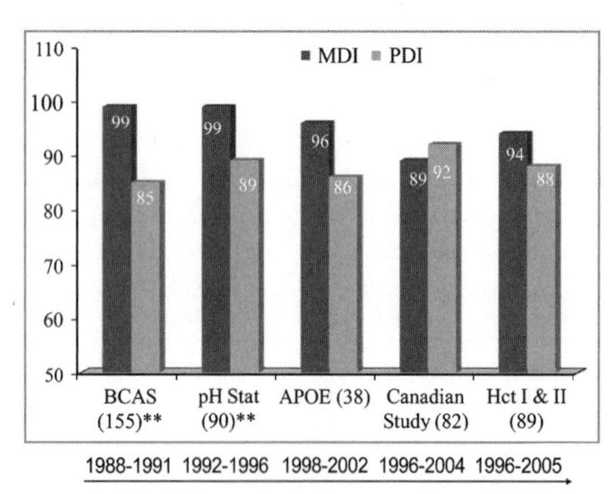

Fig. 4. The Bayley Scales of Infant Development (BSID) are shown for a single cardiac lesion (transposition of the great arteries) reported in different investigations between 1988 and 2005. The earlier studies (**) used an older format of the BSID and scores were adjusted to compare with the later studies. A total of 454 subjects are shown, across various study formats. There has been no consistent improvement in MDI or PDI scores over these surgical eras. (*Courtesy of* G. Wernovsky, MD, Philadelphia, PA.)

preassigned into comparable risk strata. A putative protection drug can thus be administered in a prospective, randomized, placebo-controlled trial before, during, and after surgery. In contrast, it is difficult to anticipate the occurrence of HIE in the term neonate, in whom a narrow 6-hour window of opportunity exists to initiate hypothermia, or in the neonate unexpectedly born prematurely.[49–51] Furthermore, the type and "dose" of the insult can be measured, including the total duration of cardiopulmonary bypass, the need for and duration of DHCA, and the need for reoperation, and other markers can be obtained. Short- and long-term endpoints of interest can be observed prospectively.

THE ALLOPURINOL NEUROCARDIAC PROTECTION TRIAL

Our center reported in 2001 the results of the allopurinol neurocardiac protection trial in 350 neonates who had congenital heart defects who needed infant heart surgery.[30] Allopurinol is one of the most potent inhibitors of xanthine oxidase, a principal source of free radical generation during ischemia followed by reperfusion, as occurs during infant heart surgery. The study group was divided into two risk strata. Those who had hypoplastic left heart syndrome (HLHS) were considered to have the highest risk for adverse events. In contrast, all the others were stratified together as "non-HLHS" and considered to be at lower risk. Allopurinol was administered intravenously before, during, and after heart surgery. Reduced measurements of serum uric acid levels confirmed xanthine oxidase inhibition. During the period of the postoperative ICU hospitalization, study subjects were prospectively observed for acute adverse events, including death, seizures, coma, or cardiac events. MRIs were performed postoperatively, before hospital discharge, to identify acute brain injuries, such as PVL or stroke. The major conclusion from this study was that allopurinol did not reduce the risk for death in either stratum (HLHS or non-HLHS). Allopurinol did provide significant protection in the higher-risk HLHS survivors with a 50% reduction in endpoints but it did not protect the lower-risk, non-HLHS survivors. MRI examinations showed PVL in 52% of the survivors, which was not reduced by allopurinol administration.

PHARMACOLOGIC CANDIDATES FOR FUTURE NEUROPROTECTION TRIALS

The spectrum of neuropathology abnormalities following infant heart surgery is complex[32,52] with a definite mixture of PVL, gray matter injury,[53] and stroke. EEG seizures arise in 11% of these children and presumably reflect cortical (gray matter) injury.[54] White matter injury, in the form of PVL, is much more common and is believed to be the basis for many of their long-term neurodevelopmental disabilities. The ideal candidate for pharmacologic trials in the CHD population would protect both gray and white matter and prevent seizures.

Neurodevelopmental outcome is the net result of a long chain of events which begins at conception and is shaped through genetic and environmental interactions in the pre-, intra-, and postoperative periods. There is no single time period to target neuroprotection intervention in infant heart surgery. The developing brain is already strained under the influence of an abnormal fetal circulation. Still, the observation that the nearly 20% PVL in preoperative MRIs increases to more than 50% postoperatively suggests that this may still be the most fruitful time period to attempt intervention.

Topiramate is an attractive candidate for pharmacologic neuroprotection in the infant heart surgery population.[55] It is an orally available anti-seizure medication that was approved by the US Food and Drug Administration to treat seizure disorders in the United States in 1996. In immature animal models of white matter injury, topiramate and its experimental analog NBQX block developmentally regulated alpha-amino-3-hydroxy-5-methyl-4-isoxazolepropionic acid receptors that are responsible for injury and death to precursors of oligodendroglia.[56–58] In models of rat hypoxia-ischemia, the administration of topiramate significantly reduced PVL and improved rat neuromotor scores. Topiramate also protects from hypoxic-ischemia gray matter injury and seizures and has been studied in a piglet model of infant heart surgery.[59]

Back and colleagues[27] have developed a model of chronic fetal rat hypoxia in which white matter precursors are delayed and easily injured. Hypoxia triggers the release of adenosine, which acts on specific targets (such as the A1 adenosine receptor) to produce PVL. This phenomenon can be prevented by the administration of caffeine, an adenosine antagonist.[60] These observations are especially interesting in light of a recent study (**Table 3**) that examined the quality of survival in premature infants administered caffeine to reduce apnea and bradycardia spells. There was a significant reduction in the rates of "death or any disability," cerebral palsy, and cognitive

Table 3
Caffeine versus placebo for apnea of prematurity

Patients	Caffeine	Placebo	*P* Value
Complete data	N = 937	N = 932	—
Dead or any disability	40.2%	46.2%	.008
Cerebral palsy	4.4%	7.3%	.009
Cognitive delay	33.8%	38.3%	.04

In a study of 2006 low birth weight infants (500–1250 g), caffeine or placebo was randomly administered for apnea of prematurity. There was a significant improvement in some outcome measures in those administered caffeine.

delays.[61] In the infant heart surgery population, it would be tempting to consider a trial of caffeine administration to the mother in the last trimester of pregnancy in those whose complex congenital heart defects were diagnosed prenatally.

Future neuroprotection trials will need to envision a broad perspective of the pathway that leads from conception through infant heart surgery and beyond. The identification of genetic variants that influence outcome will be critical. Risk stratification will assume paramount importance so that fair and balanced studies can be successfully conducted. It is conceivable that pharmacologic intervention will begin during pregnancy and continue until after the heart surgery. The endpoints of these studies must include careful neuroimaging before and after surgery and continuous EEG monitoring for seizures for several days postoperatively to ensure that the whole spectrum of perioperative neuropathology can be captured. Finally, it must be recognized that surrogate biomarkers of brain health, such as MRI and EEG examinations, are no substitute for long-term neurodevelopmental follow-up. In the end, what matters most is the successful functioning of the child within society, measured by personal, cognitive, academic, and social competence.

REFERENCES

1. Greer DM. Mechanisms of injury in hypoxic-ischemic encephalopathy: implications to therapy. Semin Neurol 2006;26(4):373–9.
2. Grow J, Barks JDE. Pathogenesis of hypoxic-ischemic cerebral injury in the term infant: current concepts. Clinics in Perinatology. Clinics in Perinatology 2002; 29(4):585–602.
3. Wernovsky G, Shillingford AJ, Gaynor JW. Central nervous system outcomes in children with complex congenital heart disease. Curr Opin Cardiol 2005;20(2): 94–9.
4. Newburger JW, Jonas JA, Wernovsky G. A comparison of the perioperative neurologic effects of hypothermic circulatory arrest versus low-flow cardiopulmonary bypass in infant heart surgery. N Engl J Med 1993;329:1057–64.
5. Bellinger D, Wypij D, duPlessis AJ, et al. Neurodevelopmental status at eight years in children with dextro-transposition of the great arteries: the Boston Circulatory Arrest Trial. J Thorac Cardiovasc Surg 2003;126:1385–96.
6. Bellinger DC, Jonas RA, Rappaport LA, et al. Developmental and neurologic status of children after heart surgery with hypothermic circulatory arrest or low-flow cardiopulmonary bypass. N Engl J Med 1995;332(9):549–55.
7. Bellinger DC, Rappaport LA, Wypij D, et al. Patterns of developmental dysfunction after surgery during infancy to correct transposition of the great arteries. J Dev Behav Pediatr 1997;18(2):75–83.
8. Bellinger DC, Wernovsky G, Rappaport LA, et al. Cognitive development of children following early repair of transposition of the great arteries using deep hypothermic circulatory arrest. Pediatrics 1991;87(5):701–7.
9. Mahle WT, et al. An MRI study of neurological injury before and after congenital heart surgery. Circulation 2002;106(Suppl I):I109–14.
10. McQuillen PS, et al. Temporal and anatomic risk profile of brain injury with neonatal repair of congenital heart defects. Stroke 2007;38(Suppl 2):736–41.
11. Licht D, Wang J, Silvestre DW, et al. Preoperative cerebral blood flow is diminished in neonates with severe congenital heart defects. J Thorac Cardiovasc Surg 2004;128:841–9.
12. Bellinger DC, et al. Eight-year neurodevelopmental status: the Boston circulatory arrest study. Circulation 2000;102:497.

13. Hovels-Gurich HH, et al. Attentional dysfunction in children after corrective cardiac surgery in infancy. Ann Thorac Surg 2007;83(4):1425–30.
14. Shillingford AJ, et al. Inattention, hyperactivity, and school performance in a population of school-age children with complex congenital heart disease. Pediatrics 2008;121(4):e759–67.
15. Perlman JM. Brain injury in the term infant. Semin Perinatol 2004;28(6):415–24.
16. Perlman JM. Intervention strategies for neonatal hypoxic-ischemic cerebral injury. Clin Ther 2006;28(9):1353–65.
17. Robertson NJ, Iwata O. Bench to bedside strategies for optimizing neuroprotection following perinatal hypoxia-ischaemia in high and low resource settings. Early Hum Dev 2007;83(12):801–11.
18. Badawi N, et al. Antepartum risk factors for newborn encephalopathy: the Western Australian case-control study. Br Med J 1998;317:1549–53.
19. Limperopoulos C, et al. Neurodevelopmental status of newborns and infants with congenital heart defects before and after open heart surgery. J Pediatr 2000; 137(5):638–45.
20. Clancy RR, et al. Allopurinol neurocardiac protection trial in infants undergoing heart surgery using deep hypothermic circulatory arrest. Pediatrics 2001;108(1):61–70.
21. Shillingford AJ, et al. Aortic morphometry and microcephaly in hypoplastic left heart syndrome. Cardiol Young 2007;17(2):189–95.
22. Licht D, et al. Brain maturation is delayed in infants with complex congenital heart defects. J Thorac Cardiovasc Surg (submitted for publication).
23. Childs AM, et al. Cerebral maturation in premature infants: quantitative assessment using MR imaging. AJNR Am J Neuroradiol 2001;22(8):1577–82.
24. Ramenghi LA, et al. Magnetic resonance imaging assessment of brain maturation in preterm neonates with punctate white matter lesions. Neuroradiology 2007; 49(2):161–7.
25. Miller SP, et al. Abnormal brain development in newborns with congenital heart disease. N Engl J Med 2007;357(19):1928–38.
26. Back SA. Recent advances in human perinatal white matter injury. Prog Brain Res 2001;132:131–47.
27. Back SA, et al. Late oligodendrocyte progenitors coincide with the developmental window of vulnerability for human perinatal white matter injury. J Neurosci 2001; 21(4):1302–12.
28. Licht DJ, et al. Reduced pre-operative cerebral vascular reativity in infants with severe congenital heart defects is associated with periventricular leukomalacia. Stroke 2006;37(2):641.
29. Wernovsky G, et al. Postoperative course and hemodynamic profile after the arterial switch operation in neonates and infants. Circulation 1995;92:2226–35.
30. Clancy RR, McGaurn SA, Goin JE, et al. Allopurinol neurocardiac protection trial in infants undergoing heart surgery utilizing deep hypothermic circulatory arrest. Pediatrics 2001;107:61–70.
31. Gerdes M, et al. Cognitive and behavioral profile of preschool children with chromosome 22q11.2 deletion. Am J Med Genet 1999;85:127–33.
32. Glauser TA, et al. Congenital brain anomalies associated with the hypoplastic left heart syndrome. Pediatrics 1990;85(6):984–90.
33. Gaynor JW, et al. Apolipoprotein E genotype and neurodevelopmental sequalae of infant cardiac surgery. J Thorac Cardiovasc Surg 2003;126:1736–45.
34. Gaynor JW, et al. Patient characteristics are important determinants of neurodevelopmental outcome at one year of age after neonatal and infant cardiac surgery. J Thorac Cardiovasc Surg 2007;133(5):1344–53, 1353 e1–3.

35. Buonocore G, Groenendaal F. Anti-oxidant strategies. Semin Fetal Neonatal Med 2007;12(4):287–95.
36. Loren DJ, et al. Maternal dietary supplementation with pomegranate juice is neuroprotective in an animal model of neonatal hypoxic-ischemic brain injury. Pediatr Res 2005;57(6):858–64.
37. Shimizu K, et al. Neuroprotection against hypoxia-ischemia in neonatal rat brain by novel superoxide dismutase mimetics. Neurosci Lett 2003;346(1–2):41–4.
38. Cai Z, et al. Minocycline alleviates hypoxic-ischemic injury to developing oligodendrocytes in the neonatal rat brain. Neuroscience 2006;137(2):425–35.
39. Caspi A, et al. Moderation of breast feeding effects on the IQ by genetic variation in fatty acid metabolism. Proc Natl Acad Sci U S A 2007;104:18860–5.
40. Clancy RR, et al. Preoperative risk-of-death prediction model in heart surgery with deep hypothermic circulatory arrest in the neonate. J Thorac Cardiovasc Surg 2000;119(2):347–57.
41. Clancy RR, et al. Risk of seizures in survivors of newborn heart surgery using deep hypothermic circulatory arrest. Pediatrics 2003;111(3):592–601.
42. Gaynor JW, et al. Increasing duration of deep hypothermic circulatory arrest is associated with an increased incidence of postoperative seizures. J Thorac Cardiovasc Surg 2005;130:1278–86.
43. Kirshbom P, et al. Late neurodevelopmental outcome following repair of total anomalous pulmonary venous connection. J Thorac Cardiovasc Surg 2005;129:1091–7.
44. Bellinger DC, et al. Developmental and neurological effects of alpha-stat versus pH-stat strategies for deep hypothermic cardiopulmonary bypass in infants. J Thorac Cardiovasc Surg 2001;121:374–83.
45. Newburger JW, et al. Randomized trial of hematocrit 25% versus 35% during hypothermic cardiopulmonary bypass in infant heart surgery. J Thorac Cardiovasc Surg 2008;135(2):347–54, 354 e1–4.
46. Wypij D, et al. The effect of hematocrit during hypothermic cardiopulmonary bypass in infant heart surgery: results from the combined Boston hematocrit trials. J Thorac Cardiovasc Surg 2008;135(2):355–60.
47. Galli KK, et al. Periventricular leukomalacia is common after neonatal cardiac surgery. J Thorac Cardiovasc Surg 2004;127(3):692–704.
48. Cho S, et al. Early EEG background prediction of seizures and short-term outcome measures following infant heart surgery. Journal of Thoracic & Cardiovascular Surgery (submitted for publication).
49. Shankaran S, Laptook A. Challenge of conducting trials of neuroprotection in the asphyxiated term infant. Semin Perinatol 2003;27(4):320–32.
50. Shankaran S, et al. Whole-body hypothermia for neonates with hypoxic-ischemic encephalopathy. [see comment]. N Engl J Med 2005;353(15):1574–84.
51. Gluckman P, et al. Selective head cooling with mild systemic hypothermia after neonatal encephalopathy: a multicentre randomized trial. Lancet 2005;365:663–70.
52. Kinney HC, et al. Hypoxic-ischemic brain injury in infants with congenital heart disease dying after cardiac surgery. Acta Neuropathol 2005;110:563–78.
53. Ferriero DM. Protecting neurons. Epilepsia 2005;46(Suppl 7):45–51.
54. Clancy RR, et al. Electrographic neonatal seizures after infant heart surgery. Epilepsia 2005;46:84–90.
55. Choi JW, Kim W-K. Is topiramate a potential therapeutic agent for cerebral hypoxic/ischemic injury? [comment]. Exp Neurol 2007;203(1):5–7.
56. Follett P, et al. Protective effects of topiramate in a rodent model of periventricular leukomalacia. Ann Neurol 2000;48:527.

57. Follett PL, Deng W, Dai W, et al. Glutamate receptor-mediated oligodendrocyte toxicity in periventricular leukomalacia: a protective role for topiramate. J Neurosci 2004;24:4412–20.
58. Follett PL, et al. NBQX attenuates excitotoxic injury in developing white matter. J Neurosci 2000;20(24):9235–41.
59. Galinkin JL, et al. The plasma pharmacokinetics and cerebral spinal fluid penetration of intravenous topiramate in newborn pigs. Biopharm Drug Dispos 2004; 25(6):265–71.
60. Back SA, et al. Protective effects of caffeine on chronic hypoxia-induced perinatal white matter injury. Ann Neurol 2006;60(6):696–705.
61. Schmidt B, et al. Long-term effects of caffeine therapy for apena of prematurity. N Engl J Med 2007;357:1893–902.

Index

Note: Page numbers of article titles are in **bold face** type.

Clin Perinatol 35 (2008) 823–831
doi:10.1016/S0095-5108(08)00105-X

U

V

W

United States Postal Service

Statement of Ownership, Management, and Circulation
(All Periodicals Publications Except Requestor Publications)

1. Publication Title	2. Publication Number	3. Filing Date
Clinics in Perinatology	0 0 1 - 7 4 4	9/15/08
4. Issue Frequency	**5. Number of Issues Published Annually**	**6. Annual Subscription Price**
Mar, Jun, Sep, Dec	4	$197.00

7. Complete Mailing Address of Known Office of Publication (*Not printer*) (*Street, city, county, state, and ZIP+4*)

Elsevier Inc.
360 Park Avenue South
New York, NY 10010-1710

Contact Person: Stephen Bushing
Telephone (Include area code): 215-239-3688

8. Complete Mailing Address of Headquarters or General Business Office of Publisher (*Not printer*)

Elsevier Inc., 360 Park Avenue South, New York, NY 10010-1710

9. Full Names and Complete Mailing Addresses of Publisher, Editor, and Managing Editor (*Do not leave blank*)

Publisher (*Name and complete mailing address*)

John Schrefer , Elsevier, Inc., 1600 John F. Kennedy Blvd. Suite 1800, Philadelphia, PA 19103-2899

Editor (*Name and complete mailing address*)

Carla Holloway, Elsevier, Inc., 1600 John F. Kennedy Blvd. Suite 1800, Philadelphia, PA 19103-2899

Managing Editor (*Name and complete mailing address*)

Catherine Bewick, Elsevier, Inc., 1600 John F. Kennedy Blvd. Suite 1800, Philadelphia, PA 19103-2899

10. Owner (*Do not leave blank. If the publication is owned by a corporation, give the name and address of the corporation immediately followed by the names and addresses of all stockholders owning or holding 1 percent or more of the total amount of stock. If not owned by a corporation, give the names and addresses of the individual owners. If owned by a partnership or other unincorporated firm, give its name and address as well as those of each individual owner. If the publication is published by a nonprofit organization, give its name and address.*)

Full Name	Complete Mailing Address
Wholly owned subsidiary of	4520 East-West Highway
Reed/Elsevier, US holdings	Bethesda, MD 20814

11. Known Bondholders, Mortgagees, and Other Security Holders Owning or Holding 1 Percent or More of Total Amount of Bonds, Mortgages, or Other Securities. If none, check box → ☐ None

Full Name	Complete Mailing Address
N/A	

12. Tax Status (*For completion by nonprofit organizations authorized to mail at nonprofit rates*) (*Check one*)
The purpose, function, and nonprofit status of this organization and the exempt status for federal income tax purposes:
☐ Has Not Changed During Preceding 12 Months
☐ Has Changed During Preceding 12 Months (*Publisher must submit explanation of change with this statement*)

PS Form 3526, September 2006 (Page 1 of 3 (Instructions Page 3)) PSN 7530-01-000-9931 **PRIVACY NOTICE**: See our Privacy policy in www.usps.com

13. Publication Title: Clinics in Perinatology
14. Issue Date for Circulation Data Below: June 2008

15. Extent and Nature of Circulation			Average No. Copies Each Issue During Preceding 12 Months	No. Copies of Single Issue Published Nearest to Filing Date
a. Total Number of Copies (*Net press run*)			4025	3900
b. Paid Circulation (By Mail and Outside the Mail)	(1)	Mailed Outside-County Paid Subscriptions Stated on PS Form 3541. (*Include paid distribution above nominal rate, advertiser's proof copies, and exchange copies*)	2178	2006
	(2)	Mailed In-County Paid Subscriptions Stated on PS Form 3541 (*Include paid distribution above nominal rate, advertiser's proof copies, and exchange copies*)		
	(3)	Paid Distribution Outside the Mails Including Sales Through Dealers and Carriers, Street Vendors, Counter Sales, and Other Paid Distribution Outside USPS®	948	818
	(4)	Paid Distribution by Other Classes Mailed Through the USPS (e.g. First-Class Mail®)		
c. Total Paid Distribution (*Sum of 15b (1), (2), (3), and (4)*) ►			3126	2824
d. Free or Nominal Rate Distribution (By Mail and Outside the Mail)	(1)	Free or Nominal Rate Outside-County Copies Included on PS Form 3541	66	68
	(2)	Free or Nominal Rate In-County Copies Included on PS Form 3541		
	(3)	Free or Nominal Rate Copies Mailed at Other Classes Mailed Through the USPS (e.g. First-Class Mail)		
	(4)	Free or Nominal Rate Distribution Outside the Mail (Carriers or other means)		
e. Total Free or Nominal Rate Distribution (Sum of 15d (1), (2), (3) and (4)			66	68
f. Total Distribution (Sum of 15c and 15e) ►			3192	2892
g. Copies not Distributed (See instructions to publishers #4 (page #3)) ►			833	1008
h. Total (Sum of 15f and g)			4025	3900
i. Percent Paid (15c divided by 15f times 100) ►			97.93%	97.65%

16. Publication of Statement of Ownership

☐ If the publication is a general publication, publication of this statement is required. Will be printed in the **December 2008** issue of this publication. ☐ Publication not required

17. Signature and Title of Editor, Publisher, Business Manager, or Owner

Jean Fanucci – Executive Director of Subscription Services — Date: September 15, 2008

I certify that all information furnished on this form is true and complete. I understand that anyone who furnishes false or misleading information on this form or who omits material or information requested on the form may be subject to criminal sanctions (including fines and imprisonment) and/or civil sanctions (including civil penalties).

PS Form **3526**, September 2006 (Page 2 of 3)

Moving?

Make sure your subscription moves with you!

To notify us of your new address, find your **Clinics Account Number** (located on your mailing label above your name), and contact customer service at:

E-mail: elspcs@elsevier.com

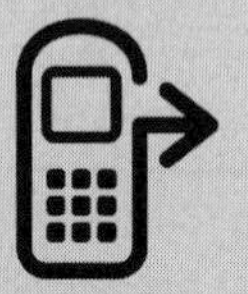

800-654-2452 (subscribers in the U.S. & Canada)
314-453-7041 (subscribers outside of the U.S. & Canada)

Fax number: 314-523-5170

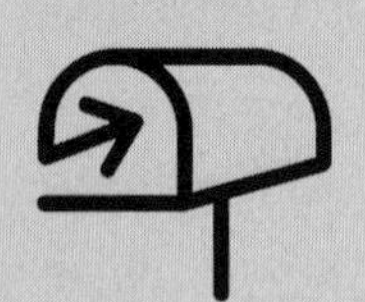

Elsevier Periodicals Customer Service
11830 Westline Industrial Drive
St. Louis, MO 63146

*To ensure uninterrupted delivery of your subscription, please notify us at least 4 weeks in advance of move.

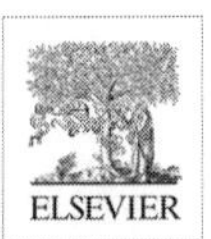